FRCEM Final OSCE:

125 OSCE Stations
Third Edition

FRCEM Final OSCE:

125 OSCE Stations
Third Edition

Kiran Somani BA (Hons) MBBS MRCP DTM&H FRCEM FACEM
Consultant in Emergency Medicine
University Hospital Southampton, UK

James Miers MBBS FACEM
Staff Specialist at Liverpool Hospital
Liverpool, NSW, Australia

London • New Delhi

© 2020 Jaypee Brothers Medical Publishers

Published by Jaypee Brothers Medical Publishers,
4838/24 Ansari Road, New Delhi, India

Tel: +91 (011) 43574357   Fax: +91 (011)43574390

Email: info@jpmedpub.com, jaypee@jaypeebrothers.com
Web: www.jpmedpub.com, www.jaypeebrothers.com

JPM is the imprint of Jaypee Brothers Medical Publishers.

The rights of Kiran Somani and James Miers to be identified as the editors of this work have been asserted by them in accordance with the Copyright, Designs and Patents Act 1988.

All rights reserved. No part of this publication may be reproduced, stored or transmitted in any form or by any means, electronic, mechanical, photocopying, recording or otherwise, except as permitted by the UK Copyright, Designs and Patents Act 1988, without the prior permission in writing of the publishers. Permissions may be sought directly from Jaypee Brothers Medical Publishers (P) Ltd. at the address printed above.

All brand names and product names used in this book are trade names, service marks, trademarks or registered trademarks of their respective owners. The publisher is not associated with any product or vendor mentioned in this book.

Medical knowledge and practice change constantly. This book is designed to provide accurate, authoritative information about the subject matter in question. However readers are advised to check the most current information available on procedures included and check information from the manufacturer of each product to be administered, to verify the recommended dose, formula, method and duration of administration, adverse effects and contraindications. It is the responsibility of the practitioner to take all appropriate safety precautions. Neither the publisher nor the authors assume any liability for any injury and/or damage to persons or property arising from or related to use of material in this book.

This book is sold on the understanding that the publisher is not engaged in providing professional medical services. If such advice or services are required, the services of a competent medical professional should be sought.

ISBN: 978-1-909836-97-6

British Library Cataloguing in Publication Data
A catalogue record for this book is available from the British Library

Library of Congress Cataloging in Publication Data
A catalog record for this book is available from the Library of Congress

Development Editor: Harsha Madan
Editorial Assistant: Keshav Kumar
Cover Design: Seema Dogra

Foreword to First Edition

Any book that helps candidates to pass an exam has to be welcomed. But this one does more than that. Not only does it prepare candidates for the FRCEM final OSCEs by describing their structure and logic and by providing multiple examples, it also explains why the subject matter is important to the practice of emergency medicine and how this knowledge will make the candidate a better emergency physician. The sections on common presentations, communication, physical examination, psychiatry, practical procedures and resuscitation all contain important information that will be valuable to all candidates for their practice as well as for the examination. This book, combined with a thorough knowledge of the curriculum and the College's own guidance for the exams, should prepare the candidate well.

Dr Mike Clancy
Past President of the Royal College of Emergency Medicine
Consultant in Emergency Medicine
University Hospital Southampton NHS Foundation Trust, UK

Dedication

This book is dedicated to Dr Nandkishor and Pramila Somani with love, gratitude and pride.

Kiran Somani

Acknowledgements

The authors wish to thank Dr Nitin Jain for his contribution to the first and second editions of this book without which this text would not have been completed.

The authors would also like to thank the following individuals for their help with providing material for this book: Dr David Connor, Dr Yulia Novytska, Dr Ka Mei Lo, Dr Elizabeth Forbes, Ross Brown and Rich Lister.

Preface to Third Edition

Completion of the Fellowship of the Royal College of Emergency Medicine (FRCEM) is the ultimate goal of all emergency medicine trainees. It is recognition that an individual has gained adequate experience, knowledge and skills to become a specialist in the field of emergency medicine. It is a badge of competency which can be worn proudly. This book has been written to assist candidates with their revision for the OSCE component of the FRCEM Final exam.

Success in any OSCE-style exam requires the candidate to have acquired the necessary knowledge and to have developed and practised the skills which will be assessed, until a proficient routine is established. It will also benefit candidates to have considered as many scenarios as possible prior to the exam as this will allow them to demonstrate familiarity and confidence in varied situations. Only through meticulous preparation will a candidate convey the level of clinical and interpersonal competence necessary to be successful.

Though there are various revision courses and individual OSCE mark sheets that some candidates acquire during their revision, there are few resources accessible to all candidates sitting the OSCE exam. Our intention when writing this book was to combine our knowledge and experience of OSCEs into a format that allows all candidates to access a high quality OSCE revision aid.

Using this book, candidates can test themselves with scenarios that reflect those used in the real exam. Furthermore we hope that candidates who read this book will be prepared for the OSCEs that commonly arise in the exam, will understand what they are being tested on and how the necessary marks in each OSCE are scored and lastly, will be able to anticipate which scenarios are likely to arise to avoid surprises. We would also like to emphasise the importance of demonstrating high quality interpersonal and communication skills as discussed in the section on non-technical skills in the following introduction. We believe this short section describes the essence of what is required to be successful in the OSCE and in your future career.

In this third edition we have added a number of new OSCE scenarios. In addition, throughout the book and particularly with reference to the extended resuscitation style OSCEs, we have focused on increasing the complexity of the scenarios to a level we feel will suitably challenge Fellowship candidates. We hope that by encouraging a wider breadth of revision, candidates will be better prepared for the variety of scenarios that may arise in their exam. To ensure our material remains current we have updated the text using the latest versions of all the national guidelines cited.

We recommend using the FRCEM curriculum to guide revision. Candidates must refer to the curriculum to ensure there are no gaps in their preparation and revision. Also, we strongly recommend that candidates check the latest exam information on the Royal College of Emergency Medicine's website.

Congratulations on choosing the most exciting and rewarding career in medicine. We wish you every success with your exams and future career!

Kiran Somani
2019

Contents

Foreword to First Edition — v
Dedication — v
Acknowledgements — v
Preface to Third Edition — vii
How to use this book — x
Introduction to the FRCEM Final OSCE examination — xi

Chapter 1	History taking	1
Chapter 2	Communication skills	95
Chapter 3	Systems examination	147
Chapter 4	Joint examination	187
Chapter 5	Psychiatry	231
Chapter 6	Practical skills and teaching	255
Chapter 7	Acute adult presentations	389
Chapter 8	Paediatric acute presentations	433
Chapter 9	Trauma presentations	471

How to use this book

The most effective way to use this book is to work though each station under exam conditions. Ideally this requires each one to be timed, allowing 1 minute to read the instructions followed by 7 minutes to complete the task. In the real exam, the stress caused by time constraints, the scrutiny of the examiner and a fear of failure can all lead to candidates performing poorly. Practising as many stations as possible in an exam-like environment is by far the best preparation.

You will find it invaluable to practise in groups of two or three, with each person taking turns to play the role of candidate, actor (if needed) and examiner (the latter two can be the same person if a third person is not available). Afterwards, time should be spent reflecting on the mark sheet, assessing the candidate's performance and identifying areas for further study and development.

If you are working alone, it is still possible to work though the practice stations. However, we encourage you to arrange to be observed by, and receive feedback from, your senior colleagues and peers on at least a few occasions prior to the exam. Without observed practise it is very difficult for a candidate to improve on their technique or to know how they will perform when being watched by an examiner during their exam.

Using this approach, you will be well prepared on the day of the exam.

Format

The majority of the stations in this book include the following information:
- Introductory text – this provides relevant background information on the topic being assessed
- Scenario – this presents the exam question or task to be completed
- Pie chart – this illustrates which areas of competence are being tested
- Mark sheet – this lists specific actions which the candidate is expected to perform. The candidate will be successful if enough of these are carried out. In most cases it is acceptable for the order of the actions to vary; however, this may have an impact on the global score (discussed later in this introduction).
- Additional guidance/observations/information – where included, these indicate important events that occur during the course of each scenario. These are particularly relevant in the resuscitation scenarios
- Instructions for actor(s) – these are intended to help candidates anticipate the different ways in which the patient or the actor may behave. These are generally included in the history, communication and teaching scenarios. However, these instructions are not provided in the examination and practical skills scenarios, as the behavior of the actor or patient is not likely to influence the candidate's actions to the same degree.
- Alternative scenarios – these have been included at the end of all of the resuscitation scenarios to highlight to candidates how the presenting case may vary. They are also provided to encourage candidates to further imagine or create their own challenging scenarios and practice their approach to them.

Introduction to the FRCEM Final OSCE examination

Aims of the examination
The Fellowship Examination of the Royal College of Emergency Medicine (FRCEM) is intended to assess the knowledge, skills and behaviours necessary for a doctor to be able to practise emergency medicine in the UK and Ireland, at the level required to be recognised as an emergency medicine specialist. It is the final hurdle which must be successfully negotiated prior to completion of higher specialist training. Successfully completing the FRCEM is recognition of all the experience, knowledge and skills a doctor has accumulated.

The clinical component of the FRCEM Final exam uses objective structured clinical examination (OSCE) stations to assess a broad range of the competences required for the evaluation and immediate management of common clinical conditions seen in the emergency department (ED) in adults and children.

The expectation is that candidates must demonstrate they have achieved a competent standard to take absolute responsibility for all clinical and non-clinical decisions made in an ED. Candidates should understand and reflect on the fact that during the examination the examiners ask themselves: 'if this doctor were one of my colleagues would they be able to manage this case (and the department) competently?', or 'would I be happy if this doctor was responsible for a member of my family?'.

Content of the exam (the curriculum)
The exam is based on the major and acute presentations listed in the curriculum (which is available from the Royal College of Emergency Medicine website). The College has clearly stated that presentations not included in the curriculum will not be assessed in the exam.

Obviously, this means the value of the curriculum as a reference during revision must not be underestimated, and for many it provides a clear framework for focusing revision. Rest assured it has also provided the framework for constructing this book.

Format of the exam
The exam consists of 18 OSCE stations which candidates rotate through over a period of approximately two and a half hours. Areas to be assessed include clinical knowledge, psychomotor ability, interpersonal skills (including communication and conflict resolution), professional behaviour and clinical decision-making skills.

Incorporated in the 18 stations there are normally two 'resuscitation-style' stations which require the candidate to manage an acute presentation. Each of these occupy two out of the total number of OSCE stations, are double the duration of the other stations, and therefore carry twice as many marks.

In addition there are usually two rest stations. During these, candidates may sometimes be given information relevant to the following station and offered the opportunity to prepare themselves.

Each OSCE station poses a scenario where specific competences are tested and the candidate's performance is observed and scored against a pre-prepared mark sheet. When rotating through the 18 stations, one minute is allowed outside each station to read the relevant instructions. In addition to the instructions, a pie chart is present which shows the general areas over which the marks for this station are distributed.

The pass mark for each station is decided for each sitting before the examination diet commences. Following the sitting, examiners are invited to confirm the pass mark after marking the exam, and further adjustment may be made in the light of the cohort performance on particular questions or stations.

Candidates must pass 14 stations to pass the whole exam.

As stated above, due to ongoing development of the curriculum and exam, we strongly recommend that candidates check the latest exam information on the Royal College of Emergency Medicine's website.

Competences tested

In each OSCE the competences being assessed are placed on a pie chart with the scenario. Candidates must be aware of where the marks lie. Without reflecting on the pie chart a candidate may mistakenly spend the majority of an OSCE performing a procedure when the marks are mainly for teaching, or spend a whole OSCE talking to a patient when the marks are for examination skills. Each OSCE in this book contains a scenario and with it a pie chart to help candidates prepare for the exam. The competences that may be tested are:

- Clinical reasoning/decision making
- Communication skills
- Examination skills
- History taking
- Dealing with conflict
- Organisation skills
- Practical skills
- Resuscitation skills
- Teaching skills
- Team leadership

How to prepare for the exam

It is vital that candidates prepare adequately for the FRCEM Final OSCE. Reviewing the curriculum and the expected competences, gaining familiarity with the exam format, practising OSCE scenarios and seeking feedback on clinical skills are all necessary for success. Already in this introduction, reference has twice been made to 'performance'. This is deliberate. The only way for the examiner to assess a candidate is based on what the candidate says and does in that OSCE station. Nothing can be assumed or inferred. In this way, an OSCE is very similar to a driving test – it is performance on the day that counts. Examiners are not looking for clever tricks, and minor faults are allowed. Candidates should remember that it is their performance which is being assessed, rather than simply their knowledge. With this in mind, many candidates find it helpful to prepare in groups. This allows them the opportunity to have their actions observed repeatedly, and to practise the same scenario repeatedly so that their performance improves. It also has the added benefit that there are enough people to play the roles of candidate, actor and examiner in each scenario.

Candidates are also strongly advised to request feedback on their clinical performance from senior colleagues within their departments and to undertake appropriate workplace-based assessments to allow them to focus their preparation for the examination.

Non-technical skills

There has been increasing acknowledgement and awareness that a senior emergency medicine clinician must possess a variety of interpersonal and cognitive skills to be effective in their role. Collectively the skills could be described as demonstrating interpersonal and situational competence. Without these skills no matter how clinically competent a clinician is, they would still struggle to provide good quality care to all patients within their department.
These skills involve:
- leadership
- teamworking
- decision-making
- situational awareness

Further examples and detail regarding non-technical skills may be found in the Global scores table below. For some individuals the development of these skills may be more challenging than learning the clinical fact-based aspects of the curriculum. To develop these skills adequately individuals must have completed workplace-based assessments and multisource feedback surveys as well as reflected on the feedback they received. They will have had to reflect on positive behaviours and skills they have witnessed in their colleagues and developed their own techniques to get the best out of everyone they interact with.

The OSCE is the best place to assess these skills as it provides the opportunity to assess the candidate's ability to engage with other individuals and their environment. Many candidates are surprised by the degree to which the OSCE focuses on scenarios that involve communication. OSCEs dealing with teaching, communication, leadership and complex decision-making should be expected.

Candidates who have trained overseas, or whose first language is not English, may find some aspects of demonstrating these abilities harder. Rather than being a competence issue this may often be due to it being harder to demonstrate or convey social or cultural awareness. We strongly recommend these candidates are observed by, and receive feedback from, senior and experienced clinicians as small changes to their approach may make a big difference to their perceived ability.

In every OSCE scenario candidates face, as well as simply answering the clinical question at hand, they should always be aiming to demonstrate a high level of awareness, sensitivity and communication skills which are appropriate to the clinical setting and the task they have been set.

Global scores

Each OSCE mark sheet includes a global score from the examiner and (if applicable) the actor or additional staff in the scenario. The global score is essentially a measure of how well the candidate has demonstrated the non-technical skills required for the scenario. The matrix below provides indicative examples in generic domains of professional behaviour. It is used by the examiners and the role players where appropriate to determine the global score. Not every domain will be applicable to every skill station. As a rough rule:

5 = mostly exemplary

4 = mix of exemplary and acceptable

3 = mostly acceptable

2 = mix of acceptable and unacceptable

Domain	Examples of unacceptable behaviour	Examples of acceptable behaviour	Examples of exemplary behaviour
Communication	No introduction, and no information about what the station is about Closed questions Not listening to the answer Gives the answer themselves Doesn't warn patient of actions Uses jargon without explanation	Attempts to introduce themselves and to inform what about to do Some open questions Invites questions Occasionally interrupts inappropriately Attempts to explain what is doing Uses jargon but then explains	Introduces and informs what the task is about Open and closed questions used appropriately Good use of silence Invites questions from patient and answers well in plain English Keeps patient involved and informed constantly
Rapport and empathy	No attempt to establish rapport No response to body language or patient distress Hurts or embarrasses patient	Adequate rapport Responds to distress but obviously uncomfortable, no eye contact Didn't offend but not always mindful of patient privacy or comfort	Excellent rapport Empathic, good eye contact Appropriate body language Ensures patient comfort
Professional competence	Appears novice No structure to task Steps in wrong order Appears over/under confident Becomes uncomfortable or irritated	Logical structure but halting and stilted Has to pause to think Appears under confident Clearly anxious but able to control	Logical sequence Looks polished Confident Appears calm and professional
Pacing	Does not complete task	Appears hurried but completes task	Completes task within time and looks comfortable
Equal opportunities/ discrimination	Appears biased – exhibits racism, sexism or ageism Stereotypes patients in questions and answers Rude or patronising	No apparent prejudice	Non-judgemental, actively accepting of patient's cultural or behavioural differences
Team skills	No involvement of helper Doesn't listen to examiners or team	Some involvement with team/ helper but works autonomously No interaction with examiner	Involves team/helper, maintains cohesive working environment Interacts well with examiner, accepting given cues

1 = mostly unacceptable

Practicalities

Candidates should make sure they arrive in plenty of time. Arriving in a rush or panic will prevent a confident, calm performance (and arriving too late may mean a candidate is not permitted to sit the exam). This may mean travelling the night before to some venues, so make sure that practical arrangements are made well in advance to reduce stress on the day of the exam. Candidates wear a variety of clothes. It is important to look professional, but there will inevitably be practical skills to be performed during the exam. Consequently, many people choose to wear 'scrubs'. Candidates who choose to wear their own clothes are advised to ensure their arms are bare below the elbows. Facilities will be provided for storage of personal belongings during the exam. It is recommended that candidates bring their own stethoscope which they are familiar with. All other equipment needed will be provided at the individual OSCE station. There will be plenty of people on hand to make sure that candidates go to the correct station at the correct time, and there should be water at the rest stations.

Candidates are usually free to leave as soon as the examination is over. Results are published online a few weeks after the exam – as a list of candidate numbers with the result for each one. Success will be confirmed by a letter from the College shortly afterwards. Those candidates who are unsuccessful will receive feedback about which stations they did well in and which stations they failed. Candidates are advised to discuss this feedback with their educational supervisor early in the process of planning a subsequent attempt.

Chapter 1

History taking

1.1 Introduction
1.2 Patient-centred history taking – falls
1.3 Abdominal pain
1.4 Rectal bleeding
1.5 Apparent life-threatening event
1.6 Back pain
1.7 Syncope
1.8 Dizziness and falls
1.9 Chest pain
1.10 Diabetes mellitus – hypoglycaemia
1.11 Dysphagia
1.12 Febrile convulsion
1.13 Traveller's diarrhoea
1.14 Haematuria
1.15 Upper gastrointestinal bleeding
1.16 Headache
1.17 Jaundice
1.18 Limping child
1.19 Palpitations

1.20 Purpuric rash
1.21 Sexual history
1.22 Breathlessness and cough
1.23 Myalgia
1.24 Transient ischaemic attack
1.25 Weight loss
1.26 Seizure
1.27 Pelvic pain
1.28 Non-accidental injury
1.29 Visual disturbance

1.1 Introduction

History taking and communication scenarios are easy to fail if not practiced in advance. In the examination, it is essential to demonstrate that you can take an adequate and focused history in the short time available and make a shared management plan with your patient. Since time is of the essence it is important to have a structure that allows your questions to flow as smoothly as possible.

The most commonly used framework for history taking is the Calgary–Cambridge framework by Kurtz et al. (**Table 1.1.1**). This describes the processes involved in a patient interview to generate a professional rapport and then exchange information. This should not be confused with the traditional model of history taking, i.e. presenting chief complaint, history of presenting complaint, past medical history, etc. which is the content of patient history.

Initiate the discussion with introductions, greetings and an explanation of what will be discussed. These seemingly straightforward things score 'easy' marks, set the tone for your interaction with the patient and allow examiners to form a positive first impression. Initially, ask open-ended questions, such as 'How can I help you today?', or 'What made you come to hospital?' Sometimes patients have more than one complaint. In this situation, it is important to negotiate the agenda at the beginning and establish the focus of the consultation.

Start gathering information with open questions, e.g. 'Tell me more about the headache', and then progress to closed questioning to clarify the details, e.g. 'Did it start suddenly, or did it come on gradually?' Summarise frequently in order to clarify the facts. For example, 'so it was the worst headache you've ever had, it came on suddenly and felt like you'd been whacked on the back of the head, but it's a little better now. Your vision has been fine all

Table 1.1.1 Approach to communication during history taking (the process in each of the columns occurs simultaneously)

Providing structure	Initiating the session	Building relationship
• Making organisation overt • Attending to flow-logical sequence and timing	• Preparation • Establishing initial rapport • Identifying the reason(s) for the consultation **Gathering information** • Exploring patient problems – use open and closed questioning techniques • Establishing patient's ideas, concerns and expectations • Background information **Explanation and planning** • Providing correct amount and type of information • Aiding accurate recall and understanding • Achieving a shared understanding – avoid jargon • Planning-shared decision making **Closing the session** • Ensuring appropriate point of closure • Forward planning	• Using appropriate non-verbal behaviour • Developing rapport, empathising • Involving the patient, explaining rationale • Demonstrating appropriate confidence

along, you don't feel sick or dizzy and your arms and legs feel completely normal.' Use silence and body language appropriately to demonstrate you are listening and encourage the patient's responses. Actively establish the patient's ideas about the condition. What is it that they are concerned about and what do they expect out of the consultation?

While explaining and planning:
- Avoid medical jargon
- Give information in small amounts, allowing time for it to be understood
- Check understanding

Always give patients an opportunity to ask questions and clarify their understanding of what you have said as you go along. At the end, make a plan, discussing the different options available and provide a 'safety-net' in case the plan is not working.

Keep the history focused to the problem at hand. In addition to asking the questions about the complaint, think about the red flag symptoms and consider a risk assessment as part of the history, e.g. chest pain assessment includes risk of ischaemic heart disease or risk of pulmonary embolism (PE); self-harm and risk of suicide; back pain and risk of cauda equina. You should then reflect back on the patient problems and address the concerns raised by the patient or their carer.

Given below is a generic plan for history taking. This should be used along with the specific mark sheets for each objectively structured clinical examination (OSCE).

Mark sheet	Achieved	Not achieved
Initiating a session		
Introduces self		
Appropriately greets the patient		
Gathering information		
Starts with appropriate opening question		
Establishes reason for attendance		
Explores presenting complaint		
Encourages patient to tell the story		
Uses open and closed questioning technique appropriately		
Listens attentively		
Confirms		
Past medical history		
Surgical and gynaecological history if appropriate		
Drug history		
Allergies		
Social history		
Explanation and planning		
Explores patient's ideas regarding their problem		
Asks about any specific concerns or expectations they have		
Summarises and confirms patient understanding		

Cont'd...

Cont'd...

Mark sheet	Achieved	Not achieved
Provides understandable information without using medical jargon		
Gives appropriate differential diagnosis		
Makes a shared management plan		
Outlines further examinations		
Outlines further investigations		
Closing the session		
Summarises and closes the session appropriately		
Invites questions and addresses any concerns		
Global score		
Global score from examiner		
Global score from patient/actor		

Focused questioning – taking a history of pain

You should mentally prepare lists of questions to ask for specific conditions or complaints. Generally, these consist of closed questions used to identify differential diagnoses and address red flag symptoms. You should have considered all presentations covered by the curriculum and be prepared with preconceived lists of questions to cover salient points. These do not need to be memorised and simply recited, but it will aid performance on the day if you have considered each presentation in the curriculum in the context of a history taking scenario.

Many presentations involve the complaint of pain as either the primary problem or a related one. A detailed history of the characteristics of the pain is fundamental to help identify the likely cause, the severity of the problem and the impact on the patient. In addition to a standard history focused (SOCRATES) questions should include:
- Site: is it generalised, in a specific area, or like a band around the body area?
- Onset: did the pain start suddenly or gradually? When did it reach its worst? Can the patient remember exactly what they were doing at the time? This often suggests an abrupt onset, and can sometimes help explain the cause.
- Character: is it sharp, aching or throbbing in nature?
- Radiation: does the pain spread or localise around a particular area?
- Associations: is there any nausea, vomiting or other localising (or systemic) features?
- Timing: is the pain related to posture or exercise?
- Exacerbating: does posture, activity, diet make it worse? Does analgesia make it better?
- Severity: how bad is it? Is it the worst pain ever?

Suggested reading

Kurtz S, Silverman J, Benson J, Draper J. Marrying Content and Process in Clinical Method Teaching: Enhancing the Calgary-Cambridge Guides. Acad Med 2003; 78:802–809.

1.2 Patient-centred history taking – falls

Ideas, concerns and expectations

Effective history taking requires the clinician not only to collect facts quickly, but also to try to find out what the patient is really thinking. Without exploring what is actually on a patient's mind, it is only possible to form a partial idea of how a problem affects an individual and it is certainly difficult to understand their point of view. There are many scenarios where patients may be embarrassed or feel inhibited about aspects of their problem and if a candidate fails to elicit these issues valuable marks will be lost.

With this in mind during every scenario the candidate must consider whether or not they have elicited the patient's ideas, concerns and expectations. Simple phrases may help get a much deeper understanding of what other factors are influencing the consultation:

- 'What do you think about...?'
- 'What do you know (or have you heard) about this condition?'
- 'Is there anything specific that worries you...?'
- 'What are you worried about?'
- 'What would you like to do about...?'
- 'What would you like us to help with?'

It is by addressing this aspect of the consultation that a clinician will gain the information to make the exchange more effective for both parties. For example, realising:

- The patient with a headache is worried about having a brain tumour
- The father accompanying his daughter is anxious because a friend's meningitis began with a sore throat
- The frail patient will struggle to cope at home with even a minor injury
- The suicidal patient has taken an overdose of which no one is aware

Social history

This is equally important in helping understand a patient's perspective on their situation. Areas to consider may include:

- Social contact: spouse, partner, family, friends, carers (and the frequency of their visits)
- Activities of daily living: who does the shopping, cooking, washing, cleaning
- Accommodation: how many floors, stairs (indoors and outdoors), lift
- Occupation (past and present), financial situation
- Alcohol intake, tobacco smoking and recreational drug use

All these factors play a significant part in placing the patient's problem in the context of their life and appreciating its impact upon them. Without addressing these points an assessment is incomplete and the final management plan may not be right for the patient in question. How much social history is required will depend on the individual patient – different questions will need to be asked of a young man who has had his first seizure (work, home life, hobbies, transport links) than will need to be asked of an older woman with new jaundice (tattoos, sexual contacts, injecting drug use, recent travel) for example. The art of emergency medicine requires careful consideration regarding what to ask to whom – in the exam the global score will certainly reflect the degree of a candidate's success in this area.

Scenario

Mr Parsons is a 76-year-old retired bus driver. He fell over at home and called an ambulance. His only injury is to his left wrist. His wrist X-ray does not demonstrate a fracture. Take a history from him and then explain your management plan to him.

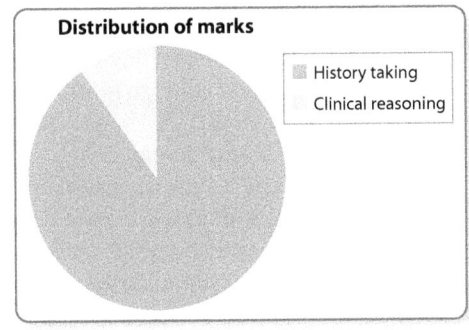

Distribution of marks
- History taking
- Clinical reasoning

Mark sheet	Achieved	Not achieved
Introduces self to patient and confirms their identity		
Checks level of comfort offers analgesia		
Establishes presenting complaint		
Specifically enquires about:		
– what patient was doing at the time?		
– any clear cause for fall?		
– any preceding symptoms?		
– did they lose consciousness – if so for how long?		
– any incontinence or tongue biting?		
– injuries sustained?		
– any witness?		
– could they get up? If so, how? If not, how long on floor?		
– any previous falls		
Past medical history		
Medications and allergies		
Social history (and illicit drug use) – alcohol, smoking, occupation		
Social history – mobility aids, type of accommodation, carers		
Elicits patient's concerns		
Explains plan: check blood pressure, blood sugar, blood tests, ECG		
Recommends falls clinic		
Recognises need for therapy-type assessment before discharge		
Discusses options: short term admission/rehabilitation bed/carers or family assistance		
Answers patient's questions appropriately		
Checks patient's understanding of diagnosis and plan		
Checks if patient has further questions		
Global mark from patient		
Global mark from examiner		

Instructions for actor

You are a 76-year-old retired bus driver called Andrew Parsons. After watching television you got up to go to the kitchen and forgot to use your walking stick. You lost your balance and fell over, landing on your left side. You could not get up, but were able to crawl to the phone and call an ambulance. You are left-handed and have a lot of pain and bruising in your wrist. You have no other injuries.

You previously had a stroke, because of which you have mild right-sided weakness but you can get around indoors using a stick in your left hand. You no longer take any regular medicines and have no allergies. You live alone in a first floor flat and have no lift. Your family visit and do your shopping for you once every fortnight. You do not go out, and you are lonely. You have no other carers. You do not think you can manage at home now you have hurt your arm. You do not want to tell the doctor this unless they ask you directly as you do not want to be a nuisance or admit you are scared of how you will manage. You feel you have been enough of a burden to everyone anyway. If the doctor does not explain what options there are to help you avoid staying in hospital, you should enquire about these.

1.3 Abdominal pain

Abdominal pain has a wide differential diagnosis. The College curriculum states that trainees should know common and serious causes and be able to differentiate between surgical, medical, gynaecological and urological causes of this presentation (**Table 1.3.1**). In addition candidates should appreciate that chest conditions like an inferior myocardial infarction or lower lobe pneumonia can also present with abdominal pain.

Candidates should aim to:
- Identify serious and common causes of abdominal pain
- Differentiate which system is likely to be involved, based on:
  - Age and gender
  - Site, onset, character, radiation, associations, type, exacerbating factors, severity of pain (SOCRATES)
  - Associated symptoms like vomiting, dysuria or weight loss
  - Duration of symptoms
  - Previous surgical/gynaecological/urological history
  - Previous such presentations
  - Pregnancy status
  - Alcohol intake
- Outline a differential diagnosis
- Make a management plan. What examination is needed and what further tests should be recommended?

Sudden, acute or delayed onset pain

Sudden onset pain is often serious. Perforation of gut or an aortic aneurysm leak can present suddenly, as can stone disease. Patients will remember what they were doing at that time and are able to give a specific time of onset. Remember though that the sudden severe pain may come with a history of a lesser background pain for a longer period of time.

Presentation over a few days is usually acute onset. Appendicitis, pyelonephritis, cholecystitis and diverticulitis are examples of conditions that usually present with a few days history.

Delayed onset over a few weeks is usually not an emergency, although suspected sub-acute bowel obstruction or cancer still needs urgent management.

Somatic and visceral pain

One of the first steps is to differentiate whether the pain is coming from intra-abdominal organs or if there is any peritoneal irritation. Visceral pain is dull and poorly localised to the upper, mid or lower abdomen depending on whether the foregut, midgut or hindgut structures are involved.

Once the parietal peritoneum is irritated due to any cause, pain becomes somatic in nature and is sharp and well localised. This is the reason why appendicitis patients initially have dull, poorly localised central abdominal pain. Once inflammation spreads to involve the peritoneum, it becomes localised to right lower quadrant.

Referred pain and radiation of pain

Referred pain is localised to an area distant from its origin. Perhaps the best example is shoulder tip pain in patients with a ruptured ectopic pregnancy or a ruptured spleen. The physiological explanation for this pain is irritation of the diaphragm from intraperitoneal blood. The nerve supply of the diaphragm is from C3,4,5 (remember 'C3,4,5 keeps the diaphragm alive') and somatic afferent nerve fibres from the shoulder also enter at the same level, hence the pain is referred to the shoulder.

Similarly, pain can radiate from front to back (e.g. pancreatitis or sometimes biliary colic) or from loin to groin (e.g. ureteric colic).

Constant or colicky pain

Distension of hollow organs (because of obstruction or pseudo-obstruction) produces colicky pain, e.g. biliary, ureteric, intestinal or fallopian. The pain comes in waves, settling down in between. Beware of colicky pain in women of child-bearing age (ectopic pregnancy).

Other symptoms

Syncope with abdominal pain is an indication of serious pathology. Ruptured ectopic pregnancy or aortic aneurysm should be excluded. Vomiting is often associated with abdominal pain and if pain started first then it is said that a surgical cause is more likely. Dysuria or other urinary symptoms suggest a renal tract cause. Abnormal vaginal discharge with lower abdominal pain raises the suspicion of pelvic inflammatory disease.

Table 1.3.1 Presentation of abdominal pain by cause

Condition	Classical presentation
Acute pancreatitis	Acute onset, constant epigastric pain radiating to the back
	History of alcohol abuse or gallstones +/− previous pancreatitis
Infected obstructed kidney	Colicky flank pain (sharp and severe) with relief in between, radiating from loin to groin, may become constant
	History of fever, dysuria, previous urolithiasis
Intestinal obstruction	Dull colicky pain, with vomiting, constipation and abdominal distension
	History of previous abdominal surgery, cancer or hernia
Mesenteric ischaemia	Sudden onset, constant, severe, poorly localised pain
	May start from periumbilical region and then becomes diffuse
	History of atrial fibrillation, elderly patient with significant cardiovascular disease
Perforated viscus	Sudden onset, constant, sharp pain, increasing with movement
	History of diverticulitis or peptic ulcer disease
Ruptured ectopic pregnancy	Acute onset lower abdomen pain localised to affected side, with radiation to shoulder or back
	Can be associated with syncope, gastrointestinal disturbance or vaginal bleeding
	History of reproductive age group, missed period or confirmed pregnancy, previous ectopic or risk factors for it

Cont'd...

Cont'd...

Leaking abdominal aortic aneurysm	Sudden onset severe pain radiating to back, flanks or legs
	Often associated with syncope or presyncope
	History of cardiovascular disease, or risk factor for it like smoking, hypertension and diabetes

Scenario

Claire Parker is a 38-year-old woman who has had abdominal pain for the last 2 days. She has been taking painkillers with no effect.

At triage her temperature was 37.7°C, pulse 90 beats per minute, blood pressure 110/70 mmHg and respiratory rate 16 breaths per minute. She was given codeine 30 mg orally for pain relief. Take a history from her and then explain a management plan to her.

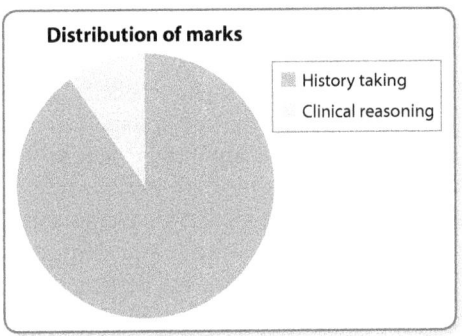

Mark sheet	Achieved	Not achieved
Introduces self to patient and confirms their identity		
Checks level of comfort offers analgesia		
Establishes presenting complaint		
Specifically enquires about:		
– duration, character, nature, site, radiation of pain		
– exacerbating or relieving factors		
– severity of pain		
Past medical history		
Past surgical history		
Past gynaecological history		
Medications and allergies		
Social history (and illicit drug use)		
Elicits patient's concerns		
Suggests appropriate differential diagnosis		
Explains plan:		
– abdominal examination		
– appropriate blood tests		
– urine dipstick for pregnancy and infection		
Answers patient's questions appropriately		
Does not agree to a scan until the patient has been examined		

Cont'd...

Cont'd...

Mark sheet	Achieved	Not achieved
Checks patient's understanding of diagnosis and plan		
Checks if patient has further questions		
Global mark from patient		
Global mark from examiner		

Instructions for actor

You are a 38-year-old woman called Claire Parker, and you have had abdominal pain for the last 2 days. You noticed it first on your way to work (office secretary), but ignored it. It feels like 'bellyache' around the belly button and around your lower right side. There is an ongoing ache but every so often you get a sharp severe pain in your groin that makes you feel sweaty and faint. It has got worse over the last 2 days. The pain does not move or radiate anywhere but is worse when you are passing urine.

You are not sure if you are passing urine more often than usual though you have felt a bit hot and cold. You tried taking paracetamol tablets, which helped on the first day but not today. Your pain is 5 out of 10 in severity but you are comfortable at the moment after being given codeine in the ED. You feel a bit sick but have not vomited and don't feel hungry at all.

You are usually healthy and well and never had this before. You have never had any abdominal surgery and don't have any abnormal vaginal discharge. Your last menstrual period was 1 month ago and you are due any time now. You have normal periods – you certainly do not have heavy bleeding. You do not take any medications and are not allergic to any medications.

You are sexually active, use contraceptive pills and have not missed any tablets. You haven't had sexual intercourse with anyone except your husband for the 12 years that you have been married and you don't think he has either. You last had sex the weekend before last. If asked, you have not recently taken any antibiotics. Nor have you had any diarrhoea or vomiting in the last few months.

You are concerned that you may have appendicitis and don't want to have an operation as your mother had a bad experience with pain when she had a knee operation. You think that you should get a scan to find out what is going on.

1.4 Rectal bleeding

Rectal bleeding is a common ED presentation. When taking the history, you are aiming to establish the anatomical location and severity of bleeding along with risk factors for a further bleed. As always, the goal of history taking is to be able to plan a focused examination and make a management plan appropriate to the severity of symptoms and the differential diagnosis.

Since large bowel cancer and colitis are important possible causes, they should be explored specifically as part of the history.

Common causes of rectal bleeding (Table 1.4.1)

In children, Meckel's diverticulum and intussusception are causes of small bowel bleeding, which can lead to rectal bleeding. Meckel's diverticulum causes dark red blood or occasionally melaena. Intussusception typically causes 'redcurrant jelly' stools.

Sometimes acute upper gastrointestinal bleeding can be so severe as to cause fresh blood per rectum or bleeding from the caecum may present as melaena. Therefore, the colour of the stool can only be considered as a guide to the origin of the bleeding.

Enquire about any change in bowel habit. Establish what is normal for the patient and what has changed. Is it a change in consistency or frequency of bowel motion? Establish what constipation and diarrhoea mean for this patient and whether there are any alternating symptoms. Various medical causes of change in bowel habit such as hypothyroidism, hypercalcaemia, diabetic neuropathy, and chronic pancreatitis may be relevant and need to be screened for in the history.

Table 1.4.1 Presentation of rectal bleeding by cause

Cause	Presentation
Haemorrhoids	Self-limiting bright red bleeding, painless, blood covering the stools
	History of constipation, bright red blood on toilet paper
Diverticular disease	Usually over 65, bleeding mixed with stools or dark red coloured stools
	History of left lower abdominal pain, constipation, bloating, diverticular disease on colonoscopy
Inflammatory bowel disease	Often relatively young patient, chronic diarrhoea presenting with blood in stools
	History of intermittent lower abdominal pain, weight loss, fever and systemic symptoms
Angiodysplasia	Usually over 65, episodes of painless bright red bleeding which may be severe
	History of renal disease, aortic stenosis, on oral anticoagulation
Colorectal cancer	Usually over 50, painless rectal bleeding, blood mixed with stools
	History of weight loss, change in bowel habit, family history of polyps or colon cancer, may experience tenesmus if rectal cancer
Ischaemic colitis	Age over 65, sudden onset lower abdominal pain or cramping and diarrhoea mixed with blood
	History of diabetes, hypertension, haemodialysis
Radiation enteropathy	Persistent or severe bleeding
	History of radiotherapy for pelvic cancer, chronic diarrhoea, rectal pain, urgency, faecal incontinence. Most commonly 2–5 months after radiotherapy

The history should cover some additional specific questions:
- The nature of the bleeding: duration, colour, mixed with stool or separate from stool and amount of bleeding
- Presence of local symptoms such as tenesmus, awareness of any external masses or blood on toilet paper
- Presence of systemic symptoms such as weight loss, dizziness, syncope, confusion, postural symptoms, abdominal pain or fever
- Risk factors:
  - Current medications, anticoagulant use, aspirin, anti-inflammatories, antibiotics
  - Alcohol use
  - Previous history of bleeding or of previous surgery or endoscopy
  - Comorbidities

Scenario

Mrs Taylor is a 68-year-old woman who noticed blood in her stools this morning. She called an ambulance and it brought her to the ED. Take a history and explain a management plan to her.

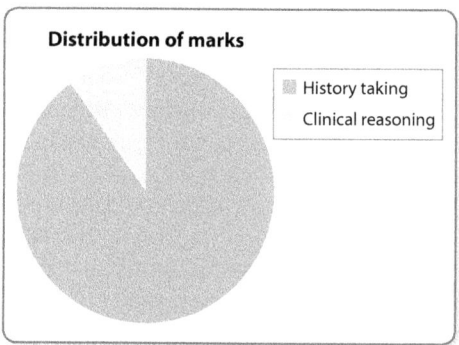

Distribution of marks
- History taking
- Clinical reasoning

Mark sheet	Achieved	Not achieved
Introduces self to patient and confirms their identity		
Checks level of comfort offers analgesia		
Establishes presenting complaint		
Specifically enquires about:		
– nature of bleeding		
– frequency of episodes		
Previous history of bleeding		
Presence of pain		
Presence of systemic symptoms		
Presence of altered bowel habit		
Past medical history		
Past surgical history		
Previous endoscopies		
Medications and allergies		
Social history (and illicit drug use)		
Elicits patient's concerns		
Offers to call daughter to help with dog		
Suggests appropriate differential diagnosis		

Cont'd...

Cont'd...

Mark sheet	Achieved	Not achieved
Explains plan:		
– abdominal (and rectal) examination		
– appropriate blood tests		
Answers patient's questions appropriately		
Checks patient's understanding of diagnosis and plan		
Checks if patient has further questions		
Global mark from patient		
Global mark from examiner		

Instructions for actor

You are a 68-year-old woman called Angela Taylor. You felt some abdominal pain this morning with an urge to go to the toilet. You initially thought you might have had an infection that is causing the bellyache. You passed a loose stool that was mainly bloody and dark red or brown in colour. It seemed like a large volume and filled the toilet bowl. When you got up you felt dizzy, light-headed, sweaty, and had to hold on to the door to avoid falling over. This has never happened before.

You felt a bit better once you lay down and then even managed to eat some breakfast. You have had a hysterectomy and are on warfarin, lisinopril and inhalers for chronic obstructive pulmonary disease (COPD). You don't know why you take these medications and have been on them for years.

You live by yourself and do your own shopping and cooking, with some help from your daughter on the weekends.

You are concerned about this episode and your dog, which is alone at home.

Suggested reading

Leal A. Lower gastrointestinal haemorhage. RCEM Learning. London: RCEM Learning 2019.
Scottish Intercollegiate Guidelines Network (SIGN). Management of acute upper and lower gastrointestinal bleeding. SIGN Guideline 105. Edinburgh: SIGN; 2008.

1.5 Apparent life-threatening event

An apparent life-threatening event (ALTE) is a presentation in infants, which has a wide differential diagnosis. It is also referred to as a brief resolved unexplained event (BRUE). The aim of the history in this station is to establish the facts around the event, enquire about the child, assess the risk of death, check for potential non-accidental injury (NAI) and handle parental anxiety.

An ALTE is defined as a sudden event, frightening to the observer in which the infant exhibits a combination of symptoms which may include a change in colour (cyanosis, pale, plethoric, redness), apnoea, change in muscle tone (floppy or rigid) with associated choking or gagging. It often provokes resuscitation attempts from the observer. The child then recovers spontaneously.

History taking (ideally from a first-hand observer) should cover:

1. **Description of the event**
   - Circumstances – e.g. was the child awake or asleep? What position (prone, supine or on side) were they in, and where were they (crib, parent's bed, cot, car seat)? What else was nearby – bedclothes, blankets, pillows, toys, siblings, animals? Who was caring and where were they? What alerted them?
   - Activity at time of the event – feeding, coughing, gagging, choking, vomiting?
   - Breathing effort – none, shallow, gasping, increased?
   - Colour – pale, red, purple, blue? In what distribution (peripheral, circumoral, whole body)
   - Movement and tone – rigid, tonic-clonic, decreased or floppy
   - Observed cough or vomiting – mucus, blood or noise (silent, cough, gag, wheeze, stridor, crying)
   - Duration of the event – length of time required to reinstate normal breathing, tone and behaviour and length and time of resuscitation required

2. **Interventions that were performed (in escalating order)**
   - None
   - Gentle stimulation
   - Blowing air in face
   - Vigorous stimulation
   - Mouth-to-mouth breathing
   - Cardiopulmonary resuscitation by medically trained personnel

3. **History of any current illness**
   - Ill in days or hours leading up to event
   - Fever
   - Poor feeding
   - Weight loss
   - Rash
   - Irritability
   - Contact with someone who is sick, medications administered, immunisation

4. **Medical history**
   - Antenatal history of mother – use of drugs, tobacco or alcohol during pregnancy
   - Small for gestational age? Prematurity?
   - Birth history – birth trauma, hypoxia, sepsis

- Feeding history – gagging, coughing, poor weight gain
  - Development history – appropriate milestones
  - Previous admissions – surgery, ALTE
  - Accidents – being dropped, tossed, possibility of NAI
5. **Family history**
   - Congenital problems, neurologic conditions, neonatal/child deaths
   - Smoking in the home
   - Cardiac arrhythmias
   - Sudden infant death syndrome

Risk assessment

There is an increased risk following an ALTE if:
- Age <28 days
- Significant prematurity
- Significant prior medical illness
- Clinically unwell
- Recurrent events before presentation
- More severe/prolonged ALTE

Risk factors indicating possibility of non-accidental injury

- Previous cyanosis, apnoea or ALTE while in the care of same person
- Age >6 months
- Previous unexpected or unexplained deaths of one or more siblings
- Previous death of infants, under the care of the same person
- Simultaneous or nearly simultaneous death of twins
- Discovery of blood on the infant's nose or mouth in association with ALTE

Common causes

Exaggerated airway protection reflexes are often the physiological basis of these episodes. In some infants, the laryngeal chemoreceptors, on coming in contact with saliva or vomitus produce apnoea with cyanosis and change in muscle tone, rather than a simple cough. This sensitivity may also be increased by upper respiratory viral infections like respiratory syncytial virus.

Gastro-oesophageal reflux disease (GORD), seizures and lower respiratory tract infections account for 50% of the diagnoses associated with ALTE.

Management plan

- Detailed physical examination of all systems, including retinal examination to check for retinal haemorrhage in suspected NAI
- Consider investigation with full blood count, urea and electrolytes, blood glucose, nasopharyngeal aspirate for viruses and pertussis and ECG to check Q-T interval. Other investigations should be tailored to the presentation
- In practice many of these patients are admitted for observation

Scenario

An ambulance has brought in Mrs Davis and her son Chris who is 2 months old. While he was asleep his mother noticed that he seemed to have choked and then stopped breathing for some time. She called an ambulance straight away. Chris is well now and is playful and active. Take a history from Mrs Davis and explain a management plan to her.

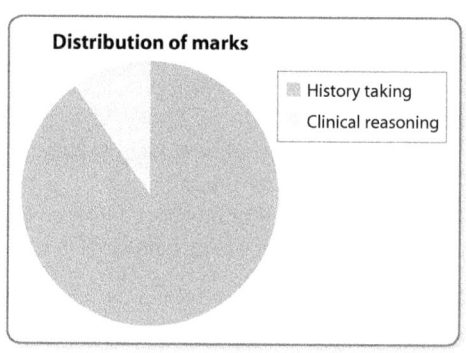

Mark sheet	Achieved	Not achieved
Introduces self, appropriately greets the patient		
Calms Mrs Davis, reassures about her son		
Starts with appropriate opening question		
Establishes presenting complaint		
Specifically enquires about:		
– location of child		
– activity at time of the event		
– breathing efforts		
– colour and its distribution		
– movement and tone		
– observed cough or vomiting		
– duration of the event		
– asks about interventions undertaken		
– any current illness		
Takes antenatal history		
Takes birth history		
Takes developmental history		
Checks immunisation status		
Takes feeding history – bottle or breastfed, volume taken		
Asks about previous admissions, previous episodes		
Asks about family history		
Asks about home environment		
Identifies duration of ALTE and of any preceding symptoms		
Offers appropriate differential diagnosis		
Outlines reasonable management plan		
Invites questions and answers any concerns		
Checks patient's understanding of diagnosis and plan		
Global score from examiner		
Global score from mother		

Instructions for actor

Your name is Julia Davis. You have come to the ED by ambulance because when putting your son Chris in his cot after feeding he coughed and seemed to go blue and stop breathing. Eventually, he started breathing after you picked him up and patted his back but was floppy for several minutes. He started crying soon after and seems to have got better now. You called an ambulance immediately and are still worried about whether Chris is going to be alright or could the same thing happen again.

He has never had anything like this before. He was born a week early by a normal delivery in hospital. You were discharged the same day. He is now 2 months old and has been gaining weight appropriate to his age and drinks approximately seven to eight bottles a day of 60 mL of formula. He was a bit snuffly yesterday, but had no fever and has been feeding as normal. He is your first child and there are no other children at home. He had his first immunisations last week. There is no family history of anything similar. You are worried this was caused by immunising Chris. If the doctor suggests you might go home now, you become distressed about the idea of the same thing happening again. If you are offered a period of observation for Chris you are reassured.

Suggested reading

Karen LH, Barry Z. Evaluation and management of apparent life-threatening events in children. Am Fam Physician 2005; 71:2301–2308.

1.6 Back pain

Most patients presenting with back pain have mechanical lumbar back pain. But one must exclude other important diagnoses like an aortic dissection, abdominal aortic aneurysm, cauda equina syndrome, epidural abscess, osteomyelitis and cancer.

Therefore, when taking a history, it is essential to ask about systemic symptoms, identify any critical neurological symptoms as well as key 'red flag' symptoms which should provoke further investigation.

Red flag symptoms:
- Age <20 or >50 years
- Thoracic pain
- Recent significant trauma or mild trauma in patients older than 50 years
- Acute onset of back, flank or testicular pain
- Constant pain worse at night or rest
- Collapse or nausea associated with back pain
- History of prolonged steroid use, osteoporosis, syncope, cancer, intravenous drug use, immunocompromised state, recent bacterial infection, morning stiffness lasting more than an hour
- Unexplained fever >38°C or unexplained weight loss
- Neurological deficit
- Spinal deformity

Specific features to ask about

1. **Character of pain**
   Pain localised to the lower back, gluteal area and thighs with varying intensity and better at rest in a patient with good health is usually mechanical back pain. Sciatica is pain originating in the lower back and radiating to the lower leg in lumbar nerve root distribution.
2. **Where is the pain and where does it radiate?**
   Thoracic pain is a red flag. Radiation to the legs and specifically below the knees or in dermatomal distribution indicates nerve root involvement. L5 and S1 pain radiates distal to the knee and is more intense than the back pain. L3 and L4 pain radiates to the front or medial aspect of the thigh and medial side of the calf or foot. Radiation to the chest or abdomen should be a prompt to look for a more serious cause. Flank pain suggests a renal cause.
3. **When did the pain start?**
   Acute onset while doing something specific suggests a mechanical cause. Sudden onset severe pain suggests a vascular event like dissection or a leaking aneurysm. Slow onset pain, gradually worsening over time unrelated to activity raises the possibility of tumour or infection.
4. **Aggravating or relieving features**
   Pain increasing with movement or cough is usually mechanical in nature. Nocturnal pain, or pain not relieved by analgesics could be tumour-related. Pain increasing with walking which radiates to the legs and eases with flexion of the back suggests lumbar canal stenosis.
5. **Neurological deficit**
   Sensory or motor weakness, loss of bladder or bowel control and perineal sensory deficit

all indicate possible cauda equina or spinal cord compression. The symptoms should be confirmed with detailed neurological examination and investigated as an emergency with an MRI.
6. **Associated history**
These should cover the red flag features like syncope, fever, intravenous drug abuse, medications like anticoagulants or steroids.
7. **Past medical history**
Ask specifically about cancer (risk of metastatic disease), inflammatory disease, intravenous drug abuse (risk of discitis), arthropathy (ankylosing spondylitis), endocrinopathy (hyperparathyroidism), bleeding disorders (retropharyngeal haematoma), osteoporosis (wedge fracture), or sickle cell disease (crisis).

Scenario

Mr Redfern is a 49-year-old man presenting with back pain. He has been taking painkillers but today he is finding it difficult to walk.

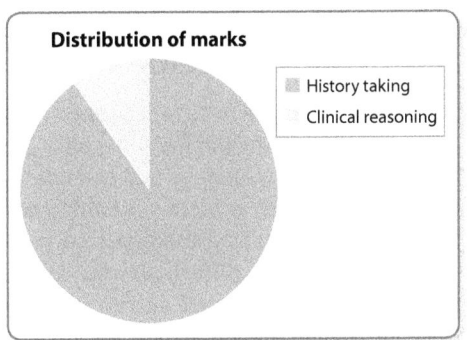

Distribution of marks
- History taking
- Clinical reasoning

Mark sheet	Achieved	Not achieved
Introduces self to patient and confirms their identity		
Checks level of comfort offers analgesia		
Establishes presenting complaint		
Specifically enquires about:		
– characteristics of pain		
– duration of symptoms		
– ability to walk		
– presence of neurological symptoms		
– presence of red flag symptoms		
– presence of systemic symptoms		
Past medical history		
Medications and allergies		
Social history (and illicit drug use)		
Elicits patient's concerns		
Suggests appropriate differential diagnosis		
Explains plan:		
– relevant examination		

Cont'd...

Cont'd...

Mark sheet	Achieved	Not achieved
– appropriate blood tests		
– bladder scan/urinary catheter		
Answers patient's questions appropriately		
Shows empathy		
Checks patient's understanding of diagnosis and plan		
Checks if patient has further questions		
Global mark from patient		
Global mark from examiner		

Instructions for actor

You are a 49-year-old man called Julius Redfern. You are a forklift operator who returned from work 3 days ago and felt some back pain. You took some paracetamol and slept. Next morning the pain was worse and you now have sharp pain in your lower back. It seemed to spread to the left leg as far as your ankle, with pins and needles in your foot. You have rested for the last 2 days, taking analgesia, 'co-something', as advised by your general practitioner (GP). You now find it difficult to walk, and today you were not able to stand up.

The pain is getting worse and now involves both legs. You can't feel your left foot and are not able to sit up due to severe pain. This morning you wet yourself without realising it. You have never been incontinent and are very anxious.

You were not able to sleep last night due to the pain. You feel nauseated, but haven't vomited and have not felt feverish. You are otherwise healthy and well, and do not take any medications. You have no allergies. You have had mild back pain in the past, but nothing like this.

You spoke to your GP again today and he advised you to go to hospital for an urgent scan of your back. You are worried that you may end up never being able to walk again.

Suggested reading

Guly H. Acute lower back pain. RCEM Learning: London: RCEM Learning; 2014.
National Institute for Health and Care Excellence (NICE). Low back pain and sciatica in over 16s. NG 59. NICE. London: NICE; 2016.

1.7 Syncope

Syncope is defined as a transient loss of consciousness due to global cerebral hypoperfusion that is characterised by a rapid onset, short duration and quick recovery leaving no sequelae. Therefore, it is important to clearly establish whether there was any loss of consciousness or not. The key features of a syncopal episode to elicit for making a diagnosis are discussed in **Tables 1.7.1** to **1.7.3**.

Table 1.7.1 Causes of syncope

Reflex syncope	Orthostatic hypotension (OH) syndromes	Cardiovascular syncope
Vasovagal episode Simple faint – emotional distress or orthostatic stress and associated typical prodrome (3 Ps – posture, prodrome, provoking factors) **Situational syncope** During or immediately following specific triggers, e.g. after micturition, straining or pain **Carotid sinus syncope** Due to carotid sinus massage **Atypical** No typical trigger but classical history	**Classical OH** >20 mmHg drop in systolic or >10 mmHg drop in diastolic pressure within 3 minutes of standing **Initial OH** Immediate drop in blood pressure of >40 mmHg on standing that corrects itself rapidly to normal **Delayed hypotension** Slow progressive decrease in systolic blood pressure on standing, usually in the elderly **Postural orthostatic tachycardia syndrome (POTS)** Usually in young women, marked heart rate increase (by >30 beats per minute or to >120 beats per minute) and instability of blood pressure Secondary autonomic failures, e.g. in Parkinson's	**Arrhythmias** Tachy-brady syndrome Sick sinus syndrome Paroxysmal atrial fibrillation Atrioventricular blocks – second or third degree Long QT syndromes Drug induced, e.g. beta-blockers, digoxin, and quinolones **Structural heart disease** Hypertrophic obstructive cardiomyopathy Arrhythmogenic right ventricular cardiomyopathy Myocardial infarction Aortic stenosis Pulmonary hypertension Prolapsed atrial myxoma **Cardiovascular collapse** Pulmonary embolism Aortic dissection

Table 1.7.2 Risk factors for cardiovascular syncope

From history	ECG features
During exertion or while supine	Persistent sinus bradycardia <40 beats per minute or sinus pause >3 seconds
Palpitations before onset	Mobitz II, complete heart block or 'trifascicular' block*
Family history of sudden cardiac death or channelopathy	Alternating LBBB and RBBB
Known structural heart disease	VT or rapid paroxysmal AF/SVT
Anaemia or electrolyte disturbance	Torsades or long or short QT
	Brugada syndrome – RBBB with ST elevation in leads V1-V3
	AVRC – Q waves in right precordial leads, epsilon waves, and ventricular late potentials

*Trifascicular block is the combination of first-degree heart block (prolonged PR interval), right bundle branch block (RSR or M pattern in V1) and left anterior (left axis deviation) or left posterior (right axis deviation) hemi block.

Table 1.7.3 Clinical features of syncope versus seizure

Feature	Syncope	Seizure
Trigger	Common	Rare
Prodrome	Presyncopal features like nausea, sweating, pallor	Aura – unpleasant smell, epigastric sensation
Onset	Gradual	Sudden
Duration	1–30 seconds	1–3 minutes
Colour	Usually pale	Cyanosed
Convulsions	May have movement after loss of consciousness (LOC)	Tonic-clonic movements, automatism, neck turned to one side
Tongue bite	Rare, usually on the tip	Common, on the side
Post event	Rapid recovery, nausea or vomiting afterwards	Confusion, aching muscles, joint dislocations

Scenario

Mr Chaudhary is a 65-year-old man who presents with a fall whilst shopping. He is well and has not had any injuries. Take a detailed history regarding the fall and make a management plan.

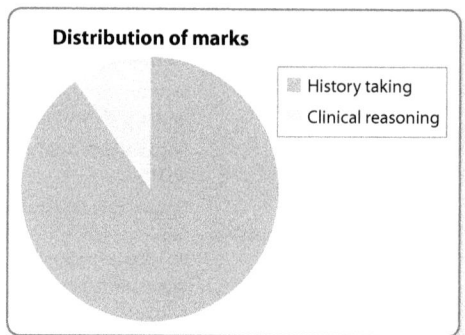

Distribution of marks
- History taking
- Clinical reasoning

Mark sheet	Achieved	Not achieved
Introduces self to patient and confirms their identity		
Checks level of comfort offers analgesia		
Establishes presenting complaint		
Specifically enquires about:		
– circumstances prior to event		
– any preceding symptoms?		
– what the patient remembers about the event?		
– did they lose consciousness – if so for how long?		
– any incontinence or tongue biting		
– any limb jerking		
– duration of event		
– injuries sustained		
– any witness?		

Cont'd...

Cont'd...

Mark sheet	Achieved	Not achieved
– history of recovery phase post event		
– any previous episodes		
Past medical history		
Medications and allergies		
Social history (and illicit drug use) – alcohol, smoking, occupation		
Social history – mobility aids, type of accommodation, carers		
Elicits patient's concerns		
Explains differential diagnosis		
Explains plan – check postural blood pressures, blood sugar, blood tests, ECG		
Recommends follow-up in appropriate setting		
Answers patient's questions appropriately		
Checks patient's understanding of diagnosis and plan		
Checks if patient has further questions		
Global mark from patient		
Global mark from examiner		

Instructions for actor

You are a 65-year-old man called Mahesh Chaudhary. You were brought to ED after falling in the street earlier in the day. You had a dental appointment this morning for a check-up. The next bus home was after an hour and you decided to take a walk around the town rather than stand at the bus stop. You sat down on a bench when you felt tired. On getting up, you felt light headed, had blurred vision and then blacked out. You tried to hold on to the bench but could not, and you cannot remember anything after that. When you regained consciousness, you were on the floor with a passer by helping you to sit up and asking you how you were. You felt a little confused but that improved soon after. You did not hurt yourself, were not incontinent and did not bite your tongue.

You did not have breakfast as you were in a hurry but are feeling hungry now. You did take your blood pressure tablet however. You live by yourself and are self-caring with shopping, cooking and cleaning. Your daughter helps out on the weekends with meals. You are usually healthy and well and are eager to go home.

Suggested reading

Dunn M. Syncope. RCEM Learning. London: RCEM Learning; 2011.
National Institute for Health and Care Excellence (NICE). Transient loss of consciousness in over 16s. CG109. NICE. London: NICE; 2010.

1.8 Dizziness and falls

Dizziness has different meanings for different patients. The first thing to do is to clarify what the patient is experiencing. They should be encouraged to describe what they feel with some input from the clinician.

Vertigo

This is the sensation of disorientation in space, with the hallucination of movement. This is often associated with nausea or vomiting. Once it is confirmed that the patient is describing vertigo, you should try to ascertain whether this is peripheral, e.g. due to a labyrinthine disorder, or central, e.g. due to a cerebellar stroke, transient ischaemic attack (TIA) or posterior fossa mass (**Table 1.8.1**).

Disequilibrium

There will not be a true sensation of vertigo, but patients may experience imbalance when standing or walking. This could be due to peripheral causes such as neuropathy or central causes like spinal cord compression.

Presyncope

Patients describe the sensation of feeling light-headed, as if going to faint. If this is related to postural change, or is happening each time the patient is getting up, they may be experiencing orthostatic hypotension. There are various other causes of syncope and they are discussed in detail in section 1.7.

Fatigue or general weakness

Anaemia, viral illness or even malignancy can make patients feel generally weak and lethargic and they may be using 'dizziness' to describe the feeling of malaise rather than true vertigo.

Table 1.8.1 Characteristics of central and peripheral vertigo

Characteristic	Peripheral	Central
Onset	Sudden	Gradual or sudden
Intensity	Severe	Mild
Duration	Usually seconds or minutes; occasionally hours or days – intermittent	Usually weeks or months (continuous) but can be seconds or minutes with vascular causes
Direction of nystagmus	One direction, horizontal or rotatory, never vertical	Different directions in different positions
Effect of head position	Worsened by position, often single critical position	Little change, associated with more than one position
Associated neurologic findings	None	Usually present
Associated auditory findings	May be present including tinnitus	None

(Adapted from Marx JA, et al. Rosen's Emergency Medicine, 7th edn. Philadelphia: Mosby, 2010)

This symptom clarification is often the most important part of the history in a patient presenting with dizziness. Once the true nature of the patient's problem is identified, further details can be asked as to the cause of their symptoms.

Elderly patients who fall

While dizziness could be a cause of falls, patients can fall for a variety of reasons. Elderly patients presenting with a fall require a detailed history of the circumstances around the fall. Remember it is unlikely that this was a simple slip or 'mechanical fall' – there is an underlying condition which led them to fall over. Always ask yourself 'Why did they trip on that rug today when they cross it successfully every day?'

Causes of falls in the elderly can be divided into causes intrinsic and extrinsic to the patient and often the cause is multifactorial. Attempts should be made to identify any reversible causes.

- Intrinsic factors:
  - Gait and musculoskeletal dysfunction
  - Foot problems
  - Cognitive or other neurological impairment
  - Cardiovascular disease or other acute illness, e.g. infections
- Extrinsic factors:
  - Environmental hazards
  - Polypharmacy
  - Use of walking stick or frame
  - Prior history of falls

Approach to history

Even though the patient may present with an injury it is essential to elicit the circumstances around the fall.

- Location of incident
- Activity at the time
- Any warning symptoms before (absence of warning is highly suggestive of cardiovascular causes)?
- Was there loss of consciousness? Do they remember hitting the ground?
- Events after fall: how did they get help? How long they stayed on the floor?
- Injuries sustained
- Are there any new symptoms like limb weakness or incontinence?
- Were there any cardiovascular symptoms such as chest pain or palpitations?

Scenario

Mr Stephens is an 83-year-old man presenting after a fall. He is complaining of left hip pain and is feeling nauseated. Take a history and discuss investigations and a management plan with him.

Distribution of marks

- History taking
- Clinical reasoning

Mark sheet	Achieved	Not achieved
Introduces self to patient and confirms their identity		
Checks level of comfort offers analgesia		
Establishes presenting complaint		
Specifically enquires about:		
– what patient was doing at the time?		
– any clear cause for fall?		
– any preceding symptoms?		
– establishes symptoms related to dizziness		
– did they lose consciousness – if so for how long?		
– any incontinence or tongue biting?		
– injuries sustained?		
– any witness?		
– could they get up? If so, how? If not, how long on floor?		
– any previous falls		
Past medical history		
Medications and allergies		
Social history (and illicit drug use) – alcohol, smoking, occupation		
Social history – mobility aids, type of accommodation, carers		
Elicits patient's concerns		
Explains plan: need to exclude hip fracture, check blood pressure, blood sugar, blood tests, ECG		
Answers patient's questions appropriately		
Checks patient's understanding of diagnosis and plan		
Checks if patient has further questions		
Global mark from patient		
Global mark from examiner		

Instructions for actor

You are an 83-year-old man called Mark Stephens. You live in a ground floor flat, by yourself and are self-caring. Your daughter helps you with shopping once a week, and cleaning at home, but you manage to take a shower and go to the toilet yourself.

You fell at home this morning when you got up to go to toilet. You felt dizzy as if you are in a whirlpool and were not able to balance yourself when you fell. You think that you lost consciousness, but are not very sure. You were not able to get up due to hip pain. You have no other injuries. You are still feeling very dizzy each time you try and move your head and are feeling nauseous and hearing a buzzing noise in your ears. The pain in your hip is still quite severe. You score it as 5 out of 10.

You got help by pressing your emergency buzzer for help. You have not fallen before, but have felt dizzy and were recently stated on a medication for it by your GP. You take medications for blood pressure, angina, leg cramps, sleeping tablets, a tablet for depression and are on warfarin for recurrent PEs.

You are worried you may have broken your hip.

1.9 Chest pain

A thorough history is essential to identify the likely cause of a complaint. Causes are divided into cardiac (which can be further subdivided into ischaemic or non-ischaemic), pulmonary, vascular, gastro-oesophageal or musculoskeletal.

Diagnoses to consider are acute coronary syndrome, pericarditis, pulmonary embolism, aortic dissection, oesophageal reflux or rupture and pneumothorax.

All of these presentations can have typical (as described below) or atypical presentations. Candidates must be aware of variation and atypical presentations associated with causes of chest pain.

Ischaemic cardiac pain

Typically, this is:
- Constricting pain in the anterior chest radiating to neck, arms, shoulder or jaw
- Exacerbated by physical exertion
- Relieved by rest or glyceryl trinitrate within approximately 5 minutes
- Associated with breathlessness, nausea or sweating

If the pain described has all the features as above, it is typical angina. If the pain has two features, it is atypical and if one or none of the above, it may be classed as non-angina pain. Features that make angina unlikely are:
- Pain is continuous or very prolonged
- Unrelated to activity
- Brought on by breathing
- Associated with symptoms such as dizziness, palpitations, tingling or difficulty in swallowing

Pleuritic pain

Pleuritic pain is typically sharp, localised, peripheral and worse with breathing. Rather than true breathlessness patients may describe shallow breathing because pain increases with deep inspiration.
- Unexplained dyspnoea, tachycardia or a history of haemoptysis in a patient, particularly with risk factors for venous thromboembolism, should prompt investigations to confirm or exclude a pulmonary embolus (PE)
- Fever, yellowish sputum and confusion could be present in a patient with pneumonia. A history of travel makes atypical pneumonia more likely
- Myalgia, prodromal illness, fever, cough, sore throat and runny nose could be feature of a viral infection with pleurisy
- A young patient that is tall and thin with associated shortness of breath or a cough could have a spontaneous pneumothorax

Aortic dissection

The typical patient is a man in his 60s with a history of hypertension and sudden onset pain, maximal at the time of onset, described as sharp, tearing or stabbing in nature. As the dissection progresses the site of pain changes from retrosternal to interscapular or even back pain. Patients may present with syncope, myocardial infarction (occlusion of coronary arteries at the ostia), hemiplegia (dissection extending to the internal carotid artery) or paraplegia (spinal cord infarction due to anterior spinal artery occlusion). Be warned that not all cases are typical, however, and this diagnosis can easily be missed particularly in its early stages.

Gastro-oesophageal reflux

This is typically retrosternal and associated with a burning sensation. The pain may be worse after eating and worse on lying down or bending forward. Symptoms may include nausea, bloating, bad breath and a cough.

Oesophageal rupture

This causes relatively sudden onset pain that is retrosternal, sharp and pleuritic in nature. It often occurs following forceful vomiting or an impacted food bolus. The patient is usually unwell and may have a history of swallowing problems or gastro-oesophageal reflux disease (GORD). Prolonged sharp pain which is worse with food and improving with antacids, associated with heartburn or dysphagia could be of oesophageal origin.

Assessing risk factors

Risk factors for the various causes of chest pain should be assessed routinely as part of the history. If cardiac pain is part of the differential diagnosis, enquire about risk factors for ischaemic heart disease and if suspecting PE, enquire about risk factors for venous thromboembolism. Candidates should be familiar with appropriate risk stratitfication scoring systems for the conditions mentioned above.

Scenario

Mr Potts is a 43-year-old man who is presenting with chest pain. He was driving to work when he felt pain in his chest. He stopped the car and decided to come to hospital and is currently pain free. Take a history and make appropriate management plan.

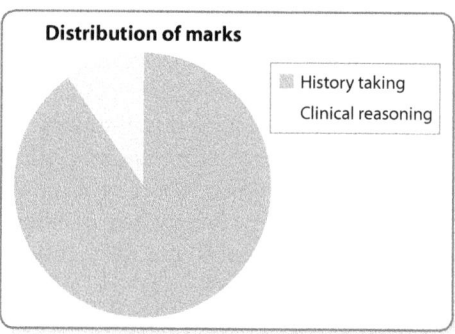

Mark sheet	Achieved	Not achieved
Introduces self to patient and confirms their identity		
Checks level of comfort offers analgesia		
Establishes presenting complaint		
Specifically enquires about:		
– characteristics of pain		
– nature of onset of pain		
– duration of pain		
– associated symptoms		
– asks about risk factors for ischaemic heart disease/PE as appropriate		
– any previous episodes		
Past medical history		
Medications and allergies		
Social history (and illicit drug use)		
Elicits patient's concerns		
Explains differential diagnosis		
Explains plan: ECG, blood tests		
Recommends follow-up in appropriate setting		
Answers patient's questions appropriately		
Checks patient's understanding of diagnosis and plan		
Checks if patient has further questions		
Global mark from patient		
Global mark from examiner		

Instructions for actor

You are a 43-year-old self-employed plumber called Marcus Potts. When driving to work this morning, you developed chest pain. You left home as usual after eating cereal and toast, and were driving to work when you felt discomfort in the chest, like indigestion. You could also feel this around your neck and shoulders. It was quite severe and you felt short of breath with it. You stopped the car, came out and felt better after taking a few deep breaths and burping. You felt as if you were sweating at the same time. You have never had this pain before, but you do feel short of breath when you walk uphill or do any heavy work. You did not feel any palpitations or back pain and although you feel pain free now, the chest still feels a bit sore. You think the episode lasted some 30–40 minutes.

You have high blood pressure and smoke 10 cigarettes a day. You don't know about family history as you were adopted. You are on a tablet for blood pressure but don't know the name. You think that this was an episode of indigestion but wanted to get checked out just in case it was to do with your heart. You want to go to work as soon as possible because you are self-employed.

Suggested reading

Kendall J. Chest pain syndromes. RCEM Learning. London: RCEM Learning; 2010.
National Institute for Health and Care Excellence (NICE). Chest pain of recent onset. Clinical guideline 95. London: NICE; 2016.

1.10 Diabetes mellitus – hypoglycaemia

Hypoglycaemia has a variety of causes and clinical presentations. The patient can present with altered mental status, confusion, delirium, suspected stroke, seizures, palpitations, anxiety, collapse or loss of consciousness. All these presentations have a wide differential diagnosis, but hypoglycaemia should always be suspected and checked with a simple bedside measure of capillary blood glucose and can be easily reversed if the blood glucose is found to be low.

The commonest cause of hypoglycaemia is in known diabetics when there is a mismatch between insulin or oral hypoglycaemic agent and ingested calories or exercise. In this group, the symptoms may develop at a relatively higher level of blood sugar if the patients are used to a degree of hyperglycaemia.

In non-diabetic patients presenting with hypoglycaemia, it is useful to remember the mnemonic **EXPLAIN**:

- Exogenous drugs (e.g. alcohol) or poisoning (e.g. beta-blockers)
- Pituitary insufficiency
- Liver failure
- Addison's disease
- Islet cell tumours, insulinoma
- Nonpancreatic insulin secreting tumours

Scenario

Mrs Desai is a 55-year-old woman. She presents with confusion and sweating. She felt tired and weak so she phoned her daughter who called an ambulance. The paramedics ascertained that her blood sugar was 2.3 mmol/L. She was given intravenous dextrose and her blood sugar now is 7.2 mmol/L. She is currently feeling much better. Take a history and explain a management plan to Mrs Desai.

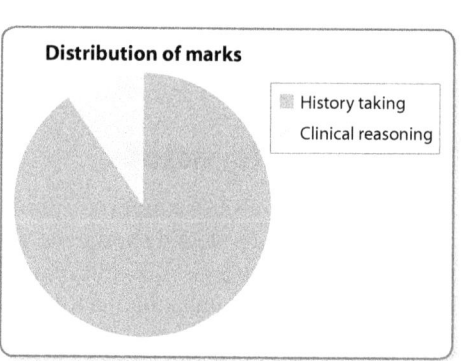

Distribution of marks
- History taking
- Clinical reasoning

Mark sheet	Achieved	Not achieved
Introduces self to patient and confirms their identity		
Checks level of comfort offers analgesia		
Establishes presenting complaint		
Specifically enquires about:		
– patient's recollection of events		
– symptoms experienced		
– nature of onset		

Cont'd...

Mark sheet	Achieved	Not achieved
– duration and severity of symptoms		
– how and when symptoms resolved		
– history of diabetes		
– use of insulin/medications		
– any unusual activity or meals during day		
– any previous episodes		
– awareness of hypoglycaemic episodes		
– symptoms of intercurrent illness		
Past medical history		
Medications and allergies		
Social history (including driving)		
Elicits patient's concerns		
Explains differential diagnosis		
Explains plan: examination, blood tests, septic screen		
Recommends follow-up in appropriate setting		
Answers patient's questions appropriately		
Checks patient's understanding of diagnosis and plan		
Checks if patient has further questions		
Global mark from patient		
Global mark from examiner		

Instructions for actor

You are a 55-year-old solicitor called Mohini Desai, who lives alone. You woke up at 7 am, but were not feeling well. You took your morning 12 units of fast-acting subcutaneous insulin as usual and 16 units of your once daily background insulin. You started feeling worse at about 8 am, and didn't think you could go to work. You called your daughter and upon her arrival, you were profoundly sweaty and feeling unwell.

You can't remember whether you had your breakfast this morning or not, or how you came to the hospital. After treatment you are feeling much better.

You have had diabetes for the last 45 years. You take a basal-bolus insulin regimen. You use fast-acting insulin at meal times and long-acting insulin every morning. This is the first 'hypo' you have had for years. You also have high blood pressure and take lisinopril.

You are otherwise well. You don't drive anymore because of vision problems. You are not allergic to anything and don't smoke, but drink a glass of wine with dinner.

Suggested reading

Jones E. Hypoglycaemia. RCEM Learning. London: RCEM Learning; 2018.

1.11 Dysphagia

Any difficulty in swallowing is termed dysphagia. Painful swallowing is termed odynophagia.
Dysphagia can either arise in the oropharyngeal or oesophageal phase of swallowing. Both have different causes and a careful history should help localise the cause.

Table 1.11.1 Localising dysphagia

Characteristic	Oropharyngeal dysphagia	Oesophageal dysphagia
Initial swallowing	Abnormal	Normal
Coughing or choking	Present	Absent
Difficulty with	Liquids	Solids
Odynophagia	Absent	Present
Reflux, dyspepsia	Absent	Present
Aspiration	Present	Absent
Causes	Neuromuscular, e.g. CVA, myasthenia, polymyositis	Structural – oesophageal stricture, cancer, external compression from mediastinal mass

(Adapted from Marx JA, et al. Rosen's Emergency Medicine, 7th edn. Philadelphia: Mosby, 2010.)

To assist with diagnosis of the underlying cause, once the initial history of the swallowing difficulties has been taken, further focused questioning is required to determine the cause. Red flag questions for malignancy, cerebrovascular and neuromuscular pathology must be asked as appropriate.

A common cause of dysphagia in the ED is food bolus obstruction. A detailed history of events can usually clarify the diagnosis. Patients often have some underlying abnormality of the oesophagus to precipitate a food bolus obstruction. These patients present with chest pain not dissimilar to angina, and therefore a careful workup with a detailed history is needed.

Sore throat

This has a variable aetiology from simple viral pharyngitis or epiglottitis to gastro-oesophageal reflux or a deep neck abscess (which is fortunately rare). Relevant features for each of these underlying conditions should be sought. Some degree of speech impairment is common with a sore throat, but presence of drooling, and muffled voice may indicate a serious infection. Enquire about systemic symptoms, fever, abdominal pain, chest pain and risk factors such as diabetes or immunosuppression.

Scenario

Mr Robinson is 87 years old. He is finding it difficult to swallow and has developed an ache in the middle of his chest. Take a history and formulate a management plan.

Distribution of marks
- History taking
- Clinical reasoning

Mark sheet	Achieved	Not achieved
Introduces self to patient and confirms their identity		
Checks level of comfort offers analgesia		
Establishes presenting complaint		
Specifically enquires about:		
– onset of symptoms		
– characteristics of dysphagia		
– severity of dysphagia		
– any previous similar episodes?		
– characteristics of pain		
– identifies association with meal		
Past medical history		
Medications and allergies		
Social history (and illicit drug use)		
Elicits patient's concerns		
Explains likely diagnosis		
Explains plan		
Answers patient's questions appropriately		
Checks patient's understanding of diagnosis and plan		
Checks if patient has further questions		
Global mark from patient		
Global mark from examiner		

Instructions for actor

You are an 87-year-old man called Benjamin Robinson. You were eating a piece of steak when you felt you could not swallow it. It felt like it was stuck in your chest. You had a tight pain just in the front of your chest that increased with movement or inspiration. Someone gave you a fizzy drink when you arrived at hospital and after a few sips the sensation settled and you are now able to swallow normally. For the past couple of months you have found it hard to swallow solid food. You have managed by eating smaller mouthfuls and chewing more. Liquids are not normally a problem. You have not weighed yourself but recently had to buy some new trousers as the older ones seemed a bit loose. You have had an endoscopy where you previously lived 10 or 15 years ago that showed 'Barratt's something' and you are taking antacid tablets. You have diabetes and hypertension and both are drug-controlled but you cannot remember the names. You feel a lot better and want to go home without a fuss because you feel there are other people more unwell than you are.

1.12 Febrile convulsion

This should be considered in conjunction with section 2.12 on febrile convulsions in the communication skills chapter. For a seizure to be classified as a febrile convulsion, it should:
- Be a generalised convulsion
- Last <5 minutes
- Occur in a child aged between 6 months and 5 years of age who is neurologically and developmentally normal
- Occur in the presence of fever
- Occur without any central nervous system (CNS) infection or alternate identifiable cause (such as hypoglycaemia or electrolyte imbalance)

Diagnostic approach

The history is best taken from someone who witnessed the event.
1. Determine whether the event was truly a seizure
   - May be confused with syncope, rigors, breath holding spells, jitteriness in neonates or normal movements
   - What was the patient doing immediately before the event? Was there any warning or aura (e.g. visual or olfactory disturbance)?
2. Determine the type of seizure
   - Was the child stiff or limp? Colour, movements, eye and head rolling, incontinence, loss of consciousness, any focality?
   - Immediately after the event – was there any postictal confusion, reduced level of consciousness or headache? Does the patient remember the episode?
3. Identify the cause
   - Recent illness, fever, trauma and new medications, not taken antiepileptic medications, rash, hypoglycaemia, electrolyte disorder
   - Risk factor for epilepsy – previous head injury, meningitis, febrile seizures, congenital anomalies or family history of epilepsy

Particularly in infants the signs of meningitis are often subtle and a septic screen (FBC, U&Es, blood cultures, MSU +/- chest X-ray and lumbar puncture) should be strongly considered before excluding meningitis. Children older than 18 months may be discharged with appropriate advice and safety-net if they:
- Have fully recovered
- Are clinically well with no signs of meningitis
- Have an identified source for their fever
- A previous history of febrile seizures and a typical story for it

Parents should be given the following information:
- Febrile seizures happen in approximately 3% of children
- Almost 30% will have a recurrence, higher in younger children
- Approximately 1% of children who have a febrile convulsion will go on to develop epilepsy

Scenario

Zak is a 4-year-old boy who has been brought in with his mother, Mrs Fiona Russell, by paramedics following a seizure at home. They checked his blood sugar on scene and it was 6.2 mmol/L. The seizure self-terminated. He is now settled and sleeping in the cot. Take a history and make a management plan.

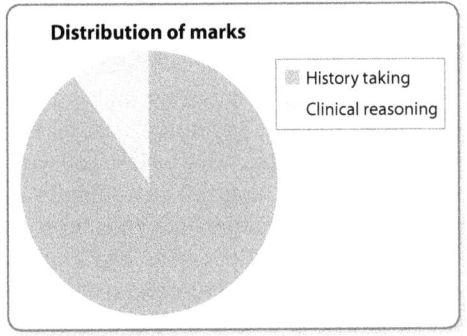

Distribution of marks
- History taking
- Clinical reasoning

Mark sheet	Achieved	Not achieved
Introduces self to mother and confirms their identity		
Checks level of comfort offers analgesia		
Establishes presenting complaint		
Specifically enquires about:		
– description of event		
– location of event		
– presence of limb jerking/body movement		
– responsiveness during event		
– duration of event		
– events during recovery		
– recent illnesses		
Takes antenatal history		
Takes birth history		
Takes developmental history		
Checks immunisation status		
Asks about previous admissions, previous episodes		
Asks about family history		
Elicits mother's concerns		
Explains likely diagnosis		
Explains plan		
Answers mother's questions appropriately		
Checks mother's understanding of diagnosis and plan		
Checks if mother has further questions		
Global mark from patient		
Global mark from examiner		

Instructions for actor

You are Mrs Fiona Russell, mother of a 4-year-old boy Zak. He has been unwell since yesterday and you did not send him to nursery today. He has had a fever overnight of 39°C. You gave him paracetamol last night and this morning, and he seemed a bit better with it. He has had a cough and runny nose. He is usually a good eater, but yesterday he ate much less. He continued to drink well so you weren't too worried. You tried to give him some breakfast this morning, but he wouldn't eat it.

He had a high temperature and looked tired and lethargic. Suddenly, you noticed that he seemed to have stiffened up and shook his head and arms, his eyes rolled back in their sockets and it looked like he was having a seizure. It lasted for a minute or two and stopped on its own. You picked him up and he seemed unaware of what was going on around him. You immediately called the ambulance and tried to keep him on his side as advised by paramedics; soon after he appeared to fall asleep.

On further questioning, you remember that Zak had a similar episode 3 years ago, when he had a high temperature. He was kept in the hospital and tests were normal.

He is otherwise well and developing normally.

He is immunised appropriately and does not take any medications. His older brother has had a cold for the last week and he is recovering from it now.

There is no family history of epilepsy and you are scared that Zak may have developed epilepsy – you ask specifically about this if the doctor invites questions.

Suggested reading

Messahel S. Paediatric seizures. RCEM Learning. London: RCEM Learning; 2018.
National Institute for Health and Care Excellence (NICE). Febrile seizure. Clinical Knowledge Summary. NICE. London: NICE; 2013.

1.13 Traveller's diarrhoea

Traveller's diarrhoea (TD) is more common in people who return to developed countries from developing countries. The history in this station should focus on the clinical presentation (fever or diarrhoea) as well as aspects related to travel which aim to elicit the patient's exposure to infectious diseases (**Table 1.13.1**).

Approach to history

Firstly, it is important to clarify the details of the clinical presentation. Is fever or diarrhoea the predominant symptom? Classical TD presents with ≥3 unformed stools in 24 hours with at least one of the following symptoms: fever, cramps, nausea, vomiting, tenesmus or bloody stools (dysentery). Mild TD does not have any systemic symptoms and patients are well.

Secondly, it is important to clarify some details related to the travel. Did the patient have any pretravel vaccination (e.g. for typhoid) or take any prophylaxis (e.g. for malaria). What preventive steps did they take during travel? Did they use mosquito nets? Where did they stay and what did they do? Were they on holiday or visiting family? Or was it a business trip, or charity work? What was their accommodation like (hotel, family home, cruise ship, rural or urban)? Did the patient take part in any particularly risky activities (freshwater swimming, unprotected sex, injected drugs)?

Next, enquire about food and drink. How careful were they about safe drinking water (did they use ice, or eat salads)? What did they eat? Did it include any uncooked or street food? Do they know if anybody else has been affected by the same symptoms?

Finally, come back to the subject of their health. Have they sought advice or taken treatment for this illness so far (if so what)? Do they have risk factors? Children warrant consideration of early antibiotic therapy but so do some adults (immunosuppression, chronic disease, pregnancy). Last of all, make sure that a broader differential diagnosis has been considered – irritable bowel syndrome, inflammatory bowel disease and *C. difficile* infection can all present in a patient who has recently travelled.

Table 1.13.1 Common pathogens in traveller's diarrhoea

Bacterial – commonest	Viral	Parasitic
- *Escherichia coli* – enterotoxic or enteroinvasive – haemorrhagic - *Shigella* - *Campylobacter* - *Salmonella* - Others such as *Vibrio*, *Yersinia*	- Rotavirus – children - Noroviruses – cruise ships	- *Giardia lambia* - *Entamoeba histolytica* - *Strongyloides stercoralis*

History taking

Scenario

Mr Sutton is a 39-year-old man who returned from Thailand this morning. He has had diarrhoea for 2 days and is now getting abdominal pain. Take a history and make a management plan.

Distribution of marks
- History taking
- Clinical reasoning

Mark sheet	Achieved	Not achieved
Introduces self to patient and confirms their identity		
Checks level of comfort offers analgesia		
Establishes presenting complaint		
Specifically enquires about:		
– type of stool		
– frequency in 24 hours		
– duration of symptoms		
– progression since onset		
– blood or mucous in stool		
– associated symptoms		
Travel history:		
– places visited		
– duration of visits		
– type of accommodation used		
– other travellers affected		
– other high risk behaviours		
– pretravel vaccinations		
Past medical history		
Medications and allergies		
Social history (and illicit drug use)		
Elicits patient's concerns		
Explains likely diagnosis		
Explains plan		
Answers patient's questions appropriately		
Checks patient's understanding of diagnosis and plan		
Checks if patient has further questions		
Global mark from patient		
Global mark from examiner		

Instructions for actor

You are a 39-year-old plumber called David Sutton You returned this morning after a holiday in Thailand. You went with your friends and spent a week in Bangkok. This was your first trip there and you ate a lot of local food. You spent most of your time in the city and stayed in a luxury hotel. You started feeling unwell just before returning and have been going to the toilet every 2 or 3 hours. You are passing watery stools, have abdominal cramps and noticed blood this morning. You are also feeling hot and cold and don't feel like eating anything.

You did not eat or drink any raw food or juice and had been peeling fruits before eating. You only drank bottled water during your stay and you did not get any vaccination before travel.

None of your friends have had any problems and they have been there before. You are usually healthy and well with no medical problems and are not on any medications. You have not had any sexual relationships for the last year and do not take drugs.

1.14 Haematuria

History taking for haematuria is focused on finding the cause and assessing how unwell the patient is.

Haematuria can be traumatic or non-traumatic. If there is any history of significant trauma and the patient presents with macroscopic haematuria, contrast-enhanced CT should be considered to investigate the extent of any kidney injury.

Causes of non-traumatic haematuria include urinary tract infection (UTI), kidney stones, bladder or renal cancer, urethritis and glomerulonephritis. While glomerulonephritis is more common in younger age groups, kidney stones are rarely seen in the young. Cancer is more common in older age. UTIs occur in both younger and older patients. Remember also that patients with coagulopathy or on warfarin can present with haematuria.

History to ascertain

- Colour of urine
- When present:
  - Initial phase of micturition suggests urethral bleeding
  - Towards the end suggests bladder neck or trigone bleeding
  - Urine mixed with blood could suggest pathology anywhere from bladder, ureter or kidneys
- Whether passing clots which suggest bladder or renal (non-glomerular) bleeding
- Whether symptoms are cyclical (endometriosis)
- Any flank pain (stone, cancer, infarction)
- Any fever, dysuria, frequency, suprapubic pain (cystitis)
- Additional urinary tract symptoms (**Table 1.14.1**)
- Additional history:
  - Trauma or vigorous exercise
  - Medication (anti-inflammatories, anticoagulants)
  - Sexual history
  - Recent bacterial or viral infection may trigger glomerulonephritides
  - Chest symptoms such as haemoptysis, dyspnoea, pleuritic chest pain, epistaxis (Wegener's)
  - Systemic symptoms such as a rash, joint aches, myalgia (possible vasculitis)
  - Family history (polycystic kidney disease, clotting disorder)

Table 1.14.1 Lower urinary tract symptoms in men

Overactive bladder	Voiding	Post micturition
• Urgency	• Hesitancy	• Post micturition dribble
• Increased day time frequency	• Straining	• Feeling of incomplete emptying
• Nocturia	• Slow stream	
• Urinary incontinence	• Intermittency	
	• Splitting or spraying	
	• Terminal dribble	

Scenario

Mr Waterston is a 53-year-old man presenting with blood in the urine. Take a history and make a management plan with him.

Distribution of marks
- History taking
- Clinical reasoning

Mark sheet	Achieved	Not achieved
Introduces self to patient and confirms their identity		
Checks level of comfort offers analgesia		
Establishes presenting complaint		
Specifically enquires about:		
– onset of blood in urine		
– progression of problem		
– timing of blood in relation to urinary stream		
– presence of pain		
– passage of clots or difficulty passing urine		
– associated symptoms		
– bleeding tendency/anticoagulation		
– any previous episodes		
Past medical history		
Sexual history		
Medications and allergies		
Social history		
Elicits patient's concerns		
Explains likely diagnosis		
Explains plan		
Answers patient's questions appropriately		
Checks patient's understanding of diagnosis and plan		
Checks if patient has further questions		
Global mark from patient		
Global mark from examiner		

Instructions for actor

You are a 53-year-old bus driver called Frank Waterston, who noted blood in the urine last night and this morning. You felt a bit uncomfortable when you went to pass urine but had no pain or burning. All the urine was dark red in colour and there were no clots that you could see. You have had problems passing urine for a few months. You find it difficult to control your bladder on long routes and notice that the stream is getting weaker. You have to wake up in the night to go to the toilet a few times and feel that you haven't emptied your bladder completely.

You have no pain, fever or weight loss. You have high blood pressure and take a water tablet for it. You have no history of kidney problems but your father had an operation for enlarged prostate.

You are worried whether this is the cause and if anything can be done about it.

Suggested reading

National Institute for Health and Care Excellence (NICE). Lower urinary tract symptoms in men. Clinical guideline 97. NICE. London: NICE; 2015.

National Institute for Health and Care Excellence (NICE). LUTS in men. Clinical Knowledge summary. NICE. London: NICE; 2018.

1.15 Upper gastrointestinal bleeding

This is a common emergency presentation. The first priority (like in many stations, but more so in someone with upper gastrointestinal bleeding) is to ensure that the patient is well and not in need of any immediate resuscitation. Usually, patients with on-going bleeding or those who have lost a significant amount of blood are unwell and need initial resuscitation before an attempt to find the cause.

Presentation

- **Haematemesis:** Iron in haemoglobin in the blood is oxidised in the stomach and develops a dark ground coffee appearance. Therefore, coffee ground vomitus usually indicates a slow bleed, unlike an actively bleeding varix or ulcer, which may present as vomiting fresh red blood
- **Melaena:** Black tarry stools result from slow passage of blood through the alimentary canal. Of note, patients can also have black stools due to iron supplementation
- **Haematochezia or bloody stools:** A large upper gastrointestinal (GI) bleed may present with bloody stools. Patients are usually very unwell, as a large amount of blood must have passed through the bowel with a very short transit time
- **Non-specific symptoms:** An upper GI bleed may not be immediately apparent as the underlying problem in a patient with syncope, angina, lethargy, confusion or abdominal pain

Upper GI bleeding can be divided in to variceal or non-variceal bleeding. In general, variceal bleeding is more concerning, because the volume is often larger and it can be difficult to control. Gastric or oesophageal varices are caused by portal hypertension usually because of underlying liver cirrhosis. This is often secondary to excess alcohol use, but can also be caused by other diseases such as hepatitis C infection and autoimmune cirrhosis.

Non-variceal haemorrhage causes include peptic ulcer disease (PUD), gastroduodenal erosions and oesophagitis. Important things to elicit in the history include previous PUD, medications (anti-inflammatories, antiplatelets or anticoagulants) or a diagnosis of hiatus hernia or chronic heartburn symptoms. Malignancy and bleeding diathesis are less common causes of bleeding, but history of constitutional symptoms (e.g. weight loss, night sweats), or a bleeding disorder should be sought. A Mallory–Weiss tear is caused by recurrent vomiting, and usually settles without the need for intervention.

The decision to discharge patients can be made objectively using the Glasgow–Blatchford score (**Table 1.15.1**). It uses clinical and biochemical indicators to identify low risk patients who can be managed safely as outpatients.

In addition there are important risk factors that should be assessed as part of the history. These risk factors help to predict adverse outcome after an upper GI endoscopy as part of the Rockall score. Enquire about congestive heart failure, ischaemic heart disease, renal failure, liver failure or metastatic cancer.

Table 1.15.1 Glasgow – Blatchford score

Admission risk marker	Score component value
Blood urea (mmol/L)	
6.0–7.9	2
8.0–9.9	3
10–25	4
≥25	6
Haemoglobin (Hb) (for men) (g/L)	
120–129	1
100–119	3
<100	6
Haemoglobin (for women) (g/L)	
100–119	1
<100	6
Systolic blood pressure (SBP) (mmHg)	
100–109	1
90–99	2
<90	3
Other markers	
Pulse ≥100/min	1
Presentation with melaena	1
Presentation with syncope	2
Hepatic disease	2
Cardiac failure	2

Score is equal to 0 if all the following are present:
- Urea <6.5
- Hb ≥130 (for men)
  ≥120 (for women)
- SBP ≥110
- Pulse <100
- Absence of melaena, syncope, cardiac or liver disease

Interpretation

A score of 0 identifies low risk patients who may be suitable for outpatient management.

A score of 6 or more is considered to indicate a greater than 50% risk of needing an intervention.

Scenario

Mr Powell is a 45-year-old man presenting with dark stools. Take a history and explain a management plan.

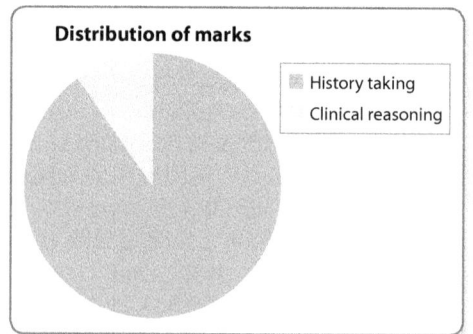

Distribution of marks
- History taking
- Clinical reasoning

Mark sheet	Achieved	Not achieved
Introduces self to patient and confirms their identity		
Checks level of comfort offers analgesia		
Establishes presenting complaint		
Specifically enquires about:		
– onset of blood in stool		

Cont'd...

Mark sheet	Achieved	Not achieved
– colour of blood		
– quantity of blood		
– progression of problem		
– timing of blood in relation to stools		
– associated symptoms		
– any previous episodes		
– bleeding tendency/anticoagulation		
Past medical history		
Medications and allergies		
Social history		
Elicits patient's concerns		
Explains likely diagnosis		
Explains plan		
Answers patient's questions appropriately		
Checks patient's understanding of diagnosis and plan		
Checks if patient has further questions		
Global mark from patient		
Global mark from examiner		

Instructions for actor

You are a 45-year-old van driver, Stewart Powell, who has noticed dark coloured stools for the last 3 or 4 days. You noticed this while you flushed the toilet and again on the toilet paper. You open your bowels once a day and your stools have been soft. It was a small amount initially but today you passed dark black almost tar-like stools, enough to make you feel concerned. You feel nauseated, but haven't vomited and feel off your food. You have felt tired and washed out for several days and don't feel like you have the energy for work.

You are usually healthy and well, and have never needed to see a doctor. You get knee pain while driving and have been taking ibuprofen for the last 2 weeks. You felt some heartburn and indigestion, but it settled once you had some food. You drink 4-5 pints of lager at the weekends and have never abused any drugs.

You don't take any other medication. You have not lost any weight. You live at home with your wife and she is on her way to the hospital. You are concerned that you may have cancer as your father died of bowel cancer.

Suggested reading

Acute Upper GI Bleeding. Clinical guideline 141. National Institute for Health and Care Excellence, London, 2012. www.nice.org.uk/CG141.

Rockall TA, Logan RF, Devlin HB, Northfield TC. Risk assessment after acute upper gastrointestinal haemorrhage. Gut 1996; 38:316–321.

Stanley AJ, Ashley D, Dalton HR, et. al. Outpatient management of patients with low-risk upper-gastrointestinal haemorrhage: multicentre validation and prospective evaluation. Lancet 2009; 373:42–47.

1.16 Headache

Knowledge of the causes of headaches and the fundamental differences in their presentation is required. As discussed in the introduction to the chapter, there is a clear set of questions that relates to any presentation where pain is a key feature. These questions, coupled with pertinent detailed enquiry into key areas, will assist the candidate in refining a differential diagnosis.

Types of headache

Subarachnoid haemorrhage

These headaches are of sudden onset. Patients usually complain of the worst-ever headache which may feel like having been hit over the head. They often occur on exertion or postural changes and may present with no additional clinical features. Vomiting, drowsiness and confusion may be present as well as focal neurology. In an acute setting, headaches of this nature with no other explanation should very rarely be dismissed without further investigation. It is also important to remember that patients often have a 'herald bleed' prior to a subarachnoid haemorrhage. This is a smaller bleed with understandably less severe symptoms. If this bleed is noticed by the astute physician, (perhaps presenting as a less severe, sudden occipital headache, or even as sudden neck pain), then much subsequent morbidity and even mortality can be avoided. Symptoms of such an episode should also be sought in the history of a patient who may have a more severe subarachnoid bleed.

Tension headaches

They are generally a bilateral ache or feeling of pressure, which is (at worst) moderately severe. The duration may vary significantly. These headaches are very common but should only be diagnosed in the ED in the absence of any sinister features.

Cluster headaches

The nature of pain with these headaches is variable but is normally severe. The pain tends to be unilateral around an eye. There may be conjunctival irritation, lacrimation, nasal congestion, eyelid swelling or drooping, facial sweating and miosis. Episodes may last 1–3 hours and occur in clusters with periods of remission in between.

Migraines

These can be unilateral or bilateral headaches of a moderate-to-severe nature (otherwise patients with known migraines rarely present). They may be triggered by exposure to specific stimuli. Often they are accompanied by a specific prodrome or associated with an aura such as visual disturbance or varied sensory symptoms. Vomiting and photophobia can both occur.

Caution should be exercised when diagnosing a migraine – particularly in patients with no relevant past history, as there are sometimes few distinguishing features between migraines and several serious pathologies.

Raised intracranial pressure

Causes include a space occupying lesion (e.g. tumour or abscess), arteriovenous malformation or idiopathic intracranial hypertension. The headache worsens with lowering the head, lying flat and coughing or sneezing. It can be associated with nausea, vomiting and blurred vision.

Temporal arteritis

This is associated with temporal tenderness and jaw claudication. It occurs usually in patients over the age of 50 years who may experience low-grade fevers, weight loss and visual disturbance that, if untreated, may result in blindness.

Other causes

Headaches may also be caused by trigeminal neuralgia, sinusitis, meningitis or be the result of medications and procedures. Coital cephalgia is a rare but severe headache that occurs during sex (including masturbation) just before orgasm. In each case a thorough history will assist in making a clear diagnosis.

Scenario

Miss Finch is a 48-year-old woman. She has attended today with a headache. Take a history from her then explain your differential diagnosis and management plan to her.

Distribution of marks
- History taking
- Clinical reasoning

Mark sheet	Achieved	Not achieved
Introduces self to patient and confirms their identity		
Offers analgesia		
Establishes presenting complaint		
Specifically enquires about:		
– onset of symptoms		
– nature and radiation of pain		
– syncope		
– vomiting		
– relieving/exacerbating factors		
– use of analgesia		
Past medical history		

Cont'd...

Cont'd...

Mark sheet	Achieved	Not achieved
Medications and allergies		
Social history including illicit drug use		
Elicits patient's concerns about managing work		
Explains differential diagnosis		
Explains plan: need for urgent investigations and likely admission		
Answers patient's questions appropriately		
Checks patient's understanding of diagnosis and plan		
Checks if patient has further questions		
Negotiates plan with patient to ensure they stay for scan		
Global mark from patient		
Global mark from examiner		

Instructions for actor

You are a 48-year-old school teacher called Caroline Finch, and have come to the ED today as you had to take the day off sick and couldn't get a general practitioner appointment.

You have had a headache for the last 2 months, which is gradually getting worse. It is mainly on the right side but also all over and feels like a general bad ache. It is worse in the morning and today it woke you up at 5 am and you felt very sick and your vision didn't seem quite right. The headache generally eases (but doesn't disappear) after you've been awake for a few hours. You have had no other symptoms. You've never had any headaches or any other medical problems in the past.

You take no medication, are a non-smoker and drink alcohol very rarely. You live alone and work full time. The headache is affecting your sleep and making you struggle with work. You have a family history of hypertension but nothing else.

You are very stressed as you are preparing for a parent's day meeting tomorrow and don't really want to stay for any tests.

Suggested reading

British Association for the Study of Headaches (BASH). BASH Guidelines (for the diagnosis and management of headache). BASH. Hull, BASH; 2010.
National Institute for Health and Care Excellence (NICE). Headache assessment. Clinical Knowledge Summary. NICE. London: NICE; 2017.
National Institute for Health and Care Excellence (NICE). Headaches in over 12s. Clinical guideline 150., NICE. London: NICE; 2012.

1.17 Jaundice

The condition refers to a raised serum bilirubin, which presents as yellowish discolouration to the conjunctiva, mucous membranes and the skin. A normal bilirubin level is considered to be <17 μmol/L. Once this rises past approximately 35 μmol/L the discolouration begins to become visible, normally at the sclera. Occasionally, patients do indeed present with this as their only symptom though more often it occurs during a pathological process with other associated symptoms.

Initially, it is worth clarifying the time course over which the jaundice has developed and if it is still progressing. It is also worth finding out if the patient has any past experience of jaundice personally or within their family.

Additional symptoms that may be present are pruritus or a change in stool and urine colour. Further associated symptoms which may point towards the underlying cause are pain (presence or absence), fever, malaise, anorexia, weight loss or gain, rash and altered mental state. Jaundice without pain suggests the cause is more likely to be related to haemolysis, primary biliary cirrhosis or malignancy (pancreatic or hepatobiliary).

The causes of jaundice are traditionally divided into prehepatic, hepatic and posthepatic.

Prehepatic jaundice

This is often caused by haemolysis – so patients may, therefore, be anaemic. There is a rise in unconjugated bilirubin, which is not water soluble and therefore does not enter the urine. Urine and stool remain their normal colour and liver enzyme tests are within the normal range.

It may be associated with a haemoglobinopathy (such as sickle cell disease) or other conditions resulting in haemolysis (e.g. malaria or haemolytic-uraemic syndrome). Gilbert's syndrome is a common inherited disorder in which there can be episodes of mild hyperbilirubinaemia which settle spontaneously. These can be precipitated by intercurrent illness or stress.

Hepatic jaundice

This is the result of hepatocellular damage and the subsequent inability of the liver to metabolise bilirubin normally. There is a rise in unconjugated and conjugated bilirubin. Causes include those for hepatitis and chronic liver disease (infection, malignancy, metabolic disorders and alcohol). These precipitating factors should become clear if a thorough history is taken. There can be a failure to excrete conjugated bilirubin normally (to the duodenum in bile) which is then excreted in the urine giving it a dark colour and leaving the patient's stools pale.

Posthepatic jaundice

Also known as cholestatic or obstructive jaundice, this occurs when there is obstruction to the outflow of conjugated bilirubin via the bile duct. The conjugated bilirubin level in the blood rises and leads to dark urine, but as less enters the bowel stools become paler. Causes include impacted gallstones in the bile duct, primary biliary cirrhosis or sclerosing cholangitis and malignancy (commonly pancreatic in origin).

Scenario

Mr Dukes is a 52-year-old journalist who has come to the ED because his wife noticed that over the weekend the whites of his eyes have begun to look yellow. He has lost his appetite in the past 2 weeks but has otherwise felt ok. Take a history and then explain your management plan to Mr Dukes.

Mark sheet	Achieved	Not achieved
Introduces self to patient and confirms their identity		
Offers analgesia		
Establishes presenting complaint		
Specifically enquires about:		
– jaundice – onset, progression		
– associated symptoms		
– previous episodes		
– contact history – foreign travel, sexual history		
Past medical history		
Medications and allergies		
Social history – alcohol, smoking, illicit drugs, tattoos, occupation		
Family history		
Elicits patient's concerns		
Explains differential diagnosis		
Explains plan: need for further investigations		
Answers patient's questions appropriately		
Checks patient's understanding of diagnosis and plan		
Checks if patient has further questions		
Global mark from patient		
Global mark from examiner		

Instructions for actor

You are a 52-year-old newspaper journalist called Stanley Dukes. You have come to the ED because your wife pointed out yesterday that your eyes looked a bit yellow and today you think they have got worse and your skin is beginning to look yellow. You have generally not been feeling great for a fortnight and have lost your appetite. You have also lost around 5 kg over the same period of time. You have had no pain at any time. Today you did notice your urine seemed very dark but didn't think to look at you stool when you had an otherwise normal bowel movement. You have had no other symptoms.

You have no other medical problems or any history of medications. You have not been abroad for years, have never had a blood transfusion and have only had one sexual partner in the last 20 years who is your wife. You drink half a bottle of wine a night and do not smoke or take drugs. You have never injected drugs.

You are worried that you are very dehydrated because your urine has become so dark but do not understand how that could be the case. You ask the doctor if they can explain what they think has happened.

Suggested reading

Reid L. Jaundice. RCEM Learning. London: RCEM Learning; 2017.

1.18 Limping child

This scenario requires the candidate to demonstrate knowledge of certain issues relating specifically to paediatrics. As well as knowing the causes for a paediatric limp it is also important to take a clear developmental history and social history. Non-accidental injury (NAI) must be a consideration for any child presenting to the ED and certain questions should be asked to address this area of concern (see section 1.28).

Always begin an assessment of a child by confirming who the adult present is. The child's safety is paramount and it is vital to know whose care they are in. It is all too easy to assume a man is a child's father (or a woman their mother) when in fact it may be another family member, friend or teacher. This information also contributes to assessing the child's social situation and can, occasionally, be a cause for concern in itself.

The next step is to take a history relevant to the presenting complaint. In the case of a limp it is logical to begin with the nature and duration of the limp itself. It is clearly important to ask about recent trauma. However, some caution should be used before attributing a limp to minor trauma as it is feasible that the trauma is coincidental and the limp represents an alternative pathology. Similarly, if a child is complaining of knee pain it is important to bear in mind that hip pathology can often cause pain that is referred to the ipsilateral knee.

Relevant questions should be asked to address each of the following common causes of a limp.

Trauma

This is clearly a common cause of a child developing a limp and a history of a specific event should be sought. After a full history is taken (regardless of whether or not there has been trauma), a full examination is needed to check for areas of tenderness or bruising (do not forget the sole of the foot). Also the rest of the child should be examined to ensure there are no other injuries to suggest NAI. A Toddler's fracture is an oblique fracture through the tibia, typically resulting from a fall in those (as the name suggests) who have recently learnt to walk. This fracture may not be apparent on initial X-rays, so if it is considered to be the likely cause of the limp then it is appropriate to immobilise the lower leg in an above-knee backslab with follow-up in fracture clinic.

Transient synovitis (irritable hip)

This is a mild inflammatory process in the joint, which commonly follows another illness, often an upper respiratory tract infection. The degree of impairment it causes is variable although it is indeed transient. The child remains systemically well and their inflammatory markers are not significantly elevated. There may be a joint effusion visible on ultrasound which can be aspirated for microscopy, culture and sensitivity (MC&S) if the diagnosis is unclear.

Septic arthritis

This usually presents with systemic features of infection, decreased range of movement in the affected joint, inability to weight-bear and raised inflammatory markers; the more of these features that are present, the more likely the diagnosis. Again a joint effusion may be visible on ultrasound and can be aspirated for MC&S. It is normally necessary for a septic joint to be washed out in theatre as an emergency.

Perthes' disease

This is avascular necrosis of the femoral head. It tends to occur between the ages of 3–10 years old and is commoner in boys. It presents with a painful limp. Inflammatory markers are normal and it is classically diagnosed on X-rays, which show a femoral head of increased density that becomes fragmented and irregular.

Slipped upper femoral epiphysis

The epiphysis of the femoral head displaces inferiorly and posteriorly. This process is most common in 10–15-year-old boys, particularly if they are obese. It again presents with hip pain or a limp and there may be limited abduction and internal rotation of the joint. X-rays are required to make the diagnosis and treatment normally requires surgical intervention.

Paediatric developmental history

For a routine developmental history a child's 'red book' is used as their health record from birth. This should be asked for and checked if available. Specific areas that should be asked about include:
- Did the pregnancy reach full term
- Complications during pregnancy or delivery
- Growth and feeding
- Immunisations
- Are developmental milestones being achieved
- Are there any siblings and if so how is there health
- What is the social situation at home, e.g. single parent family, financial situation, child-care arrangements, parental health

It is helpful to develop and practice a series of standard questions to elicit this information. Doing so will help the candidate to sound natural and relaxed, and it will allow the candidate to focus on processing the answers rather than worry about formulating the questions.

For example, if talking to the mother of an 18-month-old called Poppy, consider asking: Was Poppy born on time? And was she born normally? Did you have any problems during the birth? Did Poppy have to go to Special Care when she was born? Did you both go home the same day or the next day? Has she had to come back into hospital for any reason since then? Did she smile, rollover and sit up at the same time as other babies of the same age? Do you have any concerns about how she's developing? Has she had all the immunisations that have been recommended? Who lives at home with you? Does Poppy have any brothers or sisters? Does she go to nursery?

Safeguarding

This is an area that should be addressed in every child seen in an ED. The decision as to whether or not there are any concerns regarding the potential for child abuse should be based on the presentation, history, examination and interaction of the child with its parents/guardians and with staff in the ED. The National Institute for Health and Care Excellence (NICE) has issued guidance to assist in detecting child abuse and the Royal College of Emergency Medicine also has recommendations on how cases should be managed based on the level of concern.

Scenario

Mr Wilks has brought his nephew Jamie, a 4-year-old boy, in to the ED, because he has been limping for 2 days and does not seem to be getting better. Take a history and develop a management plan.

Distribution of marks
- History taking
- Clinical reasoning

Mark sheet	Achieved	Not achieved
Introduces self to patient and adult		
Confirms the adult's identity and who has parental responsibility		
Offers analgesia to patient		
Establishes presenting complaint		
Specifically enquires about:		
– duration of limp		
– nature of onset		
– use of analgesia		
– history of trauma		
– history of recent illness		
– any systemic symptoms now		
– any similar problems in past		
– developmental history as far as adult is aware		
Past medical history		
Family history		
Social history – who is present at home, carers, nursery		
Explains differential diagnosis		
Explains need to examine the child fully		
Explains plan: Pelvis and hip X-rays, blood tests		
Explains need to speak to parent		
Answers uncle's questions appropriately		
Checks uncle's understanding of diagnosis and plan		
Checks if uncle has further questions		
Global mark from uncle		
Global mark from examiner		

Instructions for actor

You are Stephen Wilks and you have brought Jamie, your 4-year-old nephew to the ED as he has had a limp for the past 2 days affecting his left leg. You had given it a day to see if it passed but it has not. There has not been any trauma that you are aware of and he has been well recently except for a runny nose and cough a week ago. Apart from the limp he has behaved normally with no fevers or change in his behaviour.

As far as you are aware he has had all his immunisations and there is no past medical history or family history of note. You do not have Jamie's red book. You gave him some paracetamol last night and some ibuprofen this morning but neither seemed to help. Jamie does not yet go to school, but he goes to nursery three times per week usually. He didn't go last week because he was unwell and isn't going this week as he is staying with you.

He is staying with you for the week while his parents have gone on a holiday for their wedding anniversary. You live with your wife and have no children of your own. You have his parents overseas phone number and do not mind if they are contacted.

Suggested reading

National Institute for Health and Care Excellence (NICE). When to suspect child maltreatment. Clinical guideline 89, NICE. London: NICE; 2009.
Royal College of Emergency Medicine (RCEM). Best practice for safeguarding children. London: RCEM; 2009.

1.19 Palpitations

A thorough history from someone presenting with palpitations should serve to identify the probable diagnosis and thereby risk-stratify the patient to help form a plan for further management.

Some patients are able to give very clear descriptions of the nature of their palpitations. It may be possible to ascertain whether they are regular or irregular (in which latter case atrial fibrillation or ventricular ectopic beats are likely). In addition it is useful to know if they are fast or slow. Some people suggest patients tap out the rhythm of their palpitations to better inform the clinician.

Next it is important to ask about the duration of episodes and their frequency as well as any specific precipitants or relieving factors. Palpitations may be brought on by caffeine, stimulants (including recreational drugs) or stress. In the case of supraventricular tachycardia, patients may also become aware of specific manoeuvres that terminate episodes.

To clarify the degree to which a patient's physiology is compromised by these episodes it is important to ask about associated symptoms. Do patients lose consciousness or feel light headed? The severity of breathlessness, chest tightness or pain is an important consideration. However, these factors do not necessarily indicate the type of arrhythmia as most can cause a varying degree of compromise.

Past medical history, medications and family history may all assist in the assessment. Known or as yet undiagnosed medical problems may lead to palpitations, e.g. hypertension, thyrotoxicosis and electrolyte imbalance.

Once these areas have been addressed clinical examination, blood tests and ECGs will provide further information. Subsequently a decision can be made as to whether a patient can be discharged home for outpatient investigation or needs to be admitted due to being at high risk of a significant arrhythmia or cardiac event.

Ventricular ectopic beats

These are normally benign but some patients may be aware of them to such an extent that they present to the ED. If no other abnormalities are found further investigation is rarely necessary.

Supraventricular tachycardia

Given the nature of this arrhythmia patients may describe a fast regular heart rate. It is more common in younger patients who may have had several episodes previously. These patients may be aware of manoeuvres that terminate their symptoms (vagal manoeuvres). Causes include stimulant use, Wolff–Parkinson–White syndrome or other conduction anomalies.

Atrial fibrillation/flutter

Patients are more likely to be older, describe irregular palpitations and may have one of several risk factors. These include ischaemic heart disease, hypertension, alcohol excess, thyroid disease or valve disease.

Ventricular tachycardia

This fast regular arrhythmia is more common in elderly patients and particularly those with ischaemic heart disease.

Scenario

Miss Forbes is a 26-year-old school teacher who attended the ED after palpitations earlier in the day. Take a history and explain your diagnosis and management plan to her.

Distribution of marks
- History taking
- Clinical reasoning

Mark sheet	Achieved	Not achieved
Introduces self to patient and confirms their identity		
Offers analgesia		
Establishes presenting complaint		
Specifically enquires about:		
– nature of palpitations		
– when episodes first began		
– duration of recent episode		
– frequency of episodes		
– precipitating factors		
– alleviating factors		
– associated symptoms during palpitations		
– elicits history of much lighter menstrual periods		
Past medical history		
Family history		
Medications and allergies		
Social history (and illicit drug use)		
Elicits patient's concerns		
Explains differential diagnosis		
Explains plan: need for further investigations		
Answers patient's questions appropriately		
Shows empathy		
Checks patient's understanding of diagnosis and plan		
Checks if patient has further questions		
Global mark from patient		
Global mark from examiner		

Instructions for actor

You are a 26-year-old sports teacher in a secondary school called Mary Forbes. You have come to the ED because you had 30 minutes of palpitations after break-time at work. You felt your heart beating very fast and regularly. At the same time you felt breathless but did not have any pain or feel lightheaded. The palpitations settled after you arrived in the ED. Now you feel tired but otherwise alright. This is the third similar episode in 4 months and was the worst so far.

You have no other past medical history and take no medication. Over the past months you have lost weight unexpectedly and find you feel restless and hot a lot of the time and therefore don't sleep very well. If asked specifically, you report that your periods have recently become extremely light. There have been no other symptoms.

To keep going in the day you drink three or four coffees or may have an occasional energy drink. You do not smoke or drink alcohol. There are no medical problems in your family. You are worried that you might have a heart attack or cardiac arrest, like you heard a football player did recently.

1.20 Purpuric rash

Given the association with meningococcal sepsis this type of rash can cause much anxiety. Though it is indeed imperative to exclude serious infection as a cause, there are several other causes for a purpuric rash that also need to be considered. Purpura or petechiae are caused by intradermal blood and may be caused by:
- Thrombocytopenia – Due to decreased platelet production in bone marrow or increased platelet destruction (immune or non-immune mediated)
- Leakage from vascular walls – Vasculitis or connective tissue disorders
- Trauma

The conditions in the list below (which is by no means exhaustive) represent some of those of which candidates should be aware.

Meningococcal infection

This should be considered for every child with a febrile illness and purpuric rash regardless of how well they initially look. Initially additional features may be non-specific symptoms of systemic upset such as poor feeding, lethargy, irritability or drowsiness. These may progress to headache, photophobia, neck stiffness, vomiting, seizures and collapse. The absence of any other features in a child with normal physiological markers is reassuring but discussion with someone experienced may be advisable as even sick children may initially look quite well.

Idiopathic (immune) thrombocytopenic purpura

This condition results in autoimmune mediated platelet destruction. It normally presents acutely in children, approximately a week after a viral illness. Common features are bruising spontaneously or from minimal trauma, epistaxis, and potentially bleeding from other sites. In most cases, the condition is self-limiting though immunosuppression or splenectomy may be required.

Henoch–Schönlein purpura

This is a small vessel vasculitis. It may follow a viral illness and is common in young men but can affect any age group. There may be a low-grade temperature. One of the main features is a purpuric rash, which typically develops over the extensor surfaces and the buttocks. The rash may initially be urticaria. Additional features are joint pain, micro- or macroscopic haematuria, glomerulonephritis, abdominal pain and intussusception may occur. Those with renal involvement are followed up for a period of time to ensure they do not develop any progressive renal impairment. Though rare, gastrointestinal bleeding, ileus and central nervous system involvement are all possible complications.

Trauma

Clearly this may explain what is essentially bruising and this should always be considered as a possibility. Consequently (and depending on the individual presentation), NAI is always in the differential diagnosis.

In order to assess the likely cause of a purpuric rash in a child a clinical assessment, a full blood count, clotting studies and a urine dip should normally be performed.

Scenario

Mrs Ramesh has brought her 6-year-old son to the ED because he has developed a rash on his legs. Take a history from her and answer any questions she may have.

Distribution of marks
- History taking
- Clinical reasoning

Mark sheet	Achieved	Not achieved
Introduces self to patient and parent and confirms their identity		
Offers analgesia		
Establishes presenting complaint		
Specifically enquires about:		
– onset of rash		
– associated systemic upset – fevers, vomiting, malaise		
– specific associated symptoms – joint pain, haematuria, epistaxis		
– history of trauma		
– developmental history, e.g. delivery, milestones, growth		
Past medical history		
Medications and allergies		
Social history – who is present at home, carers, school		
Acknowledges and discusses parent's concerns		
Explains differential diagnosis		
Explains need to examine the child fully		
Explains plan: Blood tests, urine dip		
Answers parent's questions appropriately		
Checks parent's understanding of diagnosis and plan		
Checks if parent or patient has further questions		
Global mark from mother		
Global mark from examiner		

Instructions for actor

You are Sunita Ramesh and you have brought your 6-year-old son to the ED because when he woke up you noticed a new rash on his body at the top of both his thighs and buttocks. He also has an ache in his right knee but is able to walk normally. Neither the rash nor the ache was present yesterday. After checking on the internet you did the 'glass test' and when you pressed on his skin the rash did not go. The internet said this meant he had meningitis so you have rushed straight to the ED. The nurse took his temperature and it was 37.1°C.

He had a cough and cold last week but got better a few days ago. He has had no fever, diarrhoea, vomiting or other symptoms and you think he seems quite well.

He has recently been well otherwise and has no ongoing medical problems. He has not missed any of his immunisations. You, your husband and 2-year-old daughter all live together and everyone else has been well.

You want to know if he has meningitis and are frustrated by the doctor asking lots of questions you do not see the need for. However, if the doctor takes time to reassure you it helps you feel calmer and you answer the questions. Once the possible diagnoses are explained you would like to know how the doctor is going to check they have the right diagnosis. Also you ask if there can be any serious consequences and how they are prevented. If blood tests are suggested you do not object but ask if they are painful for a young boy.

1.21 Sexual history

In the exam, it is common to be confronted by a station that demands candidates to ask sensitive questions of a reluctant patient. This task often takes the form of a sexual history, where the content of the history can be particularly delicate and helps examiners identify candidates with good, practised communication skills.

After an initial introduction to the patient it is important to build rapport and gain their trust by showing awareness that it is a sensitive subject. Candidates must demonstrate a high level of empathy. It is right to suggest the discussion takes place in a private room where the conversation cannot be overheard. Furthermore, a reluctant patient will be reassured if they are reminded that everything they say is confidential.

When taking a sexual history, it will be necessary to ask for very intimate information. The best approach is to begin with one or two open questions to allow the patient to explain why they have come to the ED. Having done this, further focused questions should be asked. For these it is best to explain that you need to ask some personal but very important questions, and to acknowledge that they are difficult questions. It is crucial that all questions are asked in a 'matter-of-fact' manner and that any surprise at the answers is concealed from the candidate's face and voice. It is important to confirm:

- Was the other person involved in the sexual contact male or female?
- Where were they from?
- Is the patient aware of whether or not the other person had any sexually transmitted infections (STIs) or medical problems?
- What form did the sexual contact take? (vaginal, oral, receiving or giving anal sex)
- Were condoms used?
- Was the sexual act consensual?
- Was it with a sex worker?

These questions should be asked for each sexual partner. It is also important to know if the patient has ever had a STI, and whether or not they are able to contact their sexual partners.

Following these questions it is then appropriate to continue by enquiring about the symptoms the patient is experiencing. Ask about both genitourinary and systemic symptoms. Following this, the remaining areas of a routine history should be covered. The social history should cover any further unanswered questions regarding on-going relationships.

Further management in this scenario should include a risk assessment for exposure to HIV or other STIs. This will be based on the information gathered from the history. A plan should then be discussed with the patient. It is almost always appropriate to advise or arrange follow-up as soon as possible in a genitourinary medicine (sexual health) clinic. In the clinic further tests for STIs will be performed, and further management (including contact tracing) will be initiated as necessary. Until this follow-up appointment it is wise to recommend sexual abstinence or at least that barrier contraception is used until all test results are available.

In the exam, this often leads to a discussion about whether or not to involve the patient's partner. Clearly, if they are in a relationship where they have unprotected sex they may be putting their partner at risk. The patient must be made aware of this and strongly advised not to have unprotected sex. Under these circumstances patients should also be advised to inform their partner of what has happened. This obviously needs to be done in a firm yet supportive manner, as this will likely involve some very difficult conversations for the patient.

Further considerations

In cases where there is a medium or high risk of HIV transmission, consider treatment with post exposure prophylaxis, particularly if genito-urinary medicine clinic follow-up is not available immediately. Also, when the patient is a woman, it is appropriate to discuss whether or not emergency contraception is required. This could be in the form of a levonorgestrel pill, which is considered effective for 72 hours after sexual intercourse or an intrauterine contraceptive device, which is effective for 5 days after unprotected sex.

Scenario

Mr Smith is a 32-year-old man. He told the receptionist and the triage nurse that he needed to be seen due to a 'personal problem'. Take a history from him and explain your management plan.

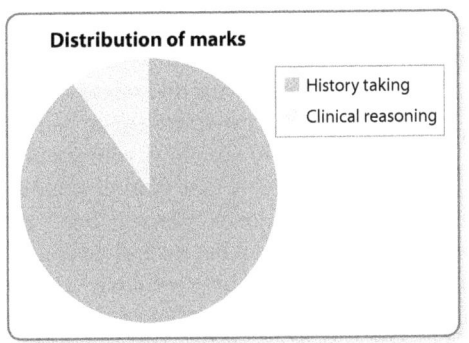

Distribution of marks
- History taking
- Clinical reasoning

Mark sheet	Achieved	Not achieved
Introduces self to patient and confirms their identity		
Checks level of comfort offers analgesia		
Comments on need for private room		
Establishes presenting complaint		
Reassures patient that discussion is confidential		
Specifically enquires about:		
– who sexual act was with?		
– where person was from?		
– any knowledge of their medical history		
– were they a sex worker?		
– nature of contact (penetrative, vaginal, anal, oral)		
– use of condom		
– any other sexual partners		
– any history of sexually transmitted infections		
Past medical history		
Medications and allergies		
Social history (and illicit drug use)		
Elicits patient's concerns		
Explains potential for infection		
Explains plan: GUM clinic, discuss telling wife		

Cont'd...

Cont'd...

Mark sheet	Achieved	Not achieved
Answers patient's questions appropriately		
Checks patient's understanding of diagnosis and plan		
Checks if patient has further questions		
Global mark from patient		
Global mark from examiner		

Instructions for actor

You are a 32-year-old married sales assistant called Richard Smith. You have attended ED today because you are worried about some penile discomfort you have had for a week. You are very reluctant to talk about your problem initially and are worried about other people overhearing or anyone else finding out. As you are embarrassed, you avoid giving specific details unless the doctor asks you direct questions.

You are concerned because while your wife was recently away you had sex with someone you met in a bar. You both went back to your house and had unprotected sex twice. They then asked you for money before they left. You had no idea you had been expected to pay and were shocked. However to avoid any further 'trouble' you did pay. If asked you reluctantly explain the person was a man who you think was around 25 years old. You both gave and received penetrative anal sex. You don't know him and have no way of contacting him.

You are worried about whether or not you have caught something and are not sure whether to tell your wife or not.

You have had no other symptoms apart from itching around your penis and have noticed some swelling in your groin. You have no past medical history, medications or allergies.

When the doctor suggests it, you become very upset at the idea of telling your wife what has happened. You are not sure she will forgive you. If the doctor understands and is sympathetic you accept that you need to think about doing this.

1.22 Breathlessness and cough

Breathlessness and cough are common symptoms for which the underlying pathology can be extremely varied. They may occur together or independently. As well as first considering primary respiratory conditions, you must also consider alternatives. These commonly include cardiac, renal, metabolic and haematological conditions, to name a few.

As always, begin with open questions and allow patients the chance to tell their story. The time frame of the presenting complaint is relevant: longer standing and progressive symptoms suggest chronic conditions such as chronic obstructive pulmonary disease (COPD), lung fibrosis or heart failure. This is in contrast to an acute or sudden onset of the problem which is suggestive of pulmonary embolism (PE) or pneumonia, for example.

Next ask about associated features which may point to an aetiology or underlying diagnosis. A cough (which may be productive of sputum or blood), or wheeze are likely to suggest respiratory diagnoses. The presence of pain, depending on its characteristics, allows consideration of cardiac causes, PE and pneumothorax. Orthopnoea, paroxysmal nocturnal dyspnoea (PND) and/or peripheral oedema are suggestive of heart failure.

With all broad presenting complaints, always ask about further general or constitutional symptoms suggestive of an associated systemic process. Identifying the presence or absence of fever, weight loss, night sweats and loss of appetite helps guide the diagnosis. They also enable a greater understanding of the impact of the problem on the patient's daily life.

There may also be relevant medical history or exposure to drugs and substances causing lung fibrosis or acute kidney injury (which may present as tachypnoea). Consider the patient's occupation in case it involves animals, feathers, dust or asbestos because these also point to specific diagnoses.

Even an isolated cough can have a significant impact on individuals in terms of disturbance to daily life, particularly sleep, and also the degree of subsequent anxiety.

The best candidates also ask pertinent questions with the aim of understanding the impact of the problem on the patient's life. If it has not already been done, ask about the patient's exercise tolerance, their ability to cope with their day-to-day tasks and discuss any further concerns they have.

Further investigations will be required. In addition, the severity of the symptoms, the ability of the patient to cope and the likely underlying diagnosis also guide the decision as to whether the patient requires admission.

Asthma

Intermittent shortness of breath, wheeze and cough are the typical symptoms of asthma. The breathlessness may be provoked by exercise, animal hair, cold air or allergens such as dust. If the cough is nocturnal it can have a significant impact on quality of sleep. Often there is a personal or family history of atopy. The patient's home circumstances may suggest a precipitant as could their occupation or work environment. Common professions to be affected are welders, spray painters and bakers.

Chronic obstructive pulmonary disease

Typical features are breathlessness, cough, sputum production and wheeze. It is usually associated with smoking but do not assume this is the case because emphysema can also be secondary to α_1-antitrypsin deficiency. Symptoms may also be related to concurrent infection or right-sided heart failure. The severity may be reflected by previous admissions to hospital, numbers of medications, use of home nebulisers or oxygen, and exercise tolerance.

Infection

In cases of an upper respiratory tract infection (usually viral), the cough may be associated with a sore throat, coryzal symptoms and conjunctival irritation. It is not unusual for the cough to persist for several weeks. With lower respiratory tract infections (more likely bacterial), there is often a more significant degree of malaise. Fevers, rigors, breathlessness, green or yellow sputum and haemoptysis may all occur. These symptoms may also be present in pulmonary tuberculosis where in addition there may be weight loss. With infective causes in mind, care should always be taken to take a contact history and a history of recent and foreign travel.

Heart failure

Causes of heart failure are varied. Symptoms depend on the underlying pathological process. Symptoms include shortness of breath which may be only exertional or progressive. Orthopnoea, paroxysmal nocturnal dyspnoea and a cough possibly productive of pinkish or frothy sputum are suggestive of left ventricular failure. Peripheral oedema and abdominal distension from ascites are suggestive of right ventricular failure.

These patients often have risk factors for hypertension or ischaemic heart disease, which are common causes. Additional clues to seek in the history are excessive alcohol use or a family history of heart failure (possibly including cardiomyopathy).

Malignancy

Features that suggest a cough is caused by malignancy include weight loss, haemoptysis, a history of smoking and a history of previous cancer.

Pleural effusion

There are few symptoms specific to this except shortness of breath and possibly pleuritic chest pain. Patients may present acutely once the effusion has accumulated to the point where they are suddenly no longer able to compensate.

Pulmonary embolism

This is a possible diagnosis if the symptoms are of sudden onset and the breathlessness is associated with pain which is typically pleuritic, possibly with haemoptysis as well. Dizziness or collapse may also form part of the presentation. There may also be symptoms of calf pain or swelling suggesting a simultaneous deep vein thrombosis. Though a cough may be present it is unlikely this would be the only symptom. Additional responses from the history help identify risk factors such as a previous venous thromboembolism, a recent operation resulting in immobility, malignancy, or a haematological disorder.

Post-nasal drip

This is a result of excessive secretions from the nasal mucosa. It can be a result of rhinitis, sinusitis and gastro-oesophageal reflux disease. The cough is often worse at night, and the patient may also complain of a sore throat.

Drug induced

Angiotensin converting enzyme inhibitors cause cough in a significant minority of patients who are commenced on this treatment. Amiodarone, phenytoin, some antimalarial and several cytotoxic drugs can also cause damage to the lungs resulting in a cough.

Scenario

Mr Logan is a 23-year-old man. He called an ambulance from work today as he had a severe cough and couldn't breathe. He was treated on the way to hospital with nebulised bronchodilators and is feeling better. Take a history and explain your management plan.

Mark sheet	Achieved	Not achieved
Introduces self to patient and confirms their identity		
Establishes presenting complaint		
Specifically enquires about:		
– onset of symptoms		
– timing of symptoms – morning, evening		
– associated symptoms – sputum, haemoptysis, fever, wheeze		
– cardiac symptoms – dyspnoea, orthopnoea, ankle swelling		
– contact history – foreign travel, tuberculosis contacts		
Past medical history – asthma, sinusitis		
Medications and allergies		
Social history (and illicit drug use)		
Elicits patient's concerns		
Explains differential diagnosis		
Explains plan: need for further investigations, outpatient follow-up		
Answers patient's questions appropriately		
Checks patient's understanding of diagnosis and plan		
Checks if patient has further questions		
Global mark from patient		
Global mark from examiner		

Instructions for actor

You are a 23-year-old man called Thomas Logan. You called an ambulance because you couldn't breathe. Your chest felt tight and it had become hard to speak. You have had a cough and felt breathless every evening lately. The cough began about 4 weeks ago. You do not think anything specific triggered it. It began at the same time as you started a new job in a bakery. You have worked as a baker for several years but changed jobs recently. There has been no fever and you are not coughing anything up.

You only have hay fever and only take antihistamine tablets when necessary. You have not been abroad for years. You live with your wife and neither of you smoke. You have no children or pets.

You are worried you may have cancer. You have seen public health advertisements saying a cough for more than 3 weeks can be serious. You don't understand why you got so breathless at work today when you spent the weekend away at the seaside feeling great. You want to know what tests you need and how they will help reach a diagnosis.

Suggested reading

The British Guideline on the management of asthma. British Thoracic Society and Scottish Intercollegiate Guidelines Network. 2014.

Chronic Obstructive Pulmonary Disease. Clinical guideline 101. National Institute for Health and Care. Excellence, London, 2010.

1.23 Myalgia

Like the last case, this objectively structured clinical examination (OSCE) begins with a non-specific presenting complaint: muscle pains. If the complaint relates to a specific region of the body this clearly points to a localised process (usually traumatic, or at least mechanical). However in cases of diffuse myalgia a more global underlying diagnosis should be sought.

Again with such non-specific presenting complaints the focus of the history can initially be unclear. The candidate must keep an open mind and allow their questions to be guided by the patient's responses. If a final diagnosis is unclear this may not be a problem as long as a sensible differential and management plan is formulated.

Aside from trauma, other common causes for myalgia are considered below.

Rhabdomyolysis

There is a triad of weakness, muscle pain and dark urine (**Figure 1.23.1**). The main diagnostic test is an elevated creatine kinase. Causes are varied, but include trauma, infection, endocrine and metabolic disorders as well as drugs (recreational and prescription). The final common pathway is cell damage with release of intracellular components into the circulation. Electrolyte disturbance and acute kidney injury follow. Myoglobin is released into the urine causing a dark brown discolouration. Treatment is based on identifying and removing or treating the cause as well as supportive therapy – the mainstay of which is intravenous fluid therapy. Sometimes renal replacement therapy is needed.

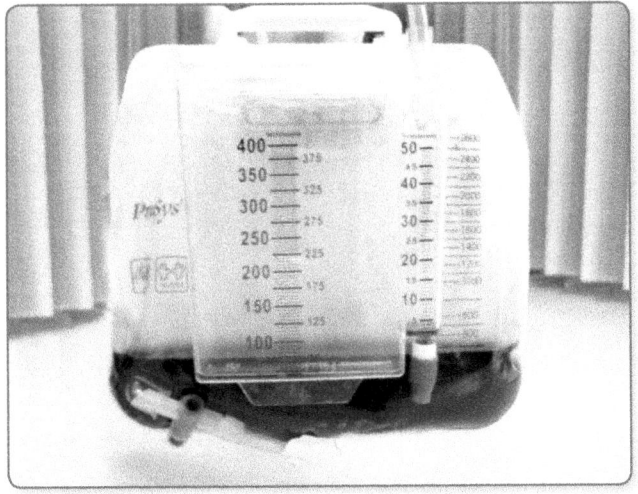

Figure 1.23.1 Myoglobinuria.

Infection

Varying degrees of acute myalgia can occur during acute infection. In the context of a normal creatine kinase level no specific treatment is required except that for the cause.

Polymyalgia rheumatica

This condition results in pain and stiffness normally occurring in the back, shoulders, neck and hips. Sufferers tend to be over 60 years of age. It is associated with giant cell arteritis but they do not always occur together. Erythrocyte sedimentation rate (ESR) is often elevated but this is not diagnostic and creatine kinase levels are usually normal. Treatment normally comprises long-term steroids.

Fibromyalgia

This is a chronic disorder of altered pain perception and processing which results in muscle pain as well as several other symptoms. This is often a diagnosis of exclusion, and not one normally made in the ED. Treatment is based on analgesia and psychological therapies.

Polymyositis (or dermatomyositis)

These conditions result in proximal muscle weakness with pain being a less prominent feature as a result of skeletal muscle inflammation. They are associated with malignancy particularly if there are cutaneous features (dermatomyositis). Diagnosis is based on elevated creatine kinase, typical findings on electromyography, antibody testing and muscle biopsy. Management involves steroids or immunosuppressants and excluding malignancy as a cause.

Scenario

Mrs Ross is a 60-year-old woman who has presented to the ED with severe, all-over-body pain, which has developed over a few days. Take a history from her and explain your differential diagnosis and plan to her.

Distribution of marks
- History taking
- Clinical reasoning

Myalgia 1.23

Mark sheet	Achieved	Not achieved
Introduces self to patient and confirms their identity		
Offers analgesia		
Establishes presenting complaint		
Asks pertinent questions regarding pain		
Specifically enquires about:		
– constitutional symptoms (fevers, night sweats, weight loss)		
– system enquiry – gastrointestinal – appetite, vomiting, bowel habit		
– system enquiry – respiratory – cough (productive), breathlessness		
– system enquiry – cardiovascular – palpitations, chest pain, ankle swelling, orthopnoea		
– system enquiry – genitourinary – polyuria, frequency, dysuria, haematuria		
– system enquiry – neurological – headache, dizziness, visual problems		
– system enquiry – musculoskeletal – limb weakness, rashes		
Past medical history		
Medications and allergies		
Family history		
Social history (and illicit drug use)		
Elicits patient's concerns		
Explains differential diagnosis		
Explains plan: need for further investigations, outpatient follow-up		
Answers patient's questions appropriately		
Checks patient's understanding of diagnosis and plan		
Checks if patient has further questions		
Global mark from patient		
Global mark from examiner		

Instructions for actor

You are a 60-year-old teacher called Jeanette Ross. You called an ambulance and came to the ED because you feel very unwell. Over the past 3 days, you have gradually developed pain in all the muscles of your body. Initially, it was a mild ache but now they are all quite painful and have become tender. You feel weak, clammy and tired. Also, if asked directly, you report that you noticed yesterday that your urine had become very dark. You have not passed urine at all today. You think this is strange, because you are drinking more water than usual in case you are dehydrated. You have had no other symptoms of note.

You are normally fit and well and have had no recent illnesses. Your only medical history is a mildly increased blood pressure and cholesterol. You also had your appendix removed when you were 17. You take ramipril and 2 weeks ago started taking simvastatin which your own doctor recommended.

You drink 2 or 3 glasses of red wine every week and do not smoke. You live with your husband who is well and have not recently been abroad.

If given the opportunity to ask questions you want to know why you feel so unwell and why your urine has become so dark.

1.24 Transient ischaemic attack

A transient ischaemic attack (TIA) is a sudden-onset, focal neurological deficit caused by disruption of part of the cerebral circulation, which resolves completely in <24 hours. In fact, most true TIAs resolve within 10 minutes, and there is an increasing school of thought, which believes that anything lasting longer than 10 minutes should be classed as a stroke.

By far the most frequent cause is an embolus in the cerebral circulation. TIAs and strokes present with the same symptoms, the only difference being the degree to which the symptoms persist. As such they occur on a continuum and following a TIA a person is at higher risk of a stroke – hence the importance of prompt diagnosis and treatment of TIAs.

The history taking of a patient who may have suffered a TIA seeks to confirm the diagnosis and risk-assess the patient so further management can be planned. Though some presentations are typical, there can be wide variation in symptoms and signs depending on the cerebral territory involved (carotid or vertebrobasilar). TIAs do not normally present with loss of consciousness or seizure activity.

Possible differential diagnoses include hypoglycaemia, migraine (which may present without a headache) or focal epilepsy.

To assist in making the diagnosis of a stroke or TIA the Recognition of Stroke in The Emergency Room (ROSIER) scale can be used. Score 1 point for each of:
- Asymmetrical facial weakness
- Asymmetrical arm weakness
- Asymmetrical leg weakness
- Speech disturbance
- Visual field defect

Subtract 1 point for each of:
- Loss of consciousness
- Seizure activity

If the total score is above 0, there is a high possibility of a stroke or TIA (once hypoglycaemia has been excluded). All of these features should be enquired about when stroke or TIA are considered.

In TIA patients with no on-going symptoms the ROSIER score is of no further benefit in terms of risk assessment. These patients should be assessed for their risk of stroke using the ABCD² score (**Table 1.24.1**).

Table 1.24.1 The ABCD² score

Parameter of ABCD² score	Score criterion	Score
Age	>60 years	1
Blood pressure	>140/90 mmHg	1
Clinical features (maximum 2 marks)	Unilateral weakness	2
	Speech disturbance	1
Duration of symptoms (maximum 2 marks)	>60 minutes	2
	10–59 minutes	1
	<10 minutes	0
Diabetes mellitus	Presence of disease	1

Patients who have had a TIA should be started on anti-platelet therapy and have admission or follow up arranged, according to local protocol. The higher the score, the higher the patient's risk of subsequent stroke, so the National Institute for Health and Care Excellence (NICE) recommends that those with a score of 4 or above are assessed by a specialist within 24 hours while those with a score of 3 or less should have this assessment within a week. Practice varies in different departments as to whether high-risk patients are admitted or followed up within 24 hours as outpatients.

This scoring system does not take into account certain other variables that should also be considered. Patients who are having recurrent TIAs or are already on antiplatelet therapy or anticoagulation are also in a higher risk group and should be assessed sooner.

Before going home, it should be explained to all patients who have had a TIA that if symptoms recur they should come straight back to the ED – and if available locally they should be given details of the hyperacute stroke unit. It is also important to advise patients that after a TIA they must inform the Driver and Vehicle Licensing Agency and not drive for at least one month – depending on the type of license they possess.

Scenario

Mr Griffin is a 61-year-old man who has been brought to the ED by his wife. He had an episode of left-sided weakness earlier in the day. His blood pressure today is 132/68 mmHg. Take a history from Mr Griffin. Then present your findings and explain your management plan to the examiner.

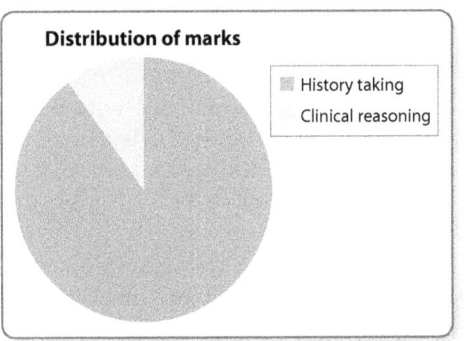

Mark sheet	Achieved	Not achieved
Introduces self to patient and confirms their identity		
Establishes presenting complaint		
Specifically enquires about:		
– symptoms		
– time of onset of symptoms		
– persistence of symptoms		
– nature of onset		
– associated symptoms		
– previous episodes		
Past medical history		
Enquires about diabetes control, blood sugar during/after episode		
Medications and allergies		
Social history – mobility aids, type of accommodation, carers		

Cont'd...

Cont'd...

Mark sheet	Achieved	Not achieved
Social history (and illicit drug use) – smoking, occupation		
Elicits patient's concerns		
Explains differential diagnosis		
Explains need to stop driving		
Explains plan: need for further investigations, outpatient follow-up		
Answers patient's questions appropriately		
Demonstrates knowledge of ABCD^2 scoring and use		
Checks patient's understanding of diagnosis and plan		
Checks if patient has further questions		
Global mark from patient		
Global mark from examiner		

Instructions for actor

You are a 61-year-old computer programmer called Harry Griffin. You have come to the ED with your wife because this morning after breakfast you suddenly found you couldn't move your left arm or leg. You had no other symptoms but struggled to stay upright in your chair. Luckily your wife was at home and you called her. Because you have type 1 diabetes mellitus she checked your blood sugar and it was 9.2 mmol/L. You waited at home to see if things would get better – your wife rang the general practitioner and left a message asking for a home visit. Your symptoms resolved within 5 minutes but when the doctor arrived he asked your wife to bring you straight to the ED.

You have been well recently and have no other medical problems apart from well-controlled hypertension. You are meticulous about controlling your blood sugar and it is normally around 7 mmol/L. You and your wife are both independent. You do not smoke; rarely drink alcohol and work from home so do not need to drive if the doctor advises you not to.

If you are asked about your concerns ask the doctor if you had (or are going to have) a stroke.

Suggested reading

Assessing fitness to drive, A guide for medical professionals. Driver's Medical Group, DVLA, Swansea.
Diagnosis and initial management of acute stroke and TIA. Clinical guideline 68. National Institute for Health and Care Excellence. London, 2008.
Scottish Intercollegiate Guidelines Network Guideline 108. Management of patients with stroke or TIA. SIGN 2008.

1.25 Weight loss

The causes of weight loss are varied, as virtually any chronic condition may be a contributing factor. However in an emergency setting there are certain causes that should be considered and excluded early. These conditions are more likely to present to the ED with weight loss as a significant feature of the presenting complaint. In addition, given their acute nature, these conditions are more likely to require early diagnosis and treatment before possibly being followed up in an outpatient setting.

With presenting complaints which are as non-specific as weight loss, it is difficult to take a focused history. Initially, it is appropriate to enquire as to whether there are any associated features and then to perform a thorough system enquiry to elicit any facts that may identify the underlying problem.

Quantifying the degree of weight loss can also be difficult if a patient has not recently been weighed. It is however easy to ask if clothes have become looser or others have commented on a change in physical appearance. Also it is always worth clarifying whether or not the weight loss has been intentional, though if it is part of the presenting complaint this is unlikely. In basic terms weight loss is caused by:
- An inadequate intake of calories
- Poor absorption in the bowel
- Poor utilisation by the body
- A state of high energy usage caused by constitutional disturbance

Weight loss, night sweats and fever are constitutional symptoms which when occurring in the context of lymphoma, are termed B symptoms. However, these features can occur in malignancy or any infective or inflammatory process. Common causes for weight loss are considered below.

Malignancy

Generalised findings may include a past history of malignancy, anorexia, fevers and fatigue. To further localise any malignancy, a systems review aims to elicit further clues and clinical examination findings are also key. With regard to lung cancer, asbestos exposure and smoking history are crucial.

Tuberculosis

Initial symptoms are anorexia, fever, night sweats and fatigue. Pulmonary tuberculosis is the commonest form and presents with a persistent cough and possibly haemoptysis. Those most at risk are in contact with people from areas where tuberculosis is endemic. The incidence is also higher in those who are homeless, alcohol dependent or immunosuppressed by medication or other illnesses.

Gastrointestinal pathology

Inflammatory bowel disease may cause altered bowel habit, the passage of rectal blood, abdominal pain and the constitutional symptoms listed above. Steatorrhoea may be present in coeliac disease or chronic pancreatitis.

Connective tissue disease

Acute flares of any connective tissue disease including vasculitis may cause weight loss. The symptoms are non-specific, but past medical history and associated findings from the history and examination may be suggestive of the underlying problem.

Diabetes mellitus

Weight loss is a common presenting feature of type 1 diabetes mellitus. It occurs with other features suggestive of hyperglycaemia such as polydipsia, polyuria, blurred vision and lethargy. There may be a family history of this or of other autoimmune/endocrine diseases.

Hyperthyroidism

In this condition, symptoms arise from the patient's increased basal metabolic rate. There is often weight loss with an increased appetite, heat intolerance, restlessness, sweating, diarrhoea, tremor and palpitations.

Scenario

Miss Stepping is a 23-year-old sales assistant. She has been brought into the ED today by her boyfriend as she is too exhausted to do anything. Take a history from her and explain your differential diagnosis and management plan to her.

Distribution of marks
- History taking
- Clinical reasoning

Mark sheet	Achieved	Not achieved
Introduces self to patient and confirms their identity		
Offers analgesia		
Establishes presenting complaint		
Specifically enquires about:		
– period and quantity of weight loss		
– constitutional symptoms		
– system enquiry – gastrointestinal – appetite, vomiting, bowel habit		
– system enquiry – respiratory – cough (productive), breathlessness		
– system enquiry – cardiovascular – palpitations, chest pain, ankle swelling, orthopnoea		
– system enquiry – genitourinary – polyuria, frequency, dysuria, haematuria		

Cont'd...

Cont'd...

Mark sheet	Achieved	Not achieved
– system enquiry – neurological – headache, dizziness, visual problems, limb symptoms		
– system enquiry – gynaecological – lower abdominal pain, menstrual cycle		
Past medical history		
Medications and allergies		
Family history		
Social history (and illicit drug use)		
Elicits patient's concerns		
Explains differential diagnosis		
Explains plan: need for further investigations and specialist opinion		
Answers patient's questions appropriately		
Shows empathy		
Checks patient's understanding of diagnosis and plan		
Discusses arranging a review with a diabetes specialist nurse		
Checks if patient has further questions		
Global mark from patient		
Global mark from examiner		

Instructions for actor

You are a 23-year-old woman called Tina Stepping, who works in a sports shop. You have been brought to the ED today by your partner. You didn't want to come, but he made you because you have been losing weight for the last month and guess you've lost at least 10 kg but you aren't sure.

Your clothes do not fit anymore. You have gradually begun to feel more and more tired and aren't sure why. You have been eating and drinking well. If asked specifically you realise you have been drinking all the time and passing urine a lot more than usual. You have even had to wake up in the night to pass urine. Your urine has been very clear and there has been no blood in it and no pain when you empty your bladder. You also feel that your vision often seems a bit blurry and you were thinking of seeing an optician soon but don't want to be told you need glasses so have avoided doing anything about it. You have otherwise felt ok. You have not been vomiting and have had no change in your bowel habit nor noticed any blood in your stools. You don't feel restless, just exhausted. You have not had any cough, fevers or sweats.

You have no past medical history and have not been abroad since going to Spain for a week 2 years ago. You live with your partner and do not smoke or take any recreational drugs. You drink 4–5 glasses of wine each week.

You are adopted so you do not know if there is any family history of medical problems.

If the doctor mentions diabetes you are upset as you have colleague at work with diabetes that now needs dialysis. You are worried this means you will need dialysis too. You want to know who will give you help and advice on what to do next.

Suggested reading

Department of Health. Immunisation Against Infectious Diseases (The Green Book), 3rd edn. London: Department of Health, 2006.

National Institute for Health and Care Excellence (NICE). Tuberculosis. Clinical guideline 117. NICE. London: NICE; 2011.

National Institute for Health and Care Excellence (NICE). Type 1 diabetes in adults. NICE guideline 17.NICE. London: NICE; 2015.

1.26 Seizure

Seizures are a common presenting complaint in the ED. The diagnosis of a seizure has significant implications for an individual in terms of lifestyle, employment, driving, insurance and possibly medication. Thus it should only be made when there is a relative certainty. History taking is key to distinguishing a seizure from other forms of collapse. The key features to consider and elicit during the history taking are described in **Table 1.7.3**. These relate to what happened before, during and after the episode in question:

- Specific precipitants can include flashing lights, exhaustion, alcohol or drug withdrawal. Prior to the event was there an aura? Auras take the form of many sensory experiences, e.g. a strange sensation in the epigastrium, a hallucination or a sense of déjà vu. Was the onset sudden or gradual? Were there other preceding symptoms suggestive of syncope?
- During the episode did the patient lose consciousness? What was the nature of any jerking movements and how long did these persist?
- Afterwards was there a postictal phase and if so how long did it last? Can the patient remember events? Were there injuries, tongue biting or incontinence?

Seizures are either unprovoked or provoked. To identify those which are provoked questions must address the risk of electrolyte disturbance, hypoglycaemia, head injury, alcohol excess/withdrawal, cerebrovascular events or intracerebral neoplasm.

Ask questions about the patient's normal activities, work and hobbies to ascertain the risk to them if further seizures occur. Clearly activities such as window cleaning or open-water swimming will be extremely risky should a further seizure occur.

Other seizure types such as absence or complex partial seizures typically occur several times before the person or family seek medical help and are often not dealt with primarily in the ED.

Early neuroimaging is required where:
- The patient has not fully recovered
- The patient has focal neurological signs
- There is focal or partial onset before generalisation
- There is a history of acute head trauma
- Malignancy is suspected
- Immunocompromise is suspected
- HIV infection is suspected or already diagnosed
- The patient is on anticoagulation

Otherwise in patients with no on-going symptoms or signs after a seizure, if baseline investigations are normal, further investigation can be on an outpatient basis, typically in a first fit clinic.

If a patient is to be discharged home for outpatient follow-up they must first be given adequate information and advice. Alcohol and a lack of sleep can lower the seizure threshold. They must inform the driver licensing authority and must not drive until their follow-up appointment. Swimming, climbing and other isolated or high-risk activities should be avoided because of the risks involved if there is a further seizure. Driving after a seizure is considered in section 2.8.

Scenario

Miss Saul is a 28-year-old woman who has been brought to the ED by ambulance after a collapse at work. Take a history from her and explain your management plan.

Distribution of marks
- History taking
- Clinical reasoning

Mark sheet	Achieved	Not achieved
Introduces self to patient and confirms their identity		
Offers analgesia, ensures patient comfort		
Establishes presenting complaint		
Specifically enquires about:		
– preceding symptoms		
– description of events		
– injuries sustained/tongue biting/incontinence		
– recovery/postictal phase		
– ongoing symptoms		
– systems enquiry		
Past medical history		
Family history – epilepsy		
Medications and allergies		
Social history (and illicit drug use)		
Asks specifically about driving		
Elicits patient's concerns		
Explains differential diagnosis		
Explains plan: need for follow-up and investigations		
Answers patient's questions appropriately		
Shows empathy		
Checks patient's understanding of diagnosis and plan		
Checks if patient has further questions		
Global mark from patient		
Global mark from examiner		

Instructions for actor

You are a 28-year-old woman called Katharine Saul. You work in a hotel reception at the front desk. You arrived in the ED by ambulance and cannot clearly remember what happened. You remember being at work and while sitting down having a strange ache in your stomach and feeling 'not right'. After that you don't remember anything until arriving in the ED. A colleague of yours accompanied you to the ED and has since told you that you had glazed over in your chair and your whole body starting shaking. This lasted around 5 minutes. Colleagues lay you on the floor and called an ambulance.

You now feel exhausted but have no other complaints. If you are asked you become aware that your tongue is very sore and you may well have bitten it. Also if asked, you reluctantly admit that you were incontinent of urine and ask why this would happen.

You have recently felt well. You have no medical problems, take no medication, do not smoke and only drink alcohol occasionally on social occasions. You have an older brother who has epilepsy and takes tablets for it. You live with your partner and don't drive. You walk to work as it is not too far.

Suggested reading

Guideline for the management of first seizure in the Emergency Department. London: Royal College of Emergency Medicine, 2009.

National Institute of Health and Care Excellence (NICE). Epilepsies. Diagnosis and management. Clinical guideline 137. NICE. London: NICE; 2012.

1.27 Pelvic pain

This is a challenging objectively structured clinical examination (OSCE) because there are several considerations which must all be managed well for a candidate to cover all relevant areas. In addition to the standard history this OSCE requires the asking of personal questions regarding gynaecological problems and a sexual history. It also requires appropriate questions to be asked to decide whether the lower abdominal symptoms are gynaecological or general surgical in nature.

Relevant questions must be asked to gain an understanding of the type of pain the patient is experiencing, as discussed in section 1.3. Low abdominal pain which radiates into the back or the legs is suggestive of a gynaecological cause. Uterine pain is often colicky and radiates to the sacrum. Ovarian pain is often located in an iliac fossa with radiation into the legs. Sudden onset pain may be related to ovarian torsion, a ruptured cyst or a vascular event. Pain that is more gradual in onset is more likely to arise from an inflammatory or infective problem.

Enquire whether the pain has any specific associations. Is it related to time of menstruation? Has the patient noticed vaginal discharge and if so what is its nature? Is the patient sexually active? If so, with whom? Based on this could she be pregnant or have been exposed to sexually transmitted infections (STIs)?

Additional areas of the history relate to the patient's menstrual cycle. These include the date of the last menstrual period, whether it was normal in nature, its duration and the regularity of the cycle, and whether the patient usually experiences pain at any particular time during the menstrual cycle. Also take a brief obstetric history to discover whether the patient has been pregnant before and, if so, the outcome of each pregnancy.

In addition to asking the correct questions to gather necessary information, another important consideration in this scenario is the nature of the information. Patients will be asked to discuss very personal and potentially embarrassing issues. These discussions must be handled in an extremely sensitive manner: this encourages the patient to be open and honest. It is helpful to say to the patient that many of the issues to be discussed are sensitive but they are important to help with correct diagnosis and management. Some related issues and taking a sexual history have already been covered in section 1.21.

Always consider pregnancy in patients who are sexually active.

Dysmenorrhoea

This is often physiological (or primary) and characterised by pain which occurs regularly at the beginning of a period. Pain commonly radiates to the back. It is crampy and in some patients is associated with nausea and vomiting. There should be no features in the history suggestive of alternative pathology. Initial treatment is anti-inflammatory drugs to reduce uterine contractions, which are due to excessive prostaglandin levels.

There are several causes for secondary dysmenorrhoea such as fibroids, endometriosis and chronic pelvic inflammatory disease.

Ovarian torsion

This results from an ovary twisting so that the respective blood vessels are occluded. Normally the arterial supply continues but venous outflow is restricted. There may be intermittent twisting and untwisting such that symptoms come and go. Pain is felt unilaterally and there is likely to be tenderness on abdominal and pelvic examination.

Pelvic inflammatory disease

This refers to infection which is ascending or spreading from the cervix. Symptoms are variable on a spectrum of acute to chronic or low-grade disease. Common symptoms include lower abdominal pain, vaginal discharge, fever, nausea and vomiting. Long-term consequences include decreased fertility and an increased risk of ectopic pregnancy.

Although in some patients pelvic inflammatory disease (PID) is secondary to instrumentation during procedures, in the vast majority it is due to STI. In addition to identifying and treating the infection, it is necessary to advise patients to refrain from sexual activity; if the cause is a sexually transmitted organism, contact tracing is likely to be required. It is advisable to refer the patient to a genitourinary medicine clinic. In sexually active women, always consider whether the patient could also be pregnant.

Ectopic pregnancy

This typically presents with unilateral lower abdominal pain, which may be followed by vaginal bleeding. The patient may experience a collapse or complain of shoulder tip pain. Risk factors relate to disruption of the normal anatomy in a way that affects the transit of the fertilised ovum. These include PID, endometriosis, previous surgery, the presence of cysts, tumours or a contraceptive device and previous ectopic pregnancy.

Endometriosis

In this condition endometrial glandular tissue occurs in areas outside the uterus. Symptoms are variable depending on the extent and areas involved. Some women experience no pain; others have significant pain. Pain may be cyclical and occur during menstruation. Additional symptoms commonly include dyspareunia and dysmenorrhoea.

Scenario

Miss Wilkes is a 26-year-old woman who has come to the ED with lower abdominal pain. Take a history from her and explain your differential diagnosis and management plan.

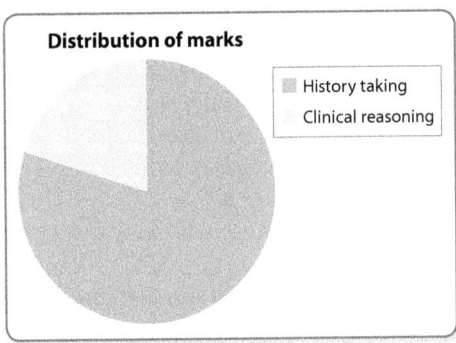

Mark sheet	Pass	Fail
Introduces self to patient and confirms their identity		
Offers analgesia, ensures patient comfort		
Establishes presenting complaint		
Specifically enquires about:		
– duration of symptoms		
– nature of pain		
– associated symptoms		
– systemic features		
– systems enquiry		
– relevant sexual history		
Gynaecological/obstetric history		
Past medical history		
Family history		
Medications and allergies		
Social history (and illicit drug use)		
Elicits patient's concerns		
Explains differential diagnosis		
Explains plan: need for further investigations		
Answers patient's questions appropriately		
Shows empathy		
Checks patient's understanding of diagnosis and plan		
Checks if patient has further questions		
Global mark from patient		
Global mark from examiner		

Instructions for actor

You are a 26-year-old primary teacher called Jenny Wilkes. You have come to see a doctor because you have been getting lower abdominal pain for several weeks and today it was worse than previously. The pain is central and constant but sometimes gets worse and other times is not so bad. For the past 2 weeks you have noticed a vaginal discharge which is continuous, light and blood stained. You've lost your appetite but have had no other symptoms. Your pain is controlled by paracetamol and dihydrocodeine but you are worried about what's causing it.

Your periods are regular, every 4 weeks, and you have not noticed any significant changes to them.

You had unprotected sexual intercourse around 10 weeks ago with a man you met at a friend's party. You have not been sexually active since and have no regular partner. You have never been pregnant.

You occasionally have migraines but have no other medical problems or medications. You are allergic to penicillin which causes a very bad rash. You smoke 10 cigarettes a day and drink 2 or 3 glasses of wine each week.

1.28 Non-accidental injury

Non-accidental injury (NAI) must be considered during every consultation that involves a child. Though there are several forms of child abuse, for example neglect or physical, sexual or emotional abuse, the following discussion and objectively structured clinical examination (OSCE) scenario relates to NAI presenting with physical injuries. The key challenge is to recognise features of the presentation that are concerning because they are suggestive of NAI, and then to be able to explain those concerns to family, carers or other staff in as non-confrontational and constructive a manner as possible.

There are specific features relating to a presentation that may indicate NAI. These are divided into those relating to the history, the examination or observed behaviour within the department. Clearly these features do not always represent NAI but their presence should increase a clinician's level of concern and prompt more thorough consideration.

Features of history suggesting potential NAI

- The history changes when retold
- The mechanism is not consistent with the injuries
- The mechanism is not consistent with the child's developmental age or ability
- There has been unreasonable delay in seeking medical attention
- There have been multiple previous attendances
- The child directly reports NAI

Features of examination suggesting potential NAI

- Burns suggesting immersion in water
- Cigarette burns
- Linear marks from belts or sticks (or fingers from slapping)
- High energy fractures not in keeping with age or mechanism
- Bruising in young or immobile children
- Injuries to the buttocks or perineum
- Retinal haemorrhages

In addition, the child's behaviour and interaction with staff and parents or guardians may also be revealing. Is the child unusually withdrawn? Does the child make eye contact? Does the child appear to have an appropriate rapport or interaction with parents/guardians?

To fully understand and evaluate any concerns, a thorough history of any incident must be taken. Ideally the history would first be taken from the child and then also discussed with whoever else is present. It is important to understand the mechanism involved. Clarify:

- Who else was present or in the vicinity at the time?
- Who identified or noticed the injury (particularly if the mechanism is unknown)?
- If there was a delay in attending hospital, was there a reasonable explanation?
- What are the circumstances at home – who lives in and visits the house?
- Has there been previous involvement with social services?

Also take a standard medical history to ensure legitimate medical pathology is not mistaken for NAI; for example, bruising or fractures may have been caused by an undiagnosed pathological process.

If a presentation causes concern regarding possible NAI, the case should be discussed with a senior doctor within the department or a member of the hospital's child protection team. If it is agreed that there is sufficient concern it will be necessary to involve social services. In the short term, hospital admission may be necessary. Remember to check if there are other children at home who could be at risk.

Discussing concerns with parents/guardians

Once possible NAI has been raised as a concern, it will be necessary to discuss this with whoever is accompanying the child. Judgement and extreme tact are required for this. It may be tempting to simply delay treatment of an injury to 'buy time' so relevant discussions can be had by staff. However, if additional staff are going to see the child or if short-term admission is required it will probably be necessary to explain what is happening and, to some extent, why. Anyone accompanying a child with a seemingly minor injury who is then told the child needs to be admitted will ask why that is necessary.

Depending on the situation it is usually best to be honest but non-confrontational. Remember that it is rarely appropriate to diagnose NAI in the ED; the task is simply to recognise that NAI is a real possibility. Hence it is reasonable to explain that what is being done is in the best interests of the child and is for the child's safety, and that further assessment by more senior or experienced staff is needed. Do not directly accuse anyone of child abuse.

The adult who has accompanied the child is likely to be upset or angry and offended; be prepared for this. Remember that even if this is truly a case of NAI, this adult may not be the person responsible for inflicting the injury. The discussion involves some elements of breaking bad news. Allow the person time to understand the situation, allow silence while they are thinking, be supportive if they are upset and remain calm if they become angry.

Treating the injury

While considering these issues ensure that any injuries are treated appropriately and without delay. Ensure the child is comfortable, pain free and receiving whatever medical treatment is required.

Female genital mutilation

This is a procedure where the female genitals are cut, injured or changed without any medical reason for doing so. It is also known as female circumcision. Female genital mutilation (FGM) is normally carried out on girls before puberty commences.

It is illegal in the UK and is recognised as a form of child abuse. As well as being a painful and potentially dangerous procedure, it can cause long term problems with pain, sexual intercourse and mental health.

It is carried out for various social, cultural and religious reasons, normally in families that originate in several North African countries.

Anyone performing or failing to protect a girl from FGM is committing an offence. There is clear guidance for health care professionals on mandatory reporting if a child has had or is felt to be at risk of FGM.

Scenario

Bobby is a 5-year-old boy who has been brought to the ED from school because he had been crying with back pain. You have already examined him and found a mark on his back which looks like a burn from an iron. He also had some linear bruising on the backs of both his thighs. He is too upset to tell you how he got them.

His mother has just arrived after being phoned by the school. Take a history from her and explain your management plan to her.

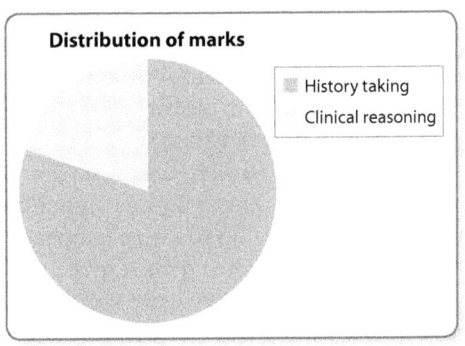

Distribution of marks
- History taking
- Clinical reasoning

Mark sheet	Achieved	Not achieved
Introduces self to mother and confirms her identity		
Explains Bobby is safe and she can see him soon		
Asks what mother knows so far		
Explains Bobby's presentation to the ED		
Enquires about his injuries		
Specifically enquires about:		
– mechanism of burn		
– who was present		
– what was done about the burn		
– reason for not seeking medical attention		
– mechanism of marks on legs		
Detailed social history – family structure, siblings, problems at home		
Ask about previous involvement of social services		
Past medical history		
Family history		
Medications and allergies		
Explains appropriate treatment for burn		
Explains concerns about cause of injuries		
Explains need to involve senior doctor/child protection team member		
Supportive communication with mother		
Explains the priority is Bobby's health/safety		
Answers mother's questions appropriately		
Shows empathy		
Checks mother's understanding of diagnosis and plan		
Checks if mother has further questions		
Global mark from mother		
Global mark from examiner		

Instructions for actor

You are a 26-year-old mother named Naomi Clark. You have come to the ED because you received a phone call from your son Bobby's school saying he had been taken to hospital because of an injury to his back. You are anxious and upset when you arrive. You want to know what happened to Bobby's back.

If prompted or asked by the doctor you realise the concern is about a burn he got from an iron 3 days ago when playing in the sitting room. You weren't there at the time but Bobby's step-sister told you what happened. She had been ironing when Bobby knocked the ironing board over and the iron landed on his back. When you came home you ran the burn under cool water and gave him some pain killers. You talked to your husband, not Bobby's father, and together decided the burn wasn't too bad and would get better. Bobby is often looked after by his older step-sister Jenny who is 15 years old. You moved in with your husband and his daughter Jenny 8 months ago.

You do not know about any marks on Bobby's legs but know he normally has some bruises from bumping into things.

Bobby has no medical problems or medicines. He is developmentally normal and otherwise well. He has no contact with his own father. You are a care worker and work shifts, so you often get his step-sister to look after him when she's not at school. Your husband works in an office as a salesman. You have never had any reason to worry about either of them looking after Bobby.

You don't see what all the fuss is about as children are bound to get some injuries from 'messing around'. Initially you are dismissive but when you realise the doctor is worried about the injuries you become angry. You feel that you are being treated as a liar and you are scared that the staff think you are a bad mother. You become very angry and defensive. You want to see Bobby and take him home. You are tearful and lose your temper.

You love Bobby and can see that looking after him is most important. Regardless you are still upset by the implication that someone has hurt him. You are also scared and angry that staff will want to take him away.

If the doctor is reassuring and explains they are trying to do the right thing for Bobby you slowly calm down. If their tone is aggressive or accusing you continue to be upset, angry and only wanting to leave.

If it has not been explained you, also ask if Bobby has been given some pain-killers, how his burn will be treated and what is going to happen next.

Suggested reading

Department of Health and Social Care. Female Genital Mutilation. Resources for healthcare staff. London: Department of Health and Social Care; 2015.

National Institute for Health and Care Excellence (NICE). When to suspect child maltreatment. Clinical guideline 89. NICE. London: NICE; 2009.

Royal College of Emergency Medicine (RCEM). Best practice for safeguarding children. RCEM. London: RCEM; 2009.

1.29 Visual disturbance

Visual disturbances represent a variety of pathologies which may be due to a local or a central problem. As always the key is to identify instances that may lead to serious outcomes such as blindness. Begin by letting the patient explain the nature of the problem and then ask specific questions that will help to identify a possible aetiology.

Clarify whether there is actual loss of vision, blurring of vision, decreased colour vision or double vision.

Nature of visual loss

- What was the speed of onset? If gradual how long has it developed over? Sudden onset disturbance may suggest a vascular cause. However, beware of the fact that someone may become aware of a problem 'suddenly' when it has gradually progressed to reach a certain threshold where it is more apparent
- Which areas of vision are involved? It may be the entirety or only a specific quadrant, half or region, such as the centre, of the visual field
- Are one or both eyes involved? Where both eyes are involved pathology is likely to be central whereas if only one eye is involved it is likely to be within the eye or optic nerve distal to the optic chiasm
- What is the timescale? Is the defect intermittent, persistent, improving or getting worse?
- Is there a loss of colour vision? This is typical of optic nerve pathology

Double vision

If double vision is present ask about the images. Are they next to or above each other? In which direction of gaze is double vision present or worst?

Pain

The presence, nature and location of pain or discomfort is important. It may be within the eye, retro-orbital or better described as a headache.

Additional symptoms

- Are there other visual symptoms such as haloes, flashing lights or strange patterns overlying images?
- Does the eye get red or watery?
- Does the eyelid seem to droop?
- Is there an associated headache?
- Are there any other focal neurological symptoms?

Migraine

Flashing lights or additional patterns such as zig-zag lines are associated with migraines, retinal detachments, or occipital lobe pathology. The onset, time course and association with headache/nausea will guide a candidate to this diagnosis. Clearly past medical history and previous episodes may also support this. Important differentials are space occupying lesions or intracerebral bleeding as discussed in section 1.16.

Giant cell arteritis

As well as transient visual loss a patient may complain of general malaise, scalp pain/tenderness and jaw claudication. The condition may progress to permanent vision loss and if not treated the other eye is also at risk. It is uncommon below the age of 50 years and is often associated with polymyalgia rheumatica.

Optic neuritis

There is progressive loss of visual acuity over a short number of days. The condition is usually painful and eye movements may hurt. Colour vision also deteriorates. This condition is associated with demyelinating diseases and diabetes. Vision may recover over a few weeks depending on the underlying cause.

Retinal detachment

This may be spontaneous or secondary to trauma. Patients experience flashes or floaters as well as loss of vision in the associated visual field and decreased visual acuity.

Papilloedema

This may result in blurring or loss of vision that lasts a few seconds. It may be monocular or binocular and symptoms may arise when activities cause raised intracranial pressure such as straining or bending down. Additional medical history or systems enquiry may indicate a systemic cause.

Glaucoma

In acute glaucoma a patient may report blurred vision or seeing haloes around lights. There may be severe pain with nausea/vomiting, decreased visual acuity and a fixed pupil.

Amaurosis fugax

This is transient visual loss which is typically described as a sensation that a curtain falls across over the visual field. It is commonly caused by a thromboembolic event but can also be caused by giant cell arteritis.

Central retinal artery or vein occlusion

These present with sudden visual loss which may only involve part of a visual field if a branch of the main retinal vessels is involved.

Scenario

Miss Murray is a 64-year-old woman who has come to see a doctor because of problems with her vision. Take a history from her and explain your management plan to her.

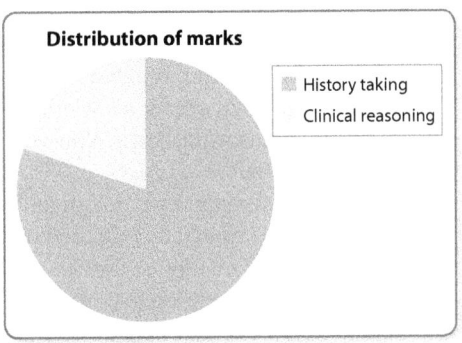

Distribution of marks
- History taking
- Clinical reasoning

Mark sheet	Achieved	Not achieved
Introduces self to patient and confirms their identity		
Offers analgesia, ensures patient comfort		
Establishes presenting complaint		
Specifically enquires about:		
– nature of vision loss		
– relevant features of vision loss		
– presence of pain		
– presence of double vision		
– associated symptoms		
– precipitating factors		
– systemic features		
– systems enquiry		
Past medical history		
Family history		
Medications and allergies		
Social history (and illicit drug use)		
Elicits patient's concerns		
Explains differential diagnosis		
Explains plan		
Answers patient's questions appropriately		
Shows empathy		
Checks patient's understanding of diagnosis and plan		
Checks if patient has further questions		
Global mark from patient		
Global mark from examiner		

Instructions for actor

You are a 64-year-old woman named Jackie Murray. You have come to the ED because of problems with your vision. While reading the paper with your breakfast this morning you lost vision in your right eye for a few minutes. It was like something had covered your eye. Gradually it got better on its own. Now your vision is back to normal. You have never had anything like this before.

You are due to see your own doctor later in the week because you haven't felt well for several weeks. You've been feeling tired with most of your body seeming to ache and have also had a headache mainly on the right side of your head which is there most of the time. You haven't noticed anything making these problems better or worse.

You are normally fit and well, take no medications and have no allergies. You live alone, don't smoke and rarely drink alcohol. You work part-time as a secretary.

Chapter 2

Communication skills

- 2.1 Introduction
- 2.2 Speaking to an angry patient, parent or relative
- 2.3 Breaking bad news
- 2.4 Clinical decisions unit handover – 1
- 2.5 Needlestick injury
- 2.6 Obtaining consent for a procedure
- 2.7 Difficult referral
- 2.8 Driving after a seizure
- 2.9 Major incident
- 2.10 Conflict resolution – request for antibiotics
- 2.11 Conflict resolution – refusing tetanus immunisation
- 2.12 Febrile convulsion
- 2.13 Difficult conversation with a colleague
- 2.14 Explaining a new diagnosis – diabetes mellitus
- 2.15 Clinical decisions unit handover – 2
- 2.16 Neonatal jaundice
- 2.17 Sexual assault

2.1 Introduction

Good interpersonal skills are fundamental for senior clinicians. These cannot be tested in other parts of the exam and subsequently form a significant part of any practical exam including the FRCEM OSCE. Tasks may include:
- Teaching or explaining a treatment or management plan
- Breaking bad news
- Managing an angry patient
- Managing a difficult colleague

Ultimately all of these scenarios require the candidate to be able to share information in an appropriate manner while demonstrating an awareness of what the other individual involved may be thinking or feeling. Effective communication will require a candidate to have considered what the task is asking them to achieve while showing a considered approach to the person they are interacting with.

Important elements to demonstrate include:
- Good use of body language, e.g. active listening or non-threatening posture
- Using terminology suited to the scenario – specifically avoiding unnecessary jargon
- Demonstrating understanding of the concerns of the other party involved
- An ability to remain calm
- An ability to build rapport with others
- An ability to use silence appropriately
- A reassuring and confident manner
- Behaving sensitively towards others

Inevitably some of these skills come more easily to some candidates than others. However with practice of different scenarios and reflection on how they should be tackled (assisted by the mark sheets provided); all candidates should be able to meet the criteria to pass these stations.

After practising some of these scenarios candidates should ideally be able to get into the role and avoid feeling awkward or inhibited by the artificial nature of some exam scenarios. As in all stations it is best to behave as if the scenario is a real one during a normal day at work.

2.2 Speaking to an angry patient, parent or relative

When dealing with someone who is angry one of the key skills is to prevent the situation from escalating. There are several things that can be done to reduce the tension during such a meeting. As with any meeting always start by introducing yourself and clarifying who it is you are speaking to. If you are in a public area it will be more appropriate to go somewhere private and possibly take another member of staff with you. Though the conversation may begin with you both standing, always suggest you continue talking while sitting down – offer the other person a seat.

It is very important that the person you are talking to feels you are taking their concerns seriously so you must show them that you are taking time to understand the problem. This is demonstrated by using appropriate body language and allowing them time to speak without interruption to show you are listening to them. With regard to an objective structured clinical examination (OSCE) station this will clearly be further reflected by the impression you make on the actor/examiner and the global marks received.

Once the angry party has explained their concerns it is important to clarify the facts as you understand them; it is appropriate to summarise events that have occurred and check any areas of misunderstanding. To do this you must have as many facts to hand as possible and it is always worth checking data in the exam, e.g. relevant notes may be available for you to read, or (more likely) X-rays may be available for you to show the complainant.

It is appropriate to apologise because someone is unhappy with the treatment they have received and this is often adequate to defuse a situation. An apology does not necessarily constitute accepting that you or your department are at fault. It simply acknowledges the other party's dissatisfaction. Having said this it is not necessary to tolerate derogatory or offensive comments about staff or the department. A balance must be reached on a case by case basis of being prepared to listen to someone who is angry and supporting your staff appropriately.

The discussion should then move onto how to deal with whatever has happened. The first priority is to ensure the individual involved is ok and that there is a safe and sensible management plan in place. This should be mutually agreed with all parties satisfied with the plan. The next priority is to explain that any concerns are taken very seriously and there are several methods that can be employed to prevent something happening again. This may involve speaking to a member of staff directly, educating staff at formal teaching sessions or discussion at departmental meetings. If someone feels their concerns are going to be dealt with to prevent similar errors occurring they will often feel reassured.

Finally if someone remains unhappy, it is important to provide them with information on how to make a formal complaint. Explain that they can receive advice and support to complain from the Patient Advice and Liaison Service (PALS). If a case is approached with a suitable amount of understanding, and is seen to be taken seriously, a formal complaint can often be avoided.

Scenario

One of the receptionists has informed you that Mrs Hill has arrived demanding to see 'whoever is in charge'. She has just received a letter stating that her daughter, who was sent home from the department 5 days ago with a sprained wrist has a fracture of her radius and should attend the outpatient department next week.

She is upset and angry with the treatment her daughter has had and the way the new information was sent to her. She is annoyed that they were treated by an 'incompetent' doctor and that it has taken so long for anyone to notice a broken bone on an X-ray. She is also worried her daughter's arm will never heal properly.

Meet Mrs Hill and discuss the issues that arise.

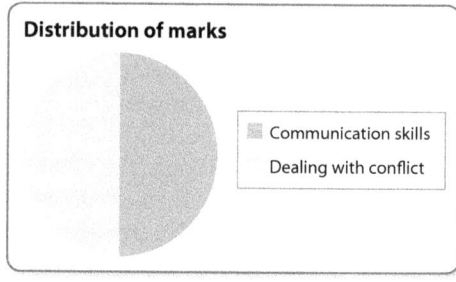

Distribution of marks
- Communication skills
- Dealing with conflict

Mark sheet	Achieved	Not achieved
Reviews notes and X-ray before speaking to mother		
Introduces self to mother appropriately		
Confirms mother and patient's identity		
Offers mother a seat		
Uses a sympathetic tone throughout the consultation		
Asks mother to explain her concerns		
Allows the mother to speak without interruption		
Apologises to mother		
Asks how her daughter is now in terms of pain and function		
Explains the diagnosis		
Offers to show mother the X-ray		
Demonstrates X-ray to mother appropriately		
Explains the events during the initial assessment chronologically		
Addresses the mother's concerns one at a time		
Does not blame the doctor involved		
Is honest about the system and potential for missed fractures		
Explains X-ray reporting to identify and recall missed fractures		
Defends the junior doctor when mother questions their ability		
Explains a plan to prevent similar incidents in the future		
Explains an appropriate plan to manage the missed fracture		
Offers the mother opportunity and information to complain formally		
Global mark from mother		
Global mark from examiner		

Instructions for actor

You are Charlotte Hill, the mother of a 9-year-old girl Debbie. You have gone to your local ED to complain about the way Debbie has been treated by one of the junior doctors. You both attended the department 5 days ago because Debbie had pain in her right wrist after a fall in the playground at school. After an X-ray you were told she had only sprained her wrist and it would get better with some rest and simple pain killers like paracetamol. Debbie has not used her wrist very much since but is starting to use it more gradually. Today you received a letter from the department saying Debbie's X-ray had shown a fracture and you have been given an appointment in a week's time (**Figure 2.2.1**).

You are very angry that the junior doctor told you the injury was only a sprain. You think they were too young and shouldn't be making such important decisions. You are upset that for the past few days you have been telling Debbie to use her arm even though it was broken. Also you feel the news of the fracture was sent in a very uncaring way.

You would like to know what is going to happen to Debbie's arm and if it will ever heal. You also want to know if the junior doctor will be reprimanded and how the department will stop this ever happening again.

Though you are initially angry if the doctor answers your concerns well you slowly calm down. You also accept that the fracture was hard to see on the X-ray if it is demonstrated to you clearly.

Figure 2.2.1 Debbie Hill's X-ray (with subtle distal radius buckle/torus fracture).

2.3 Breaking bad news

For exam purposes this specific station generally involves delivering a life-changing diagnosis or informing someone of the death of a loved one. The basic principles of this station require the ability to provide information in a sensitive and thoughtful way. Several elements can be applied to any station where the candidate is asked to provide information to an individual whether it is 'bad news', a diagnosis or a management plan.

Typical scenarios in the exam involve telling someone their loved one has died or has suffered a catastrophic event where it is not appropriate to give any interventional treatment, but simply to keep them comfortable until they die.

The setting

It is vital to ensure a quiet room where there will no interruptions. There should be comfortable seating and tissues available. In order to offer the individual ongoing support and a continuing link for communication while in the ED, another member of staff (normally an experienced nurse) should also be present.

Prior to beginning the meeting it is important to ensure familiarity with the patient's name and all events up until the present time.

Breaking the news

Before giving such life-changing news it is vital to make introductions and ensure you are speaking to the correct person. Following this, it is appropriate to offer sympathy and explain you are sorry the individual has had to come to the hospital under such difficult circumstances. Before discussing events it is always wise to discover how much the person knows about events so far. Whether they expect their loved one to be very well with minor injuries, or already expect they are likely to die, will significantly change the way the subject of bad news is introduced.

Depending on how much the individual is aware of it may be necessary to provide some brief background information as to what has happened. However, there shouldn't be significant delay before stating that you are sorry, but you have bad news. You can then explain that their loved one has died or is very ill and going to die. Though this may seem abrupt is it important that the message is clear and does not leave the person you are speaking to with any doubts or false hope. Sentences should be kept short with clear easy to understand information. We suggest one 'warning shot' (e.g. I'm sorry to say that I have some dreadful news for you), followed by the clearly-stated facts (e.g. 'Sadly Mrs Smith died shortly after arriving at the hospital'). Euphemisms (e.g. 'passed on'; 'gone to a better place') should be avoided as they can cause confusion.

Having explained this fact it is important to give the patient some time to absorb what has been said. Allowing silence is an important factor which will come more naturally to some than others. The next few moments will depend on how the individual responds to the bad news, but it is important to remain sympathetic, patient and to restate the facts if necessary.

Following this it may be necessary to explain certain events, treatments or test results. Be guided by how much it seems the person wants to know and can process as this may not be the time to go through unnecessary details.

Further support and actions

Once information has been provided and understood the task moves on to some more practical aspects. The loved one should be asked if they would like anyone else contacted. This may include family and friends, or asking a religious minister to attend the ED.

Prior to seeing the patient individuals should be warned about any disfiguring injuries and the presence of any medical equipment. Time should be taken to make the patient presentable and as soon as it is appropriate the individuals can be allowed to see and spend time with their loved one. It is common to be asked if the patient can be touched or spoken to and usually both can be encouraged.

Further practical aspects after death (paperwork, death certificate, funeral arrangements) are arranged through the hospital's bereavement office and there will normally be relevant information leaflets available which can be provided and explained.

Organ donation

In many cases, it is appropriate to enquire into the patient's wishes regarding organ donation. For example, you might ask if they carried an organ donor card.

Local guidelines vary, but in general for the purpose of exams a detailed knowledge of policies and guidelines is not necessary. In general terms if a patient is a potential donor their case should be discussed with the local transplant coordinator. The organ donor register can be checked by them and relevant issues can be discussed with the next of kin and key family members. Sufficient time will be allowed for family to come to terms with events so far and understand death is going to occur.

Caution should be used in discussing the withdrawal of life-sustaining treatment at the same time as the possibility of organ donation. It should be clear that the primary concern is the care of the patient and not the need to facilitate donation.

Once there is acceptance that the patient is going to die, it is recommended that those close to the patient should be reassured that organ donation is a normal part of end of life care, that negative or apologetic language should be avoided and that organ donation should be described positively. It should also be made clear that the standard of care received will be the same whether they give consent for organ donation or not. The extent to which information is shared initially will depend on the response of the individuals present, but it is likely that they will need some time to reflect on the situation before any decisions are made.

Scenario

You have been dealing with the case of Mr Downton who is a 66-year-old man. He was found collapsed on the pavement while walking to work and arrived in ED via ambulance with a Glasgow Coma Score of 5/15 (eyes 1, verbal 1, motor 3). He is intubated and ventilated and has returned from the CT scanner. His brain CT has been reviewed by the neurosurgical consultant who has said he will not survive from his intracerebral bleed and he should be made comfortable (**Figure 2.3.1**). His wife has just arrived alone. Explain the situation to Mrs Downton.

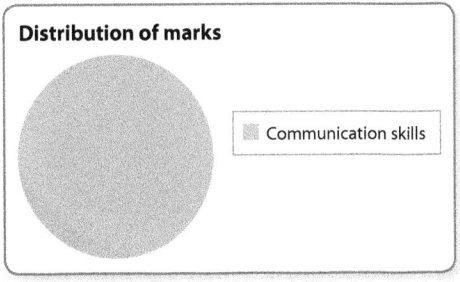

Distribution of marks

Communication skills

Mark sheet	Achieved	Not achieved
Asks if nurse is available to support patient's wife		
Introduces self to patient's wife		
Confirms wife's identity		
Asks if wife wants anyone else present		
Offers sympathy that wife has attended under stressful circumstances		
Clarifies what wife knows so far		
Explains events, CT findings and neurosurgical opinion		
Explains in clear language that husband is going to die		
Offers to show wife CT scan		
Demonstrates CT findings clearly and appropriately		
Allows silence and time for wife to reflect		
Asks if wife would like anyone else telephoned – offers to do so		
Asks regarding religious beliefs/wishes		
Explains need to involve coroner		
Asks regarding organ donation		
Suggests discussing case with transplant coordinator		
Asks if wife has any questions		
Asks if she would like to see husband		
Demonstrates appropriate level of empathy with wife		
Global mark from wife		
Global mark from examiner		

Figure 2.3.1 An image from Mike Downton's brain CT.

Instructions for actor

Your name is Jean Downton. You have been telephoned by your husband's work colleagues telling you that your husband Mike collapsed just outside his work and was taken to hospital by ambulance. You do not know what has happened but have just arrived by taxi at the local ED and been asked to wait in another room.

Your husband is normally fit and very well with no medical problems or medications. He has recently been getting headaches but hadn't seen the general practitioner yet. Both your children live abroad and you have no family locally but some good friends are nearby.

You are extremely upset and do not understand how this happened with no warning. Unless the doctor is very clear in explaining your husband is going to die you hold onto some hope he will get better and say you look forward to when he is better. If the doctor does not offer to show you the scan, you ask to see the results and have them explained to you.

Your husband was not religious. He was on the organ donor register but you forget this unless asked directly what his wishes were. Though this upsets you, you know it was important to him.

Suggested reading

National Institute for Health and Care Excellence (NICE). Organ donation for transplantation. Clinical guideline 135. NICE. London: NICE; 2011.

2.4 Clinical decisions unit handover - 1

This is a regular task in most EDs where patients who have been placed in the clinical decision unit (CDU) must be handed over and reviewed. With any handover of patient care there is the possibility of information being missed and patients not receiving appropriate and timely treatment. Doctors performing this task must be vigilant to ensure management plans are reviewed and modified as necessary. Required tasks and management plans can then be implemented as necessary whether they involve further investigations, referrals to in-hospital specialties or discharge planning. As with any ward round it also provides a valuable teaching opportunity. Remember in the exam to look carefully at the pie chart to see how the marks are distributed. For example, is the examiner's emphasis on your knowledge or your teaching?

Scenario

You are reviewing the overnight patients on the clinical decision unit. They are being presented by a capable but inexperienced junior doctor. Go through the three cases with the junior doctor, ask any relevant questions and agree an appropriate management plan. Provide appropriate teaching on the cases.

Distribution of marks
- Clinical reasoning
- Communication skills
- Teaching skills

The following information will be provided by the junior doctor with additional information available when asked for:

Case 1

This information will be presented by the junior doctor.

Tom Mitchell is a 24-year-old man who was playing football yesterday evening, when he had witnessed syncope whilst running after the ball. He was briefly unresponsive but regained consciousness and felt well by the time the ambulance arrived. He has had two similar episodes previously, has never had a medical review and is unconcerned, recalling he had not drunk much all day and feels he was dehydrated. He has no other medical history and takes no medications. The plan is for him to go home with a diagnosis of vasovagal syncope.

Additional information the junior doctor will describe if requested by the candidate:
- Full blood count, electrolytes and renal function and blood sugar are normal
- Normal cardiovascular examination
- ECG: normal sinus rhythm with 'high take-off' (ECG provided to candidate; **Figure 2.4.1**)

Figure 2.4.1 Tom Mitchell's ECG.

Case 2

This information will be presented by the junior doctor:
  Jane Hodges is an 18-year-old woman who came to the ED after a paracetamol overdose 90 minutes ago. She has no other medical problems or medication. She has just arrived in the CDU to commence an infusion of acetylcysteine and then wait for her blood paracetamol levels to be checked 4 hours after the overdose.
- Additional information the junior doctor can provide if asked by the candidate
- Overdose: 10 × 500 mg paracetamol tablets simultaneously. No other substances
- The patient is clear and precise regarding timing
- GCS 15, heart rate 68 beats per minute, blood pressure 126/68 mmHg, respiratory rate 14 breaths per minute, oxygen saturation 100% on air, blood sugar 7.1 mmol/L
- Clinical examination is normal
- ECG: normal sinus rhythm

Case 3

This information will be presented by the junior doctor:
  Eve Nicholson is a 26-year-old woman who is 30 weeks pregnant and presented with pleuritic chest pain and breathlessness and has bilateral ankle swelling. She has no other medical problems. She is on CDU waiting for a further blood sample to be taken for a D-dimer. If the D-dimer is normal she is due to go home.
Additional information the junior doctor can provide if asked by the candidate:
- GCS 15, heart rate 110 beats per minute, blood pressure 136/78 mmHg, respiratory rate 18 breaths per minute, oxygen saturation 92% on air
- Clinical examination is normal
- Chest X-ray is clear
- ECG: sinus tachycardia

Mark sheet	Achieved	Not achieved
Introduces self to junior doctor		
Confirms their level of experience		
Allows junior doctor to present first case		
Asks relevant questions to gain additional information		
Explains need for admission and investigation for Brugada syndrome		
Provides teaching on exertional syncope and ECG interpretation		
Agrees plan for patient, answers any further questions		
Allows junior doctor to present second case		
Asks relevant questions to gain additional information		
Explains need to wait for 4-hour levels before treatment		
Provides teaching regarding paracetamol levels in overdose		
Agrees plan for patient, answers any further questions		
Allows junior doctor to present third case		
Asks relevant questions to gain additional information		
Advises admission for bilateral duplex US and/or likely VQ imaging		
Provides teaching regarding use of D-dimer test in pregnancy		
Agrees plan for patient, answers any further questions		
Provides advice regarding accessing further information		
Global mark from junior doctor		
Global mark from examiner		

Instructions for actor

You are a junior doctor who has recently started work in the ED. You are presenting three patients from the CDU to your senior doctor. You provide some basic information for each case and only provide the additional information to the doctor as and when they ask for it as you are not sure what details are important. Take their advice on management plans and ask them where you can look up guidelines or policies on how to manage each of these cases.

Discussion of cases

Case 1

Candidates should be aware that the ECG is a key investigation in syncope which should always be carefully examined for abnormalities suggesting a cardiac cause. Additionally, although syncope during exercise can be benign, right ventricular dysplasia, Brugada syndrome and hypertrophic obstructive cardiomyopathy (HOCM) must be excluded because they are all associated with a high risk of sudden death.

This ECG is not normal and demonstrates the Brugada sign of coved ST segment elevation >2 mm in >1 of V1–V3 followed by a negative T wave. Associated with a syncope (or other clinical criteria), this diagnoses the patient with Brugada syndrome, which if undiagnosed has a mortality of 10% a year. This patient is likely to require an implantable cardioverter-defibrillator. The patient should be admitted to a monitored bed for cardiology assessment.

Case 2

Acetylcysteine is effective if given within 8 hours of an overdose of paracetamol. However within this period there is no further benefit from receiving the drug any earlier. Within this time frame it is standard practice to wait for a 4-hour paracetamol level to confirm treatment is truly required. This prevents unnecessary treatment and therefore minimises the frequency of hypersensitivity reactions to acetylcysteine which are relatively common.

This is, however, not the case in staggered overdoses or presentations 8 hours after an overdose.

Case 3

Pregnant women have a 4-fold increase risk of PE/DVT compared to non-pregnant women. This risk increases throughout pregnancy and is highest in the post-partum period. Physiological changes in pregnancy can cause benign dyspnoea, but pleuritic chest pain will require consideration of pulmonary embolus.

Plasma D-dimer levels rise throughout pregnancy, and although false positives are common, a negative test in a low-risk patient still carries a high negative predictive value for PE and can be used for ruling out low risk PE. It may also be possible to avoid radiation exposure by performing bilateral duplex ultrasound for DVT. If positive, this confirms the diagnosis of DVT with PE and further imaging is not required.

Imaging with ionising radiation will often be required, and candidates should be aware that the risk of inappropriate anticoagulation or missed diagnosis of PE far outweighs the risk of exposing mother and fetus to ionising radiation. CTPA and VQ imaging are both appropriate tests in pregnancy. Fetal radiation exposure is lower for CTPA (with the difference becoming less in the third trimester as the fetus enters the radiation field), but with higher maternal radiation exposure to breast tissue. Generally, VQ is preferred in the third trimester, with CTPA (with breast shielding) preferred prior to this.

The National Institute for Health and Care Excellence (NICE) offers clear guidance on the use of a D-dimer to investigate pulmonary embolism. This patient is high risk and should be imaged without D-dimer testing. This patient should be admitted, bilateral duplex ultrasound for DVT should be arranged and if negative the patient should receive a VQ scan to rule out PE.

Suggested reading

National Institute for Health and Care Excellence (NICE). Transient loss of consciousness in over 16s. Clinical Guideline 109. NICE. London: NICE; 2014.
Royal College of Emergency Medicine (RCEM). Paracetamol overdose: new guidance on the use of intravenous acetylcysteine. RCEM. London: RCEM; 2012.
Dunn M. Syncope. RCEM Learning. London: RCEM Learning; 2014.
National Institute for Health and Care Excellence (NICE). Venous thromboembolic diseases: diagnosis, management and thrombophilia testing. Clinical guideline 144. NICE. London: NICE; 2012.
Royal College of Obstetrics and Gynaecology (RCOG). Thrombosis and embolism during pregnancy and the puerperium: acute management. Green-top Guideline No. 37b. RCOG. London: RCOG; 2015.

2.5 Needlestick injury

Staff may present with needlestick injuries out of working hours when the occupational health department is closed. Occasionally, members of the public may present following needlestick injuries in the community.

These situations can be very stressful for the patient. As a senior member of the ED staff it is important to be well informed regarding their management to ensure the situation is dealt with correctly and in a manner that reassures the recipient.

Management of a needlestick injury should be initiated immediately. This involves encouraging bleeding from the site and thorough washing of the wound with soap and running water. Thorough irrigation also applies to blood splashing into the eyes, mouth or onto broken skin and in the heat of the moment it is important to ensure these basic measures are followed.

Though there are theoretically many illnesses that can be transmitted by a needlestick injury the main concerns are hepatitis B, hepatitis C and HIV. It is important to try and quantify the risk of a blood-borne virus being transmitted in each given situation, as in cases where this is high, postexposure prophylaxis (PEP) for HIV or hepatitis B may be appropriate. In cases where there is doubt as to the risk or appropriate management in a specific case it should be discussed with a specialist or based on local guidelines. Relevant history should be sought to assess this risk.

The history of the injury:
- The type of needle (hollow or solid)
- Procedure the needle had been used for
- Had the recipient been wearing gloves?
- Was appropriate first aid applied?

The donor's history:
- Known to have a blood-borne virus
- In a high-risk group for such an illness (e.g. an intravenous drug user)

The recipient's history:
- Has the recipient been immunised against hepatitis B? Do they know their antibody status?

Once basic measures have been taken to wash the wound and a risk assessment has been made further management can be considered.

Blood should be taken from the recipient and will be stored and may be tested at a later date if necessary. Similarly blood should be taken from the donor (provided they consent); after they have had the situation explained to them, and tested for hepatitis B and C, and HIV.

Regarding HIV if the risk is felt to be high the recipient should be consented and commenced as soon as possible on PEP. This normally involves combination therapy for 4 weeks. Nausea, vomiting and diarrhoea are common side effects and prepared PEP packs often contain antiemetics. A baseline set of blood tests including full blood count, urea and electrolytes and liver function tests should also be taken. If the recipient could be pregnant this should be checked and generally in high risk scenarios the benefit of PEP is felt to outweigh the risks of contracting HIV and vertical transmission.

Those who are not immunised against hepatitis B or not immune will require discussion with a local specialist and may need hepatitis B immunoglobulin and a course of immunisations commenced.

Follow-up should be advised at the occupational health department at the earliest opportunity. Occupational health will make a further risk assessment, counsel the recipient appropriately and make any necessary arrangements for follow-up testing. In the meantime recipients should use barrier contraception and avoid blood donation.

Scenario

Dr Hawkins is a newly qualified doctor on the gastroenterology ward. She has attended ED at 3 AM after a needlestick injury from a ward patient. She is very tearful and anxious at what needs to happen next. Talk to Dr Hawkins about what needs to be done.

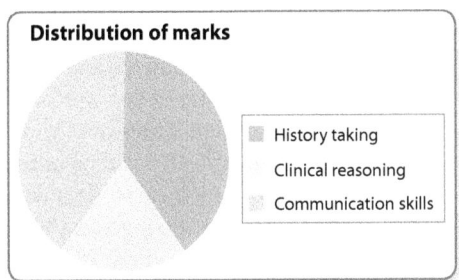

Distribution of marks
- History taking
- Clinical reasoning
- Communication skills

Mark sheet	Achieved	Not achieved
Introduces self to patient		
Confirms their identity		
Asks about events		
Comforts patient appropriately		
Ensures wound has been washed adequately		
Takes history of nature of injury		
Asks about time of injury		
Asks regarding patient's (Dr Hawkins) hepatitis B status		
Asks what is known about donor		
Explains potential for transmission of infections		
Explains need to take blood from patient		
Explains need to take blood from donor		
When patient asks for PEP explains why it is not necessary		
Advises follow-up in occupational health the next day		
Advises patient to not complete shift as very upset		
Offers to explain to patient's senior they shouldn't return to shift		
Recommends that an incident form is completed		
Is calm and reassuring towards patient		
Invites any final questions		
Global mark from patient		
Global mark from examiner		

Instructions for actor

You are a newly qualified doctor. Thirty minutes ago, you were taking blood from a ward patient to check their international normalised ratio (INR) as they are on warfarin. After taking blood you replaced the needle into the sheath and pricked your finger through your glove. You washed your finger a lot having encouraged it to bleed. The nurse on the ward told you to go to the ED. You are very upset and feel stupid. You haven't told your senior doctor what has happened as it is a busy shift and you didn't want to slow them down.

You have no medical problems and are up-to-date with all your immunisations. When you started work 1 month ago you were told you were immune to hepatitis B.

The patient in question is known to you. He is an 85-year-old man called Joseph Rogala who has a metallic heart valve and no other medical problems as far as you know.

You have heard of a medical student who caught HIV from a needlestick injury on their elective. You are worried about getting HIV and are surprised the doctor does not think you need treatment to reduce your risk of getting HIV. If they explain clearly to you why it isn't necessary you are satisfied with their answer.

Suggested reading

Royal College of Emergency Medicine (RCEM). Needlesticks: ED care of patients who have been potentially exposed to blood borne viruses. RCEM. London: Clinical Effectiveness Committee; 2013.

2.6 Obtaining consent for a procedure

With the exception of life-saving treatment in emergencies, it is the duty of all medical professionals to seek consent from a patient prior to any medical intervention. This is based on the principle of respecting the patient's right to autonomous decision making.

Where consent has not been sought the doctor (or care provider) may technically be at risk of committing battery which refers to physical violence against an individual. Furthermore in cases where consent has been obtained without the provision of adequate information the doctor may be considered to have been negligent.

Implied or express consent are both acceptable under different circumstances. Though it should never be taken for granted it is accepted that consent may be implied for certain common tasks. A simple example is when a patient offers their arm for a blood test. In other cases consent should be explicitly sought and may be verbal or written. This is more appropriate in cases where the intervention carries significant risks to the patient (it should be born in mind that different patients will understandably have different feelings as to what risks they consider significant).

For consent to be valid:
- The patient should be given all necessary information
- The patient should have capacity to give the necessary consent
- Consent should be given voluntarily

In terms of the amount of information necessary for informed consent an element of judgement is always required and it is often appropriate to ask the patient how much they would like to know. In general, however, it is a reasonable framework to explain to the patient:
- The working diagnosis
- The practicalities of the required intervention
- The indications, contraindications, aims and potential complications of the procedure
- Any alternative interventions or the likely consequences of doing nothing

In emergency settings it is accepted that patients who are unable to consent may be given life-saving treatment in their best interest unless there is a valid advance directive specifically refusing such intervention.

The General Medical Council (in the UK) has clear guidance regarding the issues of consent and capacity.

Scenario

Mr Stewart is a 33-year-old man. He fell off a ladder at home and has dislocated his left shoulder anteriorly. He has no other injuries. You have examined Mr Stewart and reviewed his X-rays (**Figure 2.6.1**). You have been asked to obtain consent from Mr Stewart for reduction of his shoulder dislocation in the ED resuscitation room under sedation.

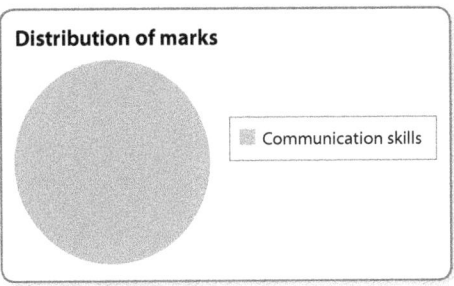

Distribution of marks

- Communication skills

Mark sheet	Achieved	Not achieved
Introduces self to patient		
Confirms their identity		
Asks what patient knows so far		
Explain diagnosis to patient		
Offers to show X-ray		
Explains need to reduce the joint		
Explains what the procedure involves		
Explains alternative methods for reduction		
Explains the risks of sedation		
Explains the risk of joint manipulation		
Checks patient understands the information provided		
Asks patient for their thoughts on the matter		
Answers patient's questions appropriately		
Shows empathy to patients anxiety		
Addresses any concerns the patient has		
Allows them time to think, avoids coercion		
Uses non-medical language appropriately		
Invites any final questions		
Asks patient to sign a consent form		
Global mark from patient		
Global mark from examiner		

Figure 2.6.1 Mr Stewart's shoulder X-ray.

Instructions for actor

You are a 33-year-old builder named Matthew Stewart. You slipped while on a ladder and fell onto your left shoulder. You have no other injuries but a severe pain in your shoulder. You have no medical problems except mild asthma. You have never had an anaesthetic before. You have a blue inhaler and no other medicines. You get a rash with penicillin and are not allergic to anything else. You last ate cereal at 8 AM and have had no food or drink since.

If the doctor does not offer, you ask if you can see your X-ray and have it explained to you. You are reluctant to have your shoulder relocated without a general anaesthetic as it is very painful. You want to know if you will be awake or if it will hurt. If you feel all your questions are answered and the doctor is reassuring you agree.

Suggested reading

Consent: patients and doctors making decisions together. General Medical Council, 2008.

2.7 Difficult referral

One of the main challenges facing ED clinicians is being able to engage the help of other colleagues to safely manage patients within the department. For a variety of reasons inpatient specialists may on occasion be reluctant to help with or take over the care of a patient.

To be able to overcome this it is often worth considering the reasons why this may be the case. Colleagues may be extremely busy, have been referred a patient without adequate explanation being given, have misunderstood the reason for referral, genuinely believe the referral is inappropriate, or generally just be having a bad day.

Bearing this in mind if you can remain non-confrontational, explain the facts and the reason for the referral, allow a colleague to also have their say and demonstrate you are willing to be helpful, it is very difficult for someone to refuse to accept a reasonable referral.

To do this an ED clinician must begin by being professional and introducing themselves appropriately. Having ensured they are in possession of the necessary facts they can then provide these to their colleague with a clear explanation of why the referral is necessary.

On occasion colleagues may for the reasons given above respond to a referral with derogatory comments or even abusive language. Though it is not acceptable for anyone to make derogatory personal comments regarding individual staff or the ED, careful judgement should be exercised before responding if a colleague does behave unprofessionally. Allowing the conversation to deteriorate into an argument is not in anyone's interests. Patient safety is the number one priority and it may be appropriate to ignore (or at least delay the response to) any inflammatory comments and stick to the facts of the referral.

Out of professional courtesy it is appropriate to acknowledge that colleagues may be busy with other patients and tasks. To help facilitate a difficult referral it can be worth considering what else can be done in the ED to offer a compromise by reducing the inpatient team's workload.

The ultimate goal is to provide the best and safest care for the patient in question. If an acceptable outcome cannot be reached it is important not to agree to an inadequate management plan. In this situation it is perfectly reasonable to close the discussion politely and explain that you feel it necessary to escalate your concerns to more senior colleagues.

Scenario

You have seen a 33-year-old woman in the resus room. Her name is Susan Kipling. She has sustained a head injury and according to friends has had 'many' alcoholic drinks and 'maybe some drugs'. Her Glasgow Coma Score (GCS) is 7 (eyes 2, verbal 2, motor 3) and she has vomited twice. Your SHO spoke to the intensive care registrar on call requesting that the they assist by intubating the patient to protect the airway before transfer to CT for a head scan. Your SHO returns and tells you the registrar they spoke

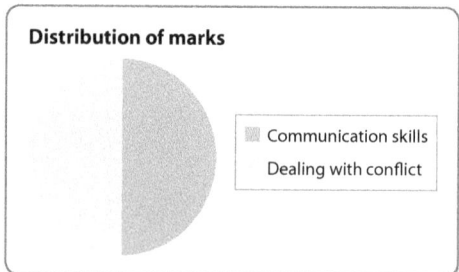
Distribution of marks
- Communication skills
- Dealing with conflict

to said they are 'too busy to be an intubation service' and the patient should go for a CT scan without being intubated.
Speak to the intensive care registrar on the phone and explain why the patient should be intubated.

Mark sheet	Achieved	Not achieved
Introduces self to ICU registrar by name and grade		
Confirms ICU registrars name and grade		
Explains wish to discuss patient		
Explains concerns regarding head injury, toxins and GCS		
Explains it is unsafe for patient not to be intubated		
Explains as the ED senior, the candidate is unable to leave the ED		
Does not react to interruptions and abrupt manner of ICU registrar		
Allows ICU registrar to explain their position		
Does not react to derogatory comments about ED referrals		
Politely asks ICU registrar to explain their lack of concern		
Reiterates concerns for patient's safety		
Acknowledges ICU registrar is busy		
Firmly asks ICU registrar to review patient in person rather than over the telephone		
Offers to prepare all equipment for airway management and patient transfer		
Remains professional and non-confrontational throughout discussion		
Achieves satisfactory conclusion to discussion		
Global mark from patient		
Global mark from examiner		

Instructions for actor

You are the intensive care registrar on call. You were called by a flustered ED junior doctor asking you to come downstairs to intubate a drunken patient with a head injury who has a GCS 'around eight'. The SHO didn't know anymore about the patient. You have been very busy with admissions to your unit all day and your own junior doctor has gone home sick. The ED doctor called you just as you were about to insert a central line in a septic patient who had deteriorated on a medical ward.

You are irritated by being asked to intubate and transfer another drunken head injury patient and want the ED to manage their own patient. The ED registrar has now bleeped you. You realise you were rude to the ED doctor that called you originally and are prepared to reconsider if the situation is explained to you reasonably. If however the registrar calls you and is not understanding of your situation or is antagonistic you will refuse to help them and ask them to call their consultant.

2.8 Driving after a seizure

A common and difficult ED scenario is advising a patient that they are no longer able to drive. This may be as a result of several conditions such as seizures, cerebrovascular or cardiovascular disease or diabetes mellitus. In many ways this scenario draws on many elements of breaking bad news. In modern life these driving restrictions require several changes to an individual's lifestyle and may therefore be difficult to accept.

The ED clinicians must be familiar with the rules regarding driving and their duty to try to persuade certain patients not to drive. Clear guidance for medical practitioners is available from national driver licensing authorities; in the UK the Driver and Vehicle Licensing Agency (DVLA) provides an at-a-glance guide to the current medical standards of fitness to drive. In addition clear guidance regarding confidentiality and reporting concerns about drivers is available from medical authorities, e.g. the General Medical Council (GMC) in the UK.

Using the UK as an example, the DVLA is legally responsible for deciding if a person is medically unfit to drive. The GMC advises that patients should be told it is their legal duty to inform the DVLA if they have been diagnosed with a condition that may prevent safe driving. Sometimes it may become clear that an individual is not willing to do this. In these cases, you can advise them to seek a second opinion, and help arrange this. The patient should still be advised not to drive until this second opinion is provided.

If a patient carries on driving despite not being fit to drive, every reasonable effort should be made to convince them to stop. In some cases it may be necessary to discuss your concerns with their relatives, friends or carers.

If the patient continues to drive you should contact the DVLA immediately and disclose any relevant medical information to the medical adviser. If possible, let the patient know you have had to decide to do this. When it has been done, write to the patient to confirm it.

Scenario

Mr Henderson is a 34-year-old man who was assessed by one of your colleagues and diagnosed as having had his first grand mal seizure. Except for having bitten his tongue his examination and investigations are normal and he was being discharged with outpatient follow-up. He has been given all the appropriate advice. From the next cubicle you overhear Mr Henderson on his mobile phone telling his boss he is fine and will be driving to meet the next client as soon as he can. Discuss driving with Mr Henderson.

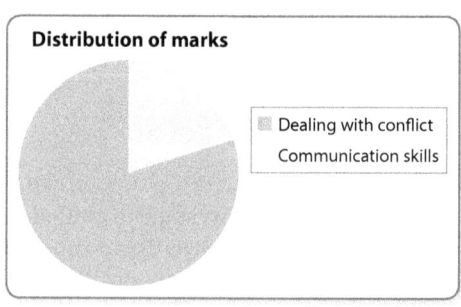

Distribution of marks
- Dealing with conflict
- Communication skills

Mark sheet	Achieved	Not achieved
Introduces self to patient		
Apologises for overhearing conversation		
Asks to discuss driving with patient		
Clarifies patient's understanding of events so far		
Clarifies patient's understanding of advice regarding driving		
Reiterates reasons for not driving to patient		
Asks patient about occupation and frequency of driving		
Advises patient that he must inform the DVLA of diagnosis		
Advises patient that his insurance may be void		
Acknowledges patient's anxieties regarding not driving		
Informs the patient they can seek a second opinion		
Explains the advice will be documented in the notes and a general practitioner letter		
Explains that if patient continues to drive his doctor is allowed to inform the DVLA		
Suggests employer may be able to provide alternative work		
Good use of silence to allow patient time to reflect		
Is appropriately sympathetic		
Asks if patient has any questions		
Summarises situation to patient – agrees outcome		
Global mark from patient		
Global mark from examiner		

Instructions for actor

You are a 34-year-old with no previous medical problems, named Mick Henderson. The doctors have said you have had a seizure and you should not drive until you have been seen by a specialist and probably not for the next one year. You feel fine and cannot believe this has happened to you. You started your new job only 2 months ago as a sales manager and you are required to drive long distances every day. You are married with a baby daughter. You cannot afford to lose your job, whatever some junior doctor has told you.

At first when the doctor starts talking to you are defensive and very upset. If they seem to understand and give you clear information you become more open to what they are telling you. If they suggest your employer may be able to change your role at work you agree that there are some jobs in the company that do not require driving.

Suggested reading

Drivers' Medical Group and Driver and Vehicle License Authority (DVLA). At a glance guide to the current medical standards of fitness to drive. DVLA. Swansea: DVLA; 2013.
General Medical Council (GMC). Confidentiality: Reporting concerns about drivers to the DVLA or DVA. GMC. GMC; 2009.

2.9 Major incident

A major incident is defined as any incident where the location, number or severity or type of live casualties requires extraordinary resources.

A major incident is generally declared by the ambulance or other emergency services. To prevent any ambiguity one of several standardised messages is used:
- Major incident standby: warns of a potential major incident declaration being imminent
- Major incident declared: requires a full major incident response
- Major incident cancelled: is used to cancel either of the above messages

Further information about the incident is communicated in a set format using one of two acronyms; **METHANE** or **CHALET**:

Major incident (standby or declared)
Exact location
Type of incident
Hazards present and potential
Access to scene and egress route
Number and severity of casualties
Emergency services present and required

or

Casualties – number and severity
Hazards present and potential
Access to scene and egress route
Location
Emergency services present and required
Type of incident

All hospitals capable of receiving casualties from a major incident have a major incident plan. Each ED will also have its own departmental plan. Though the plan may vary between different EDs there are several principles which will remain the same throughout.

Once a major incident is declared each hospital will have a protocol to ensure the message is passed to all relevant staff. This is often via the hospital switchboard which is responsible for cascading the information.

One of the first immediate tasks is to clear the ED of the current patients. Patients in the 'minors' area who are not unwell can be cleared from the department. Urgent plans for patients in the 'majors' or 'resuscitation' area can include their care being taken over by inpatient specialties with early transfer to appropriate wards.

Within the ED there will be a copy of the major incident plan and action cards for different staff. These action cards are handed out to appropriate staff and advise them of their specific duties during the major incident. Also there will be major incident documentation to be used for each patient that arrives. This commonly contains emergency hospital numbers and triage cards to record what priority has been assigned to each patient (thereby recording where and how quickly they should be seen). It is important that all patients arriving in the ED during a major incident are treated as major incident patients, whether or not they actually come from the incident itself. The plan will also contain a specific layout for the department. This will define where the triage area and different priority patients will be placed and which staff will be in each area. This plan can include the whole ED, clinical decision unit and some outpatient/ward areas. Under certain circumstances a decontamination area may also be required.

Casualties are normally triaged into one of three main categories:
- Priority 1 – requiring immediate resuscitation
- Priority 2 – have serious but non-life-threatening injuries requiring urgent treatment
- Priority 3 – have more simple injuries requiring minor or delayed treatment

In addition casualties may be triaged as dead or rarely as 'expectant' – where death is likely or resources required to prevent death will compromise the care of too many others.

Security is vital within the department to assist with crowd control and prevent media from entering clinical areas. As these situations generate a lot of curiosity (and confusion) all entrances are secured and identity cards are required by all staff.

Knowledge of major incident procedure is important for senior emergency physicians, and although this is often covered in the short answer question part of exams, it is important to be prepared for an OSCE-style test.

Scenario

A staff nurse in the department approaches you and tells you she has just taken a 'red phone' telephone call declaring a major incident after a bus crash on a local road. Injured patients are expected to start arriving in 45 minutes. She has not been involved in a major incident and asks you to explain what needs to be done next.

Distribution of marks
- Organisation skills
- Communication skills

Mark sheet	Achieved	Not achieved
Introduces self to staff nurse		
Asks for further information		
Asks if a METHANE or CHALET report was given		
Explains requirement to:		
– activate major incident cascade through switchboard		
– inform ED consultant and nurse in charge		
– inform all ED staff		
– discuss possibility of calling in off duty staff		
– assess and safely clear waiting room and minors area		
– assess and safely transfer majors/resuscitation patients to wards		
– use action cards/delegate roles to staff		
– set up triage area		
– use major incident triage cards/notes/hospital numbers		
– reassign ED areas based on major incident plan		
– document everyone in the ED		
– extra security/lock down to prevent media within the ED		
Asks staff nurse if she has any questions		
Global mark from staff nurse		
Global mark from examiner		

Instructions for actor

You are a staff nurse in the ED. You have just answered the red phone and have taken a message that a major incident has been declared and the ED should prepare for casualties to begin arriving soon. You are unsure what to do with this information and are anxious as you have not been involved in a major incident before. The nurse in charge is helping with a critically ill patient in the resuscitation room. You find one of the doctors and ask them what you need to do.

The additional information you were given is below. If the doctor asks for individual facts provide them to him. If he asks for a '**METHANE**' report, provide all the following information as below:
- Major incident declared
- Exact location is the local airport
- Type of incident is a small passenger plane has crashed on landing
- Hazards – no further information
- Access – no further information
- Number of casualties involved is approximately 26, with two more victims dead on scene
- Emergency services – no further information

Suggested reading

Major Incident Medical Management and Support. The Practical Approach in the Hospital. Advanced Life Support Group. BMJ Books: Wiley-Blackwell, 2005.

2.10 Conflict resolution – request for antibiotics

From time to time, every ED physician will be faced with a patient who is dissatisfied by the medical advice given to them. These situations can be difficult to manage while maintaining the trust and rapport required for a good doctor-patient relationship. Conflict can also occur between healthcare professionals, where there is a difference of opinion about the most appropriate management of a patient. Resolving this is clearly important for both patient care and good team working.

The priority is to ensure both parties are given opportunity to express their points of view and the thoughts that accompany these. Following this a plan for ongoing management can be negotiated.

From the ED specialist's perspective it is vital to explain and justify their opinion and provide the rationale on which it is based in language the patient can understand. A degree of judgement is required to avoid too many technical terms and yet avoid being patronising. Issues may arise when patients are unhappy with diagnoses or treatment options they are offered. Where the medical opinion is based on local or national guidelines or the results of investigations these should be explained. The difficulty is often being able to allay the patient's anxieties and it is important the clinician is seen to be confident in their judgement, without being aloof or dismissive.

It is advisable always to explore the ideas, concerns and expectations a patient may have as their anxieties may be based on misconceptions, past experience or an agenda that is initially unclear to the clinician.

In cases where it proves difficult to reassure a patient fully it may be appropriate to aim for a level of compromise. This can be achieved by:
- Suggesting early follow-up with the patient's general practitioner
- Delaying prescription of medication in some circumstances (antibiotics)
- Discussing the case with a colleague for a second opinion

One of the challenges facing the clinician is to remain calm and non-confrontational even if the other party begins to get upset or angry. Try to diffuse the other person's anger by remaining professional and making it clear you are trying to do what's best for them.

Antibiotics for tonsillitis/upper respiratory tract infections

Clinicians must have a clear idea of which patients may need antibiotics and when they should be prescribed.

The National Institute for Health and Care Excellence guidelines offer a clear pathway for managing these patients. Initially the guidelines advise history, examination and exploring the patient's ideas, concerns and expectations.

The guidelines advise immediate antibiotics for patients who:
- Are systemically very unwell
- Have symptoms and signs suggestive of serious illness and/or complications such as pneumonia or a peritonsillar abscess
- Are at high risk due to comorbidities (significant heart, lung, renal, liver, neuromuscular disease, immunosuppression or young children born prematurely)

- Are over 65 years old with acute cough and two of, or over 80 years with acute cough and one of (hospitalisation in the past 1 year, diabetes mellitus, congestive heart failure or taking oral glucocorticoids)

In addition the guidelines suggest immediate antibiotics can be considered for:
- Children younger than 2 years old with bilateral acute otitis media
- Children with otorrhoea who have acute otitis media
- Patients with acute sore throat/acute pharyngitis/acute tonsillitis with three or more Centor criteria (tonsillar exudates, tender anterior cervical lymphadenopathy, absence of cough, history of fever)

Remaining patients can be given reassurance that antibiotics are not needed immediately because they will make little difference to symptoms and may have side effects. However, delayed prescriptions can be offered if symptoms do not settle or get significantly worse. These can be provided at the time for patients to use later if needed or patients can see their own doctor for them later.

Further advice should relate to the natural course of the illness, explaining how to manage symptoms and which symptoms should prompt further medical assessment.

Scenario

James is a 3-year-old boy who has presented with his mother complaining of a painful throat, runny nose, cough and temperature. You have finished your assessment and feel James has tonsillitis which is likely to be viral in aetiology. You do not believe he needs antibiotics for this. Before he leaves his father arrives and asks to see you as he wants James to have some antibiotics.

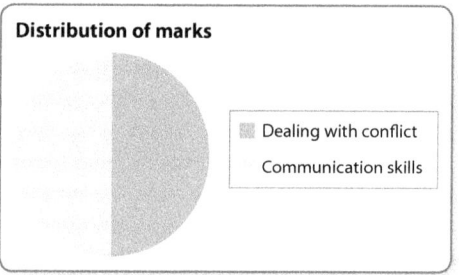

Distribution of marks

- Dealing with conflict
- Communication skills

Mark sheet	Achieved	Not achieved
Introduces self to patient's father appropriately		
Confirms father and patient's identity		
Offers father a seat		
Asks father to explain his concerns		
Allows the father to speak without interruption		
Summarises findings and diagnosis		
Explains rationale for antibiotics not being needed		
Explains existence of National Institute for Health and Care Excellence guidelines and/or Centor criteria		
Explores father's reasons for concern and desire for antibiotics		
Provides information on likely duration of illness		
Provides advice regarding managing pain		
Provides reasonable safety net advice		
Agrees further plan with father		

Cont'd...

Cont'd...

Mark sheet	Achieved	Not achieved
Acknowledges father's frustration		
Is not dismissive of father's concerns		
Maintains non-confrontational manner		
Uses clear language and minimal medical terminology		
Global mark from father		
Global mark from examiner		

Instructions for actor

You are Arthur French, the father of a 3-year-old boy called James. He has had a fever, runny nose and pain swallowing for 2 days. There were no general practitioner (GP) appointments available today so your wife brought him to the ED and you have just arrived after leaving work early.

You are frustrated that the doctor will not prescribe antibiotics for James. James' cousin Simon had a similar illness 3 years ago and suddenly became very ill and was diagnosed with meningitis. You are also very busy and it is difficult to take time off to run around visiting the GP every few days.

If the doctor explains his diagnosis of a viral infection which will get better without antibiotics you are partly reassured, but are uncertain how the doctor can be so sure. If they take the time to give you clear explanations you eventually come round to their point of view though you are still worried about what to do if James' condition persists or gets worse.

However, if you feel the doctor does not explain their findings and further plan adequately or behaves in a dismissive manner you become angry.

Suggested reading

National Institute for Health and Care Excellence (NICE). Respiratory tract infections. Clinical guideline 69. NICE. London: NICE; 2008.

2.11 Conflict resolution – refusing tetanus immunisation

ED medical staff must have a good knowledge of the tetanus vaccination to ensure they can discuss it with patients and ensure it is administered to all those who require it, without it being used excessively. A good test of this knowledge is a difficult communications scenario where an individual is concerned by the prospect of having a tetanus vaccination and asks challenging questions.

The main principal of managing the scenario is to elicit the individual's concerns and be able to explain the treatment's importance and possess the knowledge to inform the individual and reassure them. A fine balance must be reached between encouraging the patient, or parent to take the medical advice without damaging the working relationship by having to force them to agree.

Tetanus infection

Tetanus is a serious and often fatal disease. It results from infection with *Clostridium tetani*, a gram-positive bacillus, which then releases the tetanus toxin. The bacterial spores are present in soil and the environment and therefore the disease cannot be eradicated. Infection occurs when the bacteria breach the skin in various types of trauma (lacerations, puncture wounds, burns and bites).

There is an incubation period of 4–14 days before the toxin's effect on the central nervous system results in progressive stiffness and rigidity. Death is a frequent complication of the disease.

Tetanus immunisation

Tetanus vaccine is made from a cell-free purified toxin from *Clostridium tetani*. This is then treated to convert it into a toxoid with a high immunogenicity. The vaccination is prepared in various combinations containing some or all of diphtheria/polio/acellular pertussis and *Haemophilus influenzae* type B. These vaccines are not live and therefore cannot cause their respective diseases.

A primary (priming) course of immunisations should involve three doses given 1 month apart. This is then followed by two further boosters. The first should be at least 1 year after the primary course, and there should be at least a further 5-year interval before the second booster. In children where there is no reliable history of previous vaccination for any reason (e.g. they have come from an area abroad with no immunisation programme) the full UK recommendations should be followed. In the UK these five doses are typically given at:
- 2, 3, and 4 months old
- 3 years later (preschool, 3–5 years old)
- 13–15 years old

If the primary course is interrupted, the guidelines in the UK state that it should be resumed as soon as possible but not repeated.

Reactions and contraindications

The only absolute contraindication to receiving the vaccine is anaphylaxis to a previous dose or to neomycin; streptomycin or polymyxin B. True anaphylaxis is stated to occur in <3 in a million cases. During an acute illness it is advised the vaccine should not be administered to prevent symptoms incorrectly being attributed to the vaccine.
Other reactions may include:
- Fever
- Hypotonic – hyporesponsive episodes
- Prolonged crying (over 3 hours)
- A severe local reaction

Evidence demonstrates that none of these reactions are a contraindication to further doses and that there is no indication that reactions will necessarily recur or increase in severity.

With regard to pre-existing neurological conditions including seizures, administering the vaccine should only be delayed if the condition is not stable, and once stabilised and investigated vaccination can be continued. A febrile seizure may be caused by the fever caused by vaccination and this should be treated as a normal febrile seizure. A family history of seizures is not a contraindication to vaccination.

Assessing tetanus risk

Tetanus-prone wounds are:
- Puncture-type injuries acquired in a contaminated environment and likely therefore to contain tetanus spores, e.g. gardening injuries
- Wounds containing foreign bodies
- Open fractures
- Wounds or burns with systemic sepsis
- Certain animal bites and scratches (although smaller bites from domestic pets are generally puncture injuries, animal saliva should not contain tetanus spores unless the animal has been digging in soil or lives in an agricultural setting)

High-risk wounds are those contaminated with material likely to contain tetanus spores (e.g. manure), with extensive devitalised tissue (e.g. large burns) or when surgical debridement is delayed by more than 6 hours, in situations where it is required.

Management of immunisations and tetanus prophylaxis are summarised in Table 6.34.2.

Scenario

One of the ED, nurse practitioners asks if you can speak to a 4-year-old boy's mother. She is refusing to allow him to have a tetanus vaccine after a leg injury. He has never had any previous vaccinations for tetanus as far as she knows and she has asked why he needs it.

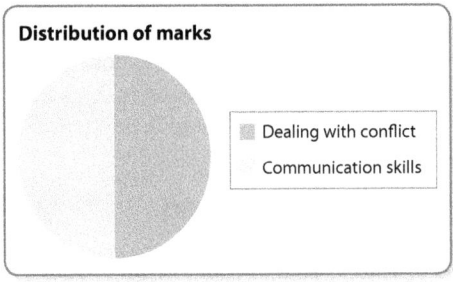

Distribution of marks
- Dealing with conflict
- Communication skills

Mark sheet	Achieved	Not achieved
Introduces self to patient's mother appropriately		
Confirms mother and patient's identity		
Establishes events regarding injury and in ED		
Checks mother's understanding of need for tetanus immunisation		
Asks mother about her concerns		
Allows the mother to speak without interruption		
Explains rationale for tetanus immunisation		
Explains serious nature of tetanus illness		
Answers mother's questions correctly:		
– what is tetanus?		
– what is in the injection?		
– is there a risk of seizures?		
– are there any other side effects?		
– can it be delayed while she thinks about it?		
Is not dismissive of mother's concerns		
Maintains non-confrontational manner		
Uses clear language and minimal medical terminology		
Ensures wound has been treated correctly		
Agrees a management plan		
Ensures mother has no further questions		
Global mark from mother		
Global mark from examiner		

Instructions for actor

Your name is Tamsin Smith. You have brought your 4-year-old son Arthur to the ED after he received a wound from scraping his leg indoors across the edge of a new metal chair earlier in the day. He has no other medical problems and is fit and well. He was born in South America and has not had any tetanus vaccines as they were not offered to him.

A nurse practitioner has seen him and treated his wound, but advised that he needs a tetanus vaccine. You know a friend's child had a seizure after a similar injection so you do not want your son to have the injection. You feel he has been fine without it so why worry now.

You have several questions about tetanus and the vaccine and if the doctor answers them clearly you are prepared to think about allowing your son to have the injection if you are offered some time to think about it.

Suggested reading

Department of Health. Chapter 30: Tetanus. In: Immunisation Against Infectious Diseases (The Green Book), 3rd edn. Department of Health; 2018.

2.12 Febrile convulsion

These are a relatively frequent cause for children's attendance to the ED. The diagnosis of a first febrile convulsion can cause significant anxiety for the parents, in terms of what the condition means for the future and how any future seizures should be managed. For all frequent presentations emergency clinicians should have a clear knowledge of the condition and be able to explain this to the parents in an informative and reassuring manner.

Febrile convulsions affect approximately 3% of children between 6 months and 5 years of age, with the peak incidence at 18 months. The seizures are normally tonic-clonic in nature, are of relatively short duration and occur in association with a fever.

In one-third of cases the child goes on to have a further febrile convulsion at a later date. For this reason parents should be given clear advice on how to manage further fits should they occur. In approximately 1% of cases sufferers go onto develop epilepsy. Although this is an increased risk compared to those who have not had a febrile seizure, it should be emphasised that the risk is still very slight.

Parents should be advised that in the future if their child is having a seizure they should:
- Lie them down and protect them from hurting themselves on surrounding objects
- Not place objects in their mouth to keep it open
- Call an ambulance if the seizure does not stop within 5 minutes
- Call an ambulance if the child does not recover fully or appears otherwise unwell

One of the main concerns is identifying the cause of the fever and excluding any serious infections such as meningitis. In cases with a clear and treatable cause for the fever where the child has recovered quickly and been observed it may be safe for them to be discharged home. In other cases children are admitted for the source of the fever to be identified and/or for a period of observation. In assessing whether or not to discharge a child after a febrile convulsion, you will also want to consider social factors. For example, what support is there for the primary carer at home? How are they coping with the stress of the situation? What other responsibilities do they have (e.g. other children)? How far away from hospital do they live?

Scenario

Freddie is a 3-year-old boy and you have diagnosed him as having had a febrile convulsion secondary to an upper respiratory tract infection. He was brought in by ambulance with his mother. He is now much better and has had a normal set of investigations. After a period of observation, a paediatric consultant has reviewed him and has said he can be discharged home. His father has just arrived and is very upset. The nurse has told him the diagnosis. Freddie's father wants to see you to find out about the diagnosis and its future implications.

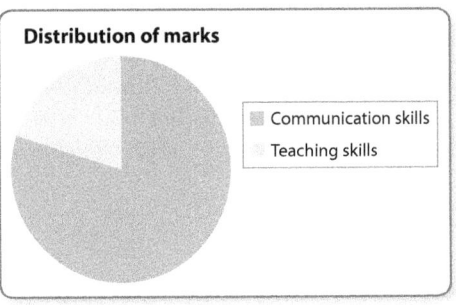

Distribution of marks
- Communication skills
- Teaching skills

Mark sheet	Achieved	Not achieved
Introduces self to father		
Checks if nurse available to support parent		
Confirms identity of father		
Acknowledges stressful nature of situation		
Confirms father's understanding of events		
Explains diagnosis		
Explains cause of fever can vary		
Explains risk of further fits		
Explains age group affected and child likely to grow out of condition		
Explains management of future febrile illnesses		
Explains management of future fits		
Explains risk of epilepsy		
Confirms father's understanding		
Asks if any further questions		
Advises reasonable follow-up plan (via GP or clinic)		
Behaves in a reassuring manner		
Avoids medical jargon		
Global mark from father		
Global mark from examiner		

Instructions for actor

Your name is Mitch Douglas. You have been called by your 3-year-old son's nursery to say Freddie became unwell with a fever and then had a seizure so was taken to the hospital. When you arrive you are very upset. The nurse tells you that Freddie has had a febrile fit and has an upper respiratory infection. No one else in the family has any medical problems. You want to ask the doctor what all of this means. Will Freddie be ok in the future? You want to be very clear about what you should do if this happens again. Will this happen every time he gets a fever? You've heard epilepsy can be dangerous and inconvenient as sufferers can hurt themselves and aren't allowed to drive. You want to know if Freddie has epilepsy and what treatment he needs. If the doctor is understanding and reassuring you will calm down and the conversation will finish with you feeling very much better because the facts are now clear to you.

2.13 Difficult conversation with colleague

This is a challenging scenario which may arise in various OSCE or interview settings and explores how to deal with a colleague who is unfit for work. The scenario could ask a candidate to speak to a clinician who appears to be intoxicated or is seen to be making dangerous clinical decisions. There is clear guidance from the General Medical Council (GMC) stating that doctors must:
- Take prompt action if they think patient safety, dignity or comfort is being or may be seriously compromised
- Protect patients from risk of harm posed by colleague's conduct, performance or health
- Be clear, honest and objective about the reason for raising a concern about a colleague's health

These situations are very challenging because the candidate is asked to confront a colleague with concerns about their behaviour. This is clearly difficult to discuss and requires as non-confrontational an approach as possible, with a view to maintaining professionalism and a working relationship. It is also vital to bear in mind that colleagues who display unprofessional behaviours are often undergoing difficult personal circumstances and may need support themselves.

When asked to discuss these concerns with a colleague the best approach is to begin with a simple opening question such as 'How are you?' This is a simple ice-breaking question to which the subject may respond by volunteering that there is a problem (which will make the conversation easier) or at the other extreme they may simply give a short closed response, e.g. 'I'm fine'. Either way it is possible to then explain why you are asking and this would lead into explaining there is a concern about the clinician's behaviour.

In a similar way to breaking bad news (see section 2.3) it is best to be honest and relatively direct about the situation. It is possible to do this while still being sensitive to the colleague. Be supportive and make it clear that you are concerned about their well-being. An accusing tone or opening comment will not lead to a constructive conversation. A statement like 'I'm sorry to have to ask you this but I am worried (or I have been told) that you have come to work smelling of alcohol' is acceptable. This sentence gets to the point quickly while acknowledging the sensitive nature of the concern. Depending on the response it may be worth explaining that you and the person you are speaking to have a duty to ensure the safety of patients.

Giving your colleague some time to accept their circumstances is important. Allow a few moments of silence if necessary. This provides them with time to think; and the fact that you are prepared to listen also demonstrates a willingness to understand their point of view. Balancing the work and personal commitments can be extremely challenging for individuals at any stage of their career. Be understanding if they admit they have been drinking alcohol prior to coming to work. If they elaborate on this allow them to do so. If they don't, ask them if this is a single episode or if it is a regular occurrence. Do they see it as a problem? If so, are they planning to do anything about it or have they already? From their response it is possible to gain an idea of their insight into the problem.

The colleague you confront does not have to tell you about any personal problems; however, they may appreciate being asked and given the opportunity to explain themselves. It is easy to end up struggling and develop a sense that nobody cares what one's problems are. If appropriate ask them if they are having any particular difficulties that have led to this situation. Is work going ok? Are they or their family having problems with financial issues or health problems?

Be supportive and try to empathise. Acknowledge that balancing the demands of work and personal life can be very difficult and stressful.

Moving on, the conversation must focus on what to do next. If you have reason to believe the colleague is under the influence of alcohol they should not be at work. Explain this is the right thing to protect patient's safety and to prevent your colleague from compromising their professional duties.

It is not acceptable just to let the colleague go home because they are 'unwell'. Though everyone does not need to know the details of what has happened, it is necessary that certain senior individuals are informed. There is probably a senior member of staff on duty who has to be informed if a member of staff is unable to work. It may also be necessary to review any clinical work done by the individual concerned during the shift to ensure no clinical mistakes were made.

Though it is understandable for your colleague to want their personal life to remain confidential, under the circumstances there is a clear duty of care to break that confidentiality.

To follow-up on the incident it is necessary that your colleague's supervisor/manager is informed. The supervisor/manager is responsible for overseeing this individual at work and should be the first point of contact. They will also be aware of any previous incidents or new ones as they arise. They will be able to discuss the circumstances leading to the current situation and help guide further actions. Depending on the circumstances, there are several options available: no further action, temporary suspension or a recommendation to involve occupational health, the colleague's own general practitioner or a specific support network through the hospital or deanery. Whenever possible constructive support will be offered to help people overcome any problems they may have.

In cases where the colleague in question is not receptive to acknowledging or discussing the concerns raised there several alternatives. In order of escalation these may include repeating that you have reason to be concerned that they should not be looking after patients and that you would like to discuss this with them, contacting a senior member of staff, asking the colleague to leave, or calling security to have the colleague removed from the workplace. Clearly, the last two alternatives are last resorts, only employed if it proves impossible to have a reasonable conversation; though these may theoretically be alternatives, they are unlikely to be required in an OSCE situation. The key principle all these alternatives illustrate, however, is that patient safety must be maintained.

Scenario

You are approached by one of the senior nurses in the ED. She tells you that Dr Bryant, one of the junior doctors has just begun his afternoon shift. When he arrived she thought she could smell alcohol on his breath. She also tells you he was 15 minutes late for his shift and when she asked him if he was ok he was very abrupt and said 'of course I am' and then went to see his first patient.

You are the senior doctor in the department and the nurse has asked you to talk to Dr Bryant.

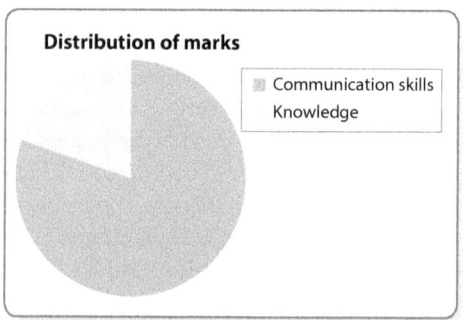

Distribution of marks
- Communication skills
- Knowledge

Mark sheet	Achieved	Not achieved
Introduces self to Dr Bryant		
Confirms Dr Bryant's identity		
Appropriately explains wish to discuss the concerns raised		
Responds calmly and professionally to Dr Bryant's initial denial		
Seeks information from Dr Bryant as to what's happened		
Explains patient safety is paramount and doctor Bryant cannot work		
Asks about personal problems Dr Bryant is experiencing		
Demonstrates empathy		
Explains there is a need to inform seniors		
Explains Dr Bryant's confidentiality will be protected as much as possible		
Explains there are systems to help support Dr Bryant		
Reaches agreement that Dr Bryant will not work his shift		
Reaches agreement that senior staff will have to be involved		
Remains professional and non-confrontational throughout discussion		
Achieves satisfactory conclusion to discussion		
Global mark from Dr Bryant		
Global mark from examiner		

Instructions for actor

You are Ross Bryant. You are a new emergency medicine trainee. You are in your first post since finishing your foundation training. You have been working in the ED for 2 months. You like the job and want to become an emergency medicine specialist.

You moved to the area 2 months ago and do not really know any of the staff yet. You've started renting a flat nearby but are unhappy as it is small and dirty. Your partner was due to move in with you but last week she told you that she had changed her mind and wants to 'break up' with you.

You've had the last 2 days off and realised you have no social contacts in this area and spent the time alone. You felt quite low in mood and have gone to the pub on your own the last two evenings. Today you were really fed up and went to the pub before starting work. Without thinking about your actions, you had four alcoholic drinks. You lost track of time and arrived for work late. One of the nurses saw you come in late and asked if you were ok. You felt terrible and didn't want to talk to them so were unintentionally rude to them.

When confronted you initially deny that you have been drinking. Eventually you admit to what has happened. You are very upset and tearful. You say that you don't want anyone to find out. As it's only a 'one-off' you ask them not to tell anyone, as you have a right to privacy. They are supportive and remind you that patient's safety come first, and you agree this is true. You're scared people will think you can't cope. Also you are worried you could lose your job and ask what will happen to you.

You have never had previous problems in your time at medical school or as a foundation doctor. Normally you would have only one or two alcoholic drinks at a social event. You have no other medical problems and have yet to register with a local general practitioner.

If the colleague is firm with you but supportive, you will be honest about the situation and agree that the best thing is for you to not work a clinical shift, acknowledging that the matter will have to be fed back to some of the senior staff, including your supervisor. If the colleague does not deal with the situation well you may become withdrawn, tearful or angry.

2.14 Explaining a new diagnosis – diabetes mellitus

A proportion of patients attending the ED are found to have their first presentation of a chronic and possibly life changing diagnosis. Clearly receiving such information is a scary and upsetting event. The nature of the information, the degree of reassurance and the tone in which it is given can have a significant impact on an individual's outlook and the degree to which they engage with their further treatment. For an emergency medicine specialist, giving a new diagnosis to a patient in a clear, sensitive and reassuring manner is a core skill.

Opening the conversation

When beginning a discussion in which new information is going to be given to someone, always begin by getting a feel for what they know so far and, in effect, what they are expecting you to say. Where the patient's expectation is in line with the facts it is possible to be relatively direct. However, if the patient is anticipating information that is very different from the facts a gentler approach is needed, e.g. delivering news to a patient who thinks the problem is a migraine but is found to have a space-occupying lesion on CT scan. In these instances, small amounts of easy-to-understand information should be supplied.

The amount of information given will need to be appropriate to the circumstances and the individual's initial responses. A distressed individual is likely to understand or retain only a few key facts. Many of the principles of breaking bad news as discussed in section 2.3 apply. Consider asking if the individual (who may be a patient, parent or relative) would like anyone else to be present. Also ask how much information they would like to be given.

Explaining the facts

By this point it should have been possible to assess how smoothly the conversation is likely to be and whether or not the person you are talking to is likely to absorb many facts or be upset. This should guide your tone and the amount of information you provide. Always avoid using medical terminology.

Consider the individual's ideas, concerns and expectations (discussed in section 1.2). At an appropriate time ask if they know much about the condition already. Also before closing the discussion, ask if they have any questions or concerns they would like to discuss. Key points to consider talking through are:
- The diagnosis
- The nature of the problem (a very simplified summary of the pathophysiology)
- Impact of diagnosis on day-to-day life
- Treatment that has been given so far
- What will happen next?
- Ongoing treatment that may be needed – where and how this will happen
- Places to seek further support/information

How much of the above is actually covered will depend on how the conversation goes. Depending on the individual's responses and their ideas, concerns and expectations, the focus may be on certain specific areas.

Closing the conversation

If the opportunity has not arisen until now check what has been understood so far (It would be easy for someone with fixed perceptions of an illness to interpret a situation to be much worse, or better, than it actually is).

Ensure there are no outstanding questions that need to be dealt with. Offer written material and/or recommendations to specific charities that offer information and support. If there is a relevant specialist nurse consider arranging for the individual to see them as well.

Scenario

You have been asked to see Sarah Underwood. She is an 18-year-old who has moved to the area to start university. She attended the ED after having several alcoholic drinks and then becoming unwell. This is on the background of recent weight loss which she had attributed to the stress of starting university. She has been diagnosed as having diabetic ketoacidosis and all appropriate treatment has begun. Her clinical condition is slowly improving. She is being treated in the resuscitation room and has begun to ask what is wrong. Explain the diagnosis of diabetes mellitus to her. You do not need to take a full history.

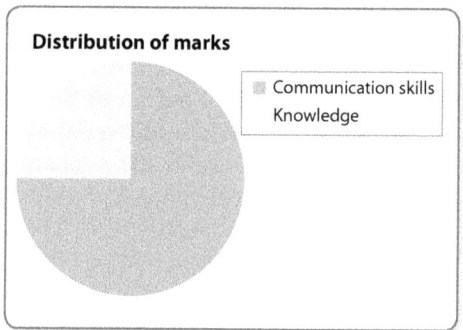

Distribution of marks
- Communication skills
- Knowledge

Mark sheet	Achieved	Not achieved
Introduces self to patient		
Confirms patients identity		
Explains reason for conversation		
Briefly revisits key points of history		
Clarifies what patients knows so far		
Provides diagnosis of diabetes mellitus		
Responds well to patient's surprise		
Explains what diabetes mellitus is		
Explains treatment so far		
Explains next steps in management		
Explores patient's ideas, concerns, expectations		
Provides reassurance appropriately		
Explains that diabetes can be managed very effectively		

Cont'd...

Cont'd...

Mark sheet	Achieved	Not achieved
Briefly discusses lifestyle adjustments – stopping smoking		
Informs patient of sources of information – leaflets, specialist nurse		
Asks if any further questions		
Offers to contact parents		
Provides appropriate amount of information		
Demonstrates appropriate level of empathy		
Global mark from patient		
Global mark from examiner		

Instructions for actor

Your name is Sarah Underwood. You are 18 years old and have just moved to the city to study business management at university. Last night you went out for a student party and had several alcoholic drinks. You've never drunk so much before and are embarrassed that you ended up in ED. You've become more lucid over the past hour and are surprised that you seem to be having various infusions. You didn't think this would be necessary for someone who gets drunk.

You have been well recently but have lost around 7 kg over the summer. You thought this was due to the pressure of studies while trying to get in to university and then the stress of moving to a new area. You have had no other symptoms. You have no medical problems and take no medications. You smoke 10 cigarettes a day and take no other recreational drugs. Your family live a 3-hour drive away.

You are not expecting to be told that you have diabetes. If this information is given to you too abruptly you become very upset and panicky. If the details are explained tactfully in easy to understand information, though you are upset, you listen and understand what is said. If medical words are used you get frustrated and ask what they mean.

You don't know much about diabetes but have an uncle with diabetes who gives himself injections. He has had one of his legs amputated. You immediately worry that this means the same will happen to you. If given the opportunity you ask if all patients with diabetes have amputations. If given the opportunity you also ask if the doctor can phone your parents and ask them to come to the hospital. If you are not given a chance to ask these questions you remain tearful.

2.15 Clinical decisions unit handover – 2

This is a regular task in most EDs whereby patients who have been placed in the clinical decisions unit (CDU) must be handed over when staff change and subsequently reviewed by the new staff. With any handover of patient care there is the possibility that information will be missed and that patients may not receive appropriate and timely treatment. Doctors performing this task must be vigilant to ensure management plans are reviewed and modified as necessary. Required tasks and management plans can then be implemented as necessary, whether they involve further investigations, referrals to in-hospital specialties or discharge planning. As with any ward round it also provides a valuable teaching opportunity. Remember in the exam to look carefully at the pie chart to see how the marks are distributed. For example, is the examiner's emphasis on your knowledge or your teaching?

Scenario

You are reviewing the overnight patients on the clinical decision unit. They are being presented by a capable but inexperienced junior doctor. Go through the three cases with the junior doctor, ask any relevant questions and agree an appropriate management plan. Provide appropriate teaching on the cases.

Distribution of marks
- Clinical reasoning
- Communication skills
- Teaching skills

The following information will be provided by the junior doctor with additional information available when asked for.

Case 1

This information will be presented by the junior doctor:

A 55-year-old woman presents with 24 hours of painless progressive right sided facial droop and the junior doctor has diagnosed a stroke so has requested a CT brain and referred the patient to the stroke team.

The patient reports increased sensitivity to sound. She feels systemically well. She has no medical history.

Additional clinical findings the junior doctor can provide if asked by the candidate are:
- The patient had viral upper respiratory tract symptoms for the preceding few days
- There is a right-sided facial nerve palsy with inability to wrinkle the forehead
- Inability to lift the corner of the mouth, unequal lid fissures, maintained ability to shut her eyes
- Cranial nerve exam was normal otherwise normal
- No other peripheral limb neurology identified
- Normal otoscopy without any visible vesicles and normal facial skin without vesicles

Case 2

This information will be presented by the junior doctor:

A 60-year-old man presents to the ED with a persistent worsening generalised headache for 3 days. The patient has a history of hypertension but no other medical problems. The patient has been observed for 4 hours and is being sent home with a diagnosis of tension headache.

Additional information the junior doctor can provide if asked by the candidate:
- Patient is systemically well with no infective symptoms
- Patient recently started on an additional blood pressure medicine (hydrochlorothiazide 25 mg OD)
- GCS 15, heart rate 65 beats per minute, blood pressure 118/78 mmHg, respiratory rate 16 breaths per minute, oxygen saturation 100% on air, blood sugar 5.2 mmol/L
- Clinical examination is normal
- Blood tests are normal other than a sodium of 118 mmol/L

Case 3

This information will be presented by the junior doctor:

A 70-year old man presents with several hours of left flank pain, the pain occurs in spasms, with intervals of dull ache. Prior to IV morphine, the pain was severe, and the patient couldn't lie still. The junior doctor suspects renal colic. The patient was initially placed in CDU for pain relief but is now referred to urology due to the severe pain.

Additional information the junior doctor can provide if asked by the candidate:
- The patient has peripheral vascular disease with no previous renal colic
- Recently well with no infective symptoms
- GCS 15, heart rate 115 beats per minute, blood pressure 151/78 mmHg, respiratory rate 20 breaths per minute, oxygen saturation 100% on air, blood sugar 6.3 mmol/L, afebrile
- Clinical examination reveals tenderness in the lower abdomen but is otherwise normal
- Urine dip is negative for haematuria, nitrites and leucocytes

Mark sheet	Achieved	Not achieved
Introduces self to junior doctor		
Confirms their level of experience		
Allows junior doctor to present first case		
Asks relevant questions to gain additional information		
Explains diagnosis of Bell's palsy and cancels CT head scan		
Provides teaching regarding management of Bell's palsy		
Agrees plan for patient, answers any further questions		
Allows junior doctor to present second case		
Asks relevant questions to gain additional information		
Explains diagnosis of severe hyponatraemia (<125 mmol/L)		
Provides teaching regarding treatment of hyponatraemia		
Agrees plan for patient, answers any further questions		
Allows junior doctor to present third case		

Cont'd...

Mark sheet	Achieved	Not achieved
Asks relevant questions to gain additional information		
Advises urgent bedside ultrasound or CT KUB		
Provides teaching regarding AAA mimicking renal colic		
Agrees plan for patient, answers any further questions		
Provides advice regarding accessing further information		
Global mark from junior doctor		
Global mark from examiner		

Instructions for actor

You are a junior doctor who has recently started work in the ED. You are presenting three patients from the CDU to your senior doctor. You provide some basic information for each case and only provide the additional information to the doctor as and when they ask for it as you are not sure what details are important. Take their advice on management plans and ask them where you can look up guidelines or policies on how to manage each of these cases.

Discussion of cases

Case 1

The patient has an acute, unilateral, idiopathic, facial nerve paralysis (Bell's palsy). There is no preceding pain or rash to suggest herpes zoster as a cause (Ramsay Hunt syndrome). Inability to wrinkle the forehead and lack of other nerve involvement confirms a lower motor neuron lesion. Alterations in taste and hyperacusis may also occur. A CT head is not required to make the diagnosis. Maximum facial weakness develops within 2 days, and the person should be reassured that the prognosis is good: most people with Bell's palsy make a full recovery within 9 months.

Care should be taken to exclude other causes of facial nerve palsy (HIV, Lyme disease, sarcoidosis) by carrying out a thorough history and examination.

The affected eye should be lubricated with drops during the day and ointment at night. If the cornea remains exposed after attempting to close the eyelid, an urgent referral to ophthalmology should be arranged and the eye should be taped closed at bedtime using microporous tape. For people presenting within 72 hours of the onset of symptoms, prednisolone 60 mg a day should be prescribed for 5 days. Antiviral treatment is not recommended, either alone or in combination with prednisolone.

If the paralysis shows no sign of improvement after 1 month, an urgent referral to ENT should be arranged to consider suspicion of a serious underlying diagnosis (e.g. cholesteatoma, parotid tumour, malignant otitis externa).

Case 2

The patient presents with severe hyponatraemia (Na$^+$ <125 mmol/L) and is symptomatic (confusion, headache, vomiting, seizure or reduced GCS). Treatment requires eliminating the cause and sodium correction while balancing risks of cerebral oedema and myelinolysis. Symptomatic patients should be admitted. About 1-2 mL/kg of 3% saline over 10-60 minutes can be administered to symptomatic patients to reduce the risk of seizure by increasing the sodium level acutely by 2-3 mmol/L.

After immediate treatment the cause should be eliminated (e.g. stop causative medication) and free water intake should be restricted to 1 L in 24 hours. Sodium can then be replaced at a rate <12 mmol/L/day. Ideally, patients with a sodium of <125 mmol/L should be admitted even if asymptomatic.

Case 3

Symptomatic or ruptured aortic aneurysm can mimic renal/ureteric colic (particularly in those older than 50 years of age with a first presentation of pain or syncope). Older patients require imaging to exclude this life-threatening diagnosis. This can be either an urgent CT kidney, ureters and bladder or bedside ultrasound by an experienced provider (provided the aorta can be visualised from diaphragm to bifurcation).

CT or ultrasound diagnosis of an aortic abdominal aneurysm (>3 cm) should prompt vascular consult for consideration of urgent surgical repair.

Suggested reading

National Institute for Health and Care Excellence (NICE). Clinical Knowledge Summaries: Bell's Palsy. NICE. London: NICE; 2012.
National Institute for Health and Care Excellence (NICE). Clinical Knowledge Summaries: Hyponatraemia. NICE. London: NICE; 2015.
National Institute for Health and Care Excellence (NICE). Clinical Knowledge Summaries: Renal Colic. NICE. London: NICE; 2015.
Royal College of Emergency Medicine (RCEM). Renal colic in adults. Clinical Standards for Emergency Departments. RCEM. London: RCEM; 2014.

2.16 Neonatal jaundice

Hyperbilirubinemia results in jaundice (yellow skin discolouration) in 60% of term and 80% of preterm babies in the first week of life. At 1 month 10% of breastfed babies are still jaundiced. For most babies, jaundice is not an indication of an underlying disease, and this early 'physiological jaundice' is a simple byproduct of fetal haemoglobin breakdown, immature mechanisms and breastfeeding.

Bilirubin is produced from the breakdown of red blood cells in an unconjugated (or 'indirect') form. This is then metabolised in the liver to produce conjugated (or 'direct') bilirubin which is largely excreted in stool. In neonates, unconjugated bilirubin can penetrate the blood–brain barrier and is potentially toxic to neural tissue (brain and spinal cord), causing both short- and long-term neurological dysfunction (kernicterus). Kernicterus occurs at high bilirubin levels or, in preterm babies, at lower levels of bilirubin.

Causes

The pathological causes of neonatal jaundice are sepsis, haemolysis, liver disease, metabolic disorders and dehydration.

The age of a jaundiced neonate may suggest the cause: jaundice with onset in the first 24 hours of life is always pathological. Strongly consider sepsis and haemolysis [rhesus or ABO incompatibility, red cell enzyme defects (G6PD deficiency), red cell membrane defects (spherocytosis), subgaleal bleeding].

Jaundice with onset between 24 hours and 14 days from birth is most often related to poor feeding or exaggerated physiological jaundice. However, sepsis; haemolytic disorders; hepatic disease; and Toxoplasmosis, Other (syphilis, varicella-zoster, parvovirus B19), Rubella, Cytomegalovirus (TORCH) infections are also potential causes.

Prolonged jaundice (onset >14 days) is most commonly due to exclusive breastfeeding (breast milk jaundice), or immature neonatal mechanisms and prematurity. However, these are diagnoses of exclusion. Haemolysis, sepsis, hypothyroidism, hepatic enzyme disorders and liver disease causing conjugated jaundice must be excluded. The most common cause of neonatal liver disease causing conjugated jaundice is biliary atresia and surgical management is required within the first few weeks of life.

Assessment

The assessment of jaundice starts with a history, looking for abnormalities and clues to the cause of the jaundice:
- When was the jaundice noticed?
- Has treatment been initiated?
- Is the child well or lethargic (not waking for feeds), poorly feeding, floppy or irritable?
- Feeding: breast (duration and frequency); bottle (volume and frequency)
- Hydration: 4 or 5 wet nappies a day is normal
- Stools (normal green/yellow or pale and chalky) and urine (normal or dark in nappy)
- Maternal history: maternal blood group and sensitising events requiring anti-D
- Pregnancy history: length of the gestation, US scans and follow up
- Birth history: date and time of birth (to plot bilirubin), delivery type (bleeding or bruising), risk factors for sepsis (prolonged rupture of membranes, maternal Group B *Streptococcus* status, maternal infection at birth), vitamin K given at birth (bleeding)

- Postnatal history: neonatal complications (fever), Guthrie metabolic screening normal (day 5)
- Drugs and past medical history: is the neonate on any medications or do they have any known medical conditions?
- Family history: jaundice, blood disorders, liver disorders, cystic fibrosis, metabolic disease

A full set of observations and weight measurement should be performed at triage. The weight should be plotted against birthweight on a growth chart, followed by an examination to look for:
- Jaundice: how far down the body is the jaundice evident (progresses downwards from face)?
- Tone and alertness: does this look like a well or sick baby?
- Pallor and signs of bleeding: bruising, subgaleal haemorrhage
- Hydration status: capillary refill, anterior fontanelle, mucous membranes
- Examine the chest and pulses for features of congenital heart disease
- Examine the abdomen for hepatosplenomegaly
- Check the nappy for evidence of stool or urine colour

After assessment, babies with suspected jaundice require measurement of bilirubin level. A transcutaneous bilirubinometer (TCB) is adequate in non-premature neonates >24 hours old. Otherwise, or if the TCB reading is greater than 250 µmol/L, a serum bilirubin is required by heel prick. All babies with a serum bilirubin level above the treatment line on a threshold graph require referral to the paediatrician, and need blood tests for:
- Split bilirubin
- Full blood count and film
- Blood packed cell volume
- Blood group (mother and baby) and direct antiglobulin test (Coombs' test).

Also consider the following additional tests when clinically indicated:
- Urea, electrolytes and a blood sugar level (if poor feeding or dehydration is suspected)
- Microbiological cultures of blood, urine and/or cerebrospinal fluid (if infection is suspected)
- Blood glucose-6-phosphate dehydrogenase levels (if the neonate is of African, Asian or Mediterranean origin)
- Conjugated bilirubin (if neonate is >14 days old)
- Urine culture (if neonate is >14 days old)
- Thyroid function tests (>14 days old)
- Guthrie metabolic screening (must be carried out >14 days old)

Scenario

A junior doctor has just assessed Luca, a 12-day old boy presenting with his mother, Maria Penco. The mother is concerned that Luca has begun to appear yellow over the last 3 days. The doctor has taken a history and examined Luca, but he is not confident in his history taking and is unsure of how to interpret his findings.

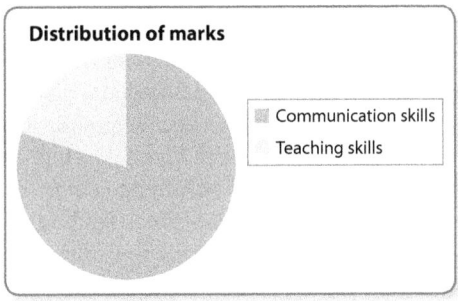

Distribution of marks
- Communication skills
- Teaching skills

Take the neonatal history again yourself from Maria, then discuss the examination findings and blood results with the junior doctor. Explain the likely diagnosis, formulate a management plan and demonstrate a framework for assessing neonatal jaundice. You do not need to re-examine Luca.

These are the test results that junior doctor provides to you:
- Transcutaneous bilirubinometer 280 µmol/L
- Bilirubin 290 µmol/L (direct or conjugated fraction 18 µmol/L)
- White cell count 8.0×10^9/L, haemoglobin 170 g/L, platelet count 300×10^9/L, packed cell volume 55%, reticulocytes 1%, mean corpuscular volume 98, blood film normal
- Blood groups: mother A +ve, neonate A +ve, Coombs' test -ve
- Blood sugar level 4.0, creatinine 50 ummol/L, urea 10.0, sodium 149, potassium 4.5
- Blood G6PD level: normal

Mark sheet	Achieved	Not achieved
Introduces self to junior doctor and mother		
Takes history of presenting complaint		
Takes history of feeding and output		
Takes prenatal, birth and postnatal history		
Takes maternal history		
Takes family history		
Asks for weight, vital signs and birth weight		
Confirms jaundice on examination and exam findings		
Asks for screening TCB and then relevant blood tests – considers G6PD and requests testing given background		
Confirms clinical picture excludes serious pathology – sepsis Haemolysis or Liver disease		
Concludes jaundice most likely due to inadequate oral intake due to painful breastfeeding		
Admits child for phototherapy and breastfeeding support – lactation consult, nipple shield, formula top ups		
Explains approach to jaundice to junior doctor		
Global score from examiner		
Global score from junior doctor		

Instructions for actor

The candidate is expected to demonstrate understanding of the assessment of neonatal jaundice, with a structured neonatal history, requests for focused examination findings and relevant blood tests. Luca's jaundice in this scenario has been caused by problems with breastfeeding due to Maria developing painful cracked nipples which limits feeding time. The candidate is expected to come to this conclusion and admit the child for light phototherapy and provide breastfeeding support, whilst explaining why more serious causes are less likely. Provide the following information to the candidate as they ask you questions:

1. Luca is Maria's first child (G1P1). Luca has been unsettled and jaundiced for 3 days. He is exclusively breastfed every 3 hours, limited to 10 minutes in the last 3 days due to his mother having painful, cracked nipples. He is producing 2 straw-yellow wet nappies a day and 1 mustard stool. Apart from the pain of feeding, Maria is otherwise well and has no medical problems and no sensitizing events in pregnancy.
2. Luca had a term vaginal delivery. Vitamin K was given and there were no complications pre- or postnatally. Luca is of Mediterranean background with no known medical conditions in the family.
3. Luca's observations are in the normal range (respiration rate 35 breaths per minute, heart rate 150 beats per minute, temperature 37°C). He was born at 3.5 kg and his current weight is 3.6 kg. He is jaundiced down to the umbilicus, alert and crying, with normal tone. Luca's nappy, which has been on for 8 hours, is only a little wet. His examination is otherwise normal.

Suggested reading

National Institute for Health and Clinical Excellence (NICE). Jaundice in newborn babies under 28 days. CG98. NICE. London: NICE; 2010.

2.17 Sexual assault

Sexual assault may result in physical injuries, sexually transmitted infections (including HIV and hepatitis B), unwanted pregnancy and significant psychological symptoms.

Victims may not disclose acts of sexual assaults initially. You should be vigilant in cases of potential domestic violence and with patients requesting emergency contraception. Assessment should be conducted in a non-judgemental, confidential and supportive manner.

Assess patients reporting sexual assault for physical injuries that require treatment, with treatment of life-threatening injuries taking priority over forensic examination. After the ED has managed acute injuries, it is best practise to encourage patients to attend a Sexual Assault Referral Centre (SARC), although this may not be available in all regions.

At a SARC, victims of sexual assault may receive a forensic examination, emergency contraception, postexposure prophylaxis (PEP), psychological counselling, legal advice and other support, from professionally trained staff. Victims can choose to be dealt with anonymously if they do not wish police involvement. If unwilling to attend a SARC, ED staff should respect that decision, assess the patient and manage emergency contraception and sexually transmitted infection risks.

When assessing sexual assault patients in the ED a choice of gender of the doctor should be provided where possible. Take a history of the assault, including time and location, characteristics of the assailant(s), physical violence, sexual acts (vaginal, oral, anal, penile/digital penetration). Examine for bruising, abrasions, and lacerations and any patterns such as fingertip marks. Document examination findings clearly as you may be asked to produce a statement later or go to court if the victim decides to press charges.

Do not conduct a pelvic examination unless there is significant bleeding, as this may disrupt forensic evidence. Generally, evidence can be collected up to 7 days after a sexual assault or rape. Evidence should not be collected in the ED unless the patient requires admission due to their injuries, and in this case many SARCs will arrange for a forensic medical examiner to attend the hospital.

Prior to forensic examination, advise victims to avoid showering, brushing teeth and to preserve the clothes worn until they have been examined.

The risk of pregnancy should be addressed; offer emergency contraception to the victim. Assessing the risk of exposure to STIs may be limited by lack of information and testing of the assailant. Seek expert advice from the relevant on-call service, and take baseline blood tests for hepatitis B, hepatitis C and HIV. Accelerated hepatitis B vaccination with a first dose in the ED should be considered if the perpetrator is not known to be hepatitis B negative. Postexposure prophylaxis after sexual exposure (PEPSE) for HIV should be considered, especially in cases where: the assailant is known to carry an STI, has risk factors for HIV, anal rape, assault with multiple assailants or bleeding. Prophylactic antibiotics for bacterial sexually transmitted infections should also be offered.

If the victim does not attend a SARC, they may need further referral to Social Services, Victim Support, a Community Safety Unit or other organisations which can offer support after the assault. Patients should be offered police involvement, but any decision not to involve the police should be respected.

Clinical information should be regarded as confidential unless a child or a person without capacity is felt to be at risk or violence with a knife or a gun has been used against the victim. In these exceptional situations information should be shared with the police and statutory agencies as appropriate. This should be discussed with the patient where possible and clearly documented.

Scenario

Michelle is a 24-year-old woman who reports falling yesterday whilst taking shopping out of the car landing heavily on her right hand. She has attended because she is worried her hand may be broken and asking for a 'doctor's letter' as she is unable to attend an exam due to her hand injury.

A junior doctor has assessed Michelle. Her wrist is swollen without bony tenderness and the X-ray taken in advance of your assessment shows no fractures. She has decided against a splint for support and pain relief. Whilst assessing Michelle the junior doctor notices she has fingerprint bruising on her neck and upper arm with bilateral subconjunctival haemorrhages. She has no other injuries. He is suspicious Michelle's injuries do not fit the described mechanism and has asked for your help as the senior doctor. Discuss a treatment plan. There is no need to examine Michelle.

Distribution of marks

- Communication skills

Mark sheet	Achieved	Not achieved
Introduces self to patient		
Confirms treatment plan for wrist injury		
Confirms provision of a work certificate for tomorrow's exam		
Ask opening questions to explore mechanism of injury		
Describes junior doctors' concerns		
Ensures confidentiality outside extraordinary circumstances		
Acknowledges stressful situation, and desire to help patient		
Asks if patient has been assaulted physically or sexually		
Listens to patient without interruption		
Acknowledges physical and sexual assault		
Takes history of assault		
Non-judgemental, confidential and supportive manner		
Advises police and forensic medical examiner involvement, respects patient decision to decline		
Discusses and provides emergency contraception. Explains effectiveness cannot be guaranteed and follow-up with GP or family planning clinic is therefore required		
Recognises no additional HIV risk		
Recognises no additional risk of hepatitis B		
Recognises no additional risk of bacterial STIs		
Assess whether patient feels unsafe at home		
Offers additional staff to support patient – nurses/social worker		

Cont'd...

Mark sheet	Achieved	Not achieved
Inform about available sources of psychosocial support (GP, social worker)		
Documents accurately		
Global mark from patient		
Global mark from examiner		

Instructions for actor

You are a 24-year-old full-time personal assistant called Michelle Browning. You are also studying for a law degree in your spare time and have an exam tomorrow. You have been married to John, a 28-year-old accountant for 2 years. You have no children but have planned to start a family after your degree.

John has been increasingly unhappy since the death of his father 6 months ago, he has been drinking regularly in the evenings and can become angry and aggressive when drunk.

He has hit you twice whilst drunk in the last few months when you have tried to address his problem and stop him drinking. Last night John was drunk and verbally abusive to you when you refused to sleep with him, he forced himself on you, holding you tight around the neck. You were terrified and unable to breathe. You struggled to get free and hurt your hand. John had non-consensual vaginal intercourse with you.

In the morning John left for work leaving you feeling lost and desperate. You attend the ED for a work certificate because you will be unable to sit your exam. You do not admit the cause of your injury initially but will be willing to discuss it if questioned in a supportive way.

You do not wish to get pregnant in this situation. You have no concerns about sexually transmitted disease, and do not wish any police involvement. You wish to return home as soon as possible.

Suggested reading

Royal College of Emergency Medicine (RCEM). Management of adult patients who attend emergency departments after sexual assault or rape. Best Practice Guideline. RCEM. London: 2015.

Chapter 3

Systems examination

3.1 Introduction
3.2 Cardiovascular examination
3.3 Abdominal examination
3.4 Upper limb neurology examination
3.5 Lower limb neurology examination
3.6 Cranial nerve examination
3.7 Respiratory examination
3.8 Thyroid examination
3.9 Eye examination

3.1 Introduction

Your ultimate goal for these objective structured clinical examinations (OSCEs) is, of course, to score as many marks as possible. The areas where marks are scored can be divided into three (opening the station, the examination itself and closing the station). By focusing on each of these areas individually, you should be able to maximise your score.

Opening the station

Several basic things are required to start the station. You must always introduce yourself to the patient, confirm their identity and explain what you intend to do. You should always ask the patient if they are in pain and if appropriate offer them some painkillers and remember to exercise caution when examining any painful areas. It will detract from your global score if you cause undue pain to the patient. Finally before touching the patient you should always clean your hands and seek their permission for the examination.

The examination

This should be a well-rehearsed routine. A candidate who must stop between steps of the examination to think about what they need to do next is unlikely to do very well. It also means they are unable to concentrate on the clinical findings that they elicit, and may also run out of time. From the examiner's and patient's point of view it makes the candidate seem at best nervous and at worst inexperienced with what are fundamental examinations.

In this chapter each examination is outlined in full and should be thoroughly rehearsed so that steps become second nature. Each is based on the principles of inspect, palpate, percuss then auscultate. It is best to practice these in small groups of two or three to allow you to grow accustomed to being observed while examining and also provides an opportunity for feedback on your technique.

It might be the case that you will be asked to talk through the steps in your examination while performing it. This may not suit all candidates so it is worth practicing. If there is any doubt as to whether or not this is expected of you it is acceptable to ask the examiner at the start of the station if they would like you to talk through your examination or not.

Closing the station

Having finished the examination, you should always thank the patient and offer them help getting redressed. The OSCE will usually require the candidate to present their findings in a particular way. It is important that attention is paid to this – and the style required. Some OSCEs require a management plan to be explained to (and agreed with) the patient, whereas others may simply require presentation of findings to the examiner. You should be clear which is required. It is always tempting when presenting your findings to look from the examiner to the patient. However this causes the presentation to be fragmented and can make a candidate seem uncertain of their clinical findings.

It is likely that a diagnosis (or at least a differential diagnosis) will be expected as well as an appropriate management plan.

3.2 Cardiovascular examination

Begin by introducing yourself, washing your hands, confirming the name of the patient and asking for permission to examine them.

Ask if the patient has any pain and offer analgesia if appropriate.

The patient will often already be appropriately positioned. If not, they should be positioned at 45°, naked from the waist up. In the examination, this patient will usually be a man. If they are a woman, it is appropriate to tell the examiner that ideally you would expose the whole of their chest for some parts of the examination, but to ask whether you may preserve their dignity in the examination by leaving a bra or sports top in place.

General inspection

Stand at the end of the bed and perform a general inspection. The main features to note are:
- The patient's general appearance and level of comfort
- Is the patient breathless?
- Are there any scars indicating previous interventions (e.g. a scar below the left clavicle from a pacemaker or internal defibrillator, a midline sternotomy scar which may indicate valve replacement or a coronary artery bypass or a left thoracotomy scar from a valvotomy for mitral stenosis)?
- The presence of any medical equipment or medication (oxygen, glyceryl trinitrate spray, tablets)

Hand inspection

The next step is to inspect the hands for:
- Clubbing (present in cyanotic congenital heart disease or subacute bacterial endocarditis)
- Splinter haemorrhages suggest endocarditis. Also look for Osler's nodes (tender nodules in the finger pads) and Janeway lesions (purpuric macules on the palms)
- Tar staining of the finger tips indicating a significant smoking history
- Nail bed pulsation of aortic regurgitation (Quincke's sign)

Pulses and blood pressure

Palpate the radial pulse to determine the rate and rhythm.

Then move on to palpate the brachial artery for a collapsing pulse of aortic regurgitation. A collapsing pulse feels like a sudden unusually powerful upstroke followed by a palpable 'whoosh' as the blood rushes away and pours back through the incompetent aortic valve into the left ventricle. Continue to move up the arm and comment on the need to check the patient's blood pressure (or lying and standing blood pressures if relevant). This could be mentioned once your examination is complete but the examiner may give you a blood pressure reading if you mention it at this stage. A wide pulse pressure raises the possibility of aortic regurgitation and a narrow one aortic stenosis. Hypotension or a postural drop will be relevant if there is a history of collapse, dizziness or new medication. Also if it is left until the end you may forget to mention the blood pressure (or run out of time).

Head and neck examination

Move up to the patient's face and examine the eyes for:
- Conjunctival pallor (suggesting anaemia)
- Cholesterol deposits (xanthelasma) in the skin below the eyes or corneal arcus, both suggesting hyperlipidaemia

Next examine the tongue for central cyanosis.

Examine the internal jugular vein in the neck to assess the patient's jugular venous pressure (JVP). This is measured with the patient at 45° and is reported as how many centimetres above the sternal angle the JVP can be seen, as shown in **Figure 3.2.1**. Unlike the carotid pulse the JVP is biphasic and not palpable. To help identify the JVP gentle pressure can be applied over the liver which causes increased venous return and distension of the neck veins. This hepatojugular reflux then subsides as a healthy heart is able to accommodate the increased venous return by increasing cardiac output. In patients with congestive cardiac failure the venous distension may persist as the cardiac output cannot increase adequately.

Observe and palpate the carotid pulse. A forceful carotid pulse associated with the ear lobes moving may suggest aortic regurgitation (Corrigan's sign). A slow rising pulse may be due to aortic stenosis.

Figure 3.2.1 Measuring the jugular venous pressure, with the patient at 45° to the horizontal.

Precordium examination

Palpate the precordium. Begin by locating the apex beat and determine its position with reference to both the rib space it lies within and the clavicle (the normal position is in the fifth intercostal space in the mid-clavicular line). Next rest your hand over each valve area feeling for any heaves or thrills (palpable murmurs) associated with valve disease. Consider palpating below the lateral part of the left clavicle to demonstrate or exclude the presence of a cardiac device implanted under the skin.

Auscultation

Perform auscultation while palpating the carotid or brachial pulse upstroke to time the first heart sound. The first heart sound is caused by the mitral and tricuspid valves closing, while the second heart sound is the aortic and pulmonary valve closing. Identify these and any added sounds.

Auscultate the:
- Apex with the diaphragm
- Apex with the bell while positioning the patient on their left side in expiration (for mitral stenosis – the bell is used for low pitched sounds)
- Left axilla for radiation of a mitral regurgitation murmur
- Remaining three valve areas (**Figure 3.2.2**) with the diaphragm
- Carotids for radiation of an aortic stenosis murmur (or a carotid bruit)
- Left sternal edge while leaning forward in full expiration (for aortic regurgitation)

While the patient is sitting up, auscultate the lung bases for crackles signifying left ventricular failure and palpate for sacral oedema.

Finally expose the lower legs and palpate for pedal oedema, you may also note scars from saphenous vein harvesting for bypass.

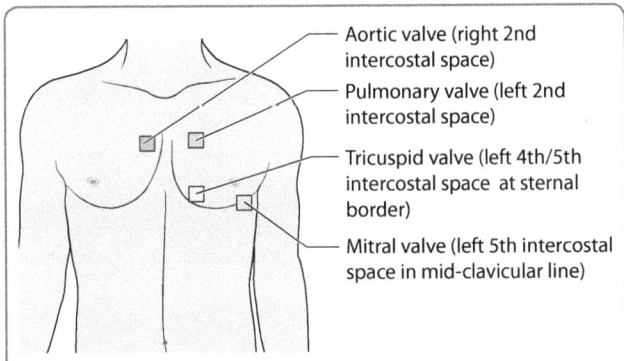

Figure 3.2.2 Auscultation positions for heart valves.

Ending the examination

Thank the patient, offer to help them redress and ensure they are comfortable.
Tell the examiner you would like to:
- Examine the peripheral pulses (and check for radiofemoral delay)
- See an ECG
- See a urine dip to exclude haematuria/proteinuria (as immune complex deposition in endocarditis may lead to glomerulonephritis)

Common cases

Aortic stenosis

The pulse may be slow rising. The apex beat will normally be undisplaced with a possible systolic thrill palpable over the aortic area. There will be a harsh ejection systolic murmur loudest in the aortic area radiating into the neck. There may be a narrow pulse pressure (**Figure 3.2.3**).

Mitral regurgitation

The rhythm may be atrial fibrillation. The apex beat may be thrusting and displaced inferiorly and/or laterally with a possible systolic thrill. The murmur is pansystolic and usually radiates into the axilla (**Figure 3.2.3**).

Aortic regurgitation

The pulse is collapsing in character with a wide pulse pressure. The apex beat may be thrusting and displaced inferiorly and towards the axilla. There is an early diastolic murmur audible at the left sternal edge. It is best heard with the patient leaning forward in full expiration.

The large volume pulse of aortic regurgitation is associated with many additional signs such as Quincke's (nail bed pulsation), de Musset's (head nodding) and Corrigan's (carotid pulsation causing the ear lobe to twitch) (**Figure 3.2.3**).

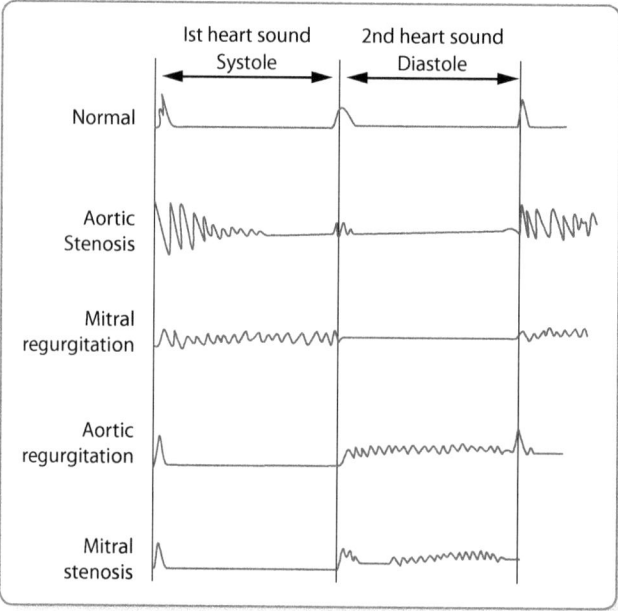

Figure 3.2.3 Heart sounds in valve pathology.

Mitral stenosis

There may be a malar flush or a left thoracotomy scar from a mitral valvotomy. The rhythm may be atrial fibrillation. The apex will typically be undisplaced. The murmur is a mid-diastolic rumbling (hence best heard with the bell) sound over the mitral area and is most easily picked up with the patient rolled to their left (**Figure 3.2.3**).

Prosthetic valves

There may be a midline sternotomy scar (although an increasing number of patients are having aortic valves replaced endovascularly). Bruising may be apparent if the patient is anticoagulated (routine with an artificial valve). A clicking sound may be audible even without a stethoscope.

A click (artificial valve) or loud (tissue valve) first heart sound and a diastolic flow murmur suggest a mitral valve replacement.

A normal first heart sound, a systolic flow murmur and click or loud second heart sound suggest an aortic valve replacement.

A normal examination

If you have failed to identify any abnormal clinical signs, don't be afraid to say so. A normal examination is always a possibility.

Scenario

Mrs Hall has attended after a collapse. You see her in the major's area of the ED. Examine her cardiovascular system and then explain your diagnosis and management plan to her.

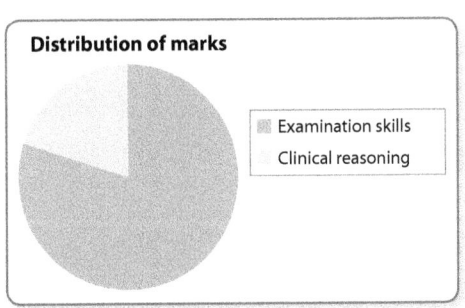

Distribution of marks
- Examination skills
- Clinical reasoning

Mark sheet	Achieved	Not achieved
Introduces self to patient appropriately		
Confirms patient identity		
Explains reason for examination and obtains consent		
Enquires regarding presence of pain and offers analgesia if needed		
Cleans hands appropriately		
Positions and exposes patient correctly		
Performs initial inspection from end of bed		
Inspects hands and fingernails		
Palpates radial pulse and determines heart rate and rhythm		
Examines for a collapsing pulse		

Cont'd...

Cont'd...

Mark sheet	Achieved	Not achieved
Comments on the need to check blood pressure		
Inspects eyes for cholesterol deposits/pallor and mouth for cyanosis		
Examines jugular venous pressure		
Palpates carotid pulse		
Palpates apex beat and determines its position		
Palpates for heaves/thrills over precordium		
Auscultates all four valve areas		
Uses correct manoeuvres for mitral stenosis and aortic regurgitation		
Auscultates for radiation to axilla and carotids		
Auscultates lung bases		
Palpates for sacral and pedal oedema		
Comments on need to examine peripheral pulses		
Thanks patient and offers to help patient dress		
Correctly identifies clinical signs		
Correctly states diagnosis		
Describes appropriate management plan		
Global mark from patient		
Global mark from examiner		

3.3 Abdominal examination

Begin by introducing yourself, washing your hands, confirming the name of the patient and asking for permission to examine them.

Ask if the patient has any pain and offer analgesia if appropriate.

The patient should be positioned flat with a pillow under their head and their arms relaxed by their sides. Their upper body should be exposed from the level of the pubis symphysis upwards.

General inspection

Stand at the end of the bed and perform a general inspection. The main features to note are:
- The presence of pallor, jaundice, spider naevi, gynaecomastia, abdominal distension, visible swellings and dilated veins on the abdominal wall
- The presence of any scars/stomas/catheters/drains (**Figure 3.3.1**)

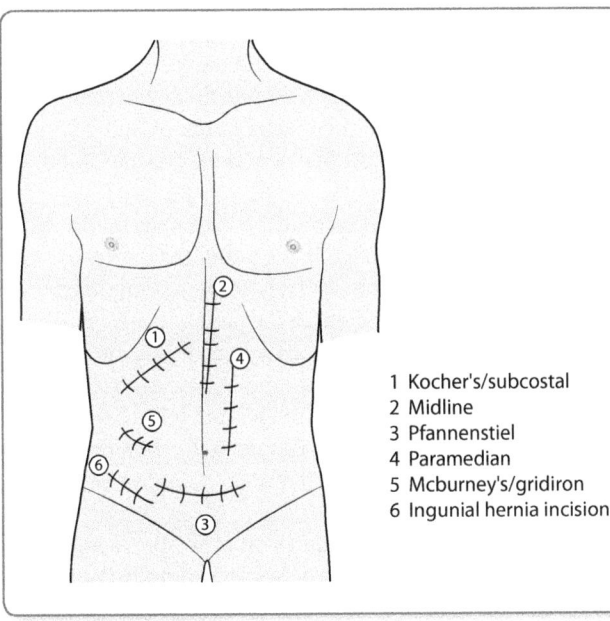

Figure 3.3.1 Common abdominal scars.

1. Kocher's/subcostal
2. Midline
3. Pfannenstiel
4. Paramedian
5. Mcburney's/gridiron
6. Inguinal hernia incision

Hand inspection

The next step is to approach the patient and examine both hands for:
- Clubbing (can be present in cirrhosis, inflammatory bowel disease, malignancy and malabsorption)
- Leukonychia (white nails due to hypoalbuminaemia)
- Palmar erythema
- Dupuytren's contracture

Ask the patient to hold their hands in front of them and observe for asterixis (liver flap)

Inspect the patient's arms for fistulae related to dialysis. If a fistula is present palpate it to note whether or not it is functioning.

Head and neck examination

Move up to the patient's face and examine for:
- Conjunctival pallor suggesting anaemia
- Oral mucosal ulceration
- Examine the tongue for central cyanosis

If the patient is able to do so comfortably ask them to sit up and palpate their neck for cervical lymphadenopathy. A hard palpable lymph node in the left supraclavicular fossa (Virchow's node) suggests gastrointestinal malignancy and if lymph nodes are present in the neck, the axillae and groin should also be examined. While they are sitting up inspect their back for spider naevi and for any scars that you would otherwise miss e.g. over the loins.

Abdominal examination

Return the patient to the supine position and note relevant signs on their chest:
- Gynaecomastia
- Spider naevi

Take a further opportunity to inspect the abdomen to ensure no scars or other signs are missed. Ensure inspection includes looking round to the patient's left flank. Then begin palpating the abdomen with light palpation only. Great care should be taken not to hurt the patient. Palpation should be performed using the pulp of the fingers rather than the finger tips and the patient's face should be observed for any signs of discomfort. The abdomen should then be examined again with deeper palpation.

Next, focus on the liver, spleen and kidneys in turn. To palpate the liver, start in the right iliac fossa and palpate towards the right hypochondrium while the patient takes deep breaths (**Figure 3.3.2**). If a liver edge is felt gently try to assess if it is smooth or nodular. Tenderness in the right hypochondrium with inspiration, where the patient stops breathing in, 'catches' their breath and winces represents a positive Murphy's sign. This is most commonly caused by cholecystitis.

For the spleen, begin again in the right iliac fossa and while the patient takes deep breaths palpate towards the left hypochondrium. If the spleen is not felt the patient should be asked to roll onto their right hand side and the left subcostal margin palpated for a splenic tip, which is found in mild splenomegaly.

Each kidney should then be examined bimanually. Candidates must be able to identify or at least form an appropriate differential diagnosis for any masses they identify (**Box 3.3.1** and **Box 3.3.2**).

Then percuss over the liver and spleen to assess the size from their upper to lower border and palpate in the midline for an abdominal aortic aneurysm.

Shifting dullness of ascites should be assessed for. First percuss the flanks for stony dullness. If this is present ask the patient to roll onto their side and assess whether the level of stony dullness has shifted.

Finally auscultate the abdomen to check for normal bowel sounds and the presence of bruits over the aorta and renal arteries.

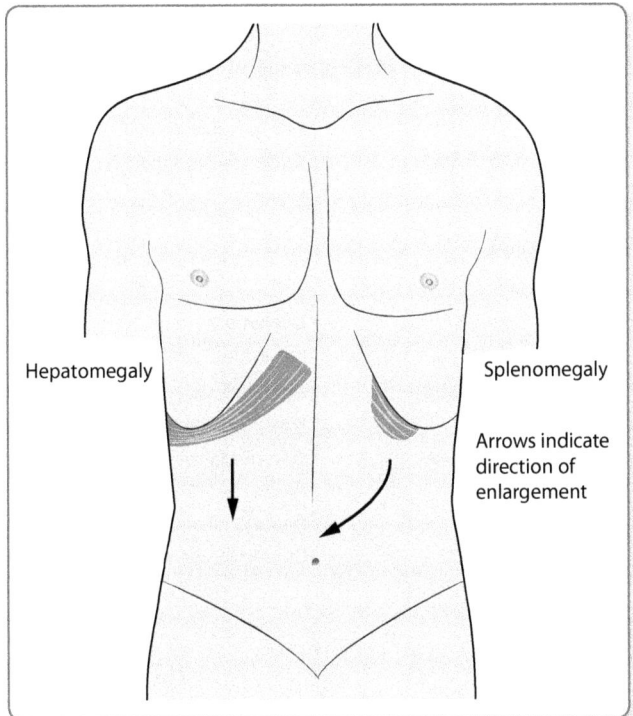

Figure 3.3.2 Hepatomegaly and splenomegaly.

Ending the examination

Thank the patient, help them redress and ensure they are comfortable.
Tell the examiner you would like to:
- Examine the external genitalia and hernial orifices
- Perform a rectal examination
- See the result of a urine dip analysis

Box 3.3.1 Distinguishing spleen from kidney

Unlike the kidney, the spleen:
- is not bimanually palpable (ballotable)
- does not have a palpable upper border (you can't get above it)
- moves down on inspiration
- is dull to percussion
- has a notch on its lower medial border

> **Box 3.3.2** Abdominal masses by site. On occasion it may simply be necessary to give a differential diagnosis for an abdominal mass and a plan for investigation and management. This table offers a differential list based on the position of any mass

Right hypochondrium	Epigastrium	Left hypochondrium
Liver (causes as below)	Pancreatic cyst/pseudocyst/malignancy	Spleen (causes as below)
Kidney	Lymphoma	Kidney
	Gastric malignancy	
	Aortic aneurysm	
Right lumbar	**Umbilical**	**Left lumbar**
Kidney	Aortic aneurysm	Kidney
Right Iliac fossa	**Hypogastric (suprapubic)**	**Left Iliac fossa**
Caecal malignancy	Bladder	Transplanted kidney
Crohn's disease	Uterine fibroids/malignancy/pregnancy	Colon malignancy
Transplanted kidney		Faeces
Tuberculosis mass		Ovarian cyst/malignancy
Ovarian cyst/malignancy		Diverticular abscess

Common cases

Chronic liver disease

Causes:
    Alcohol
    Viral hepatitis
    Autoimmune hepatitis
    Primary biliary cirrhosis
    Deposition disorders (Haemochromatosis: a disorder of iron metabolism leading to deposition in many organs and causing grey pigmentation of the skin. Wilson's disease: where copper accumulates in the liver and central nervous system sometimes causing pathognomonic Kayser–Fleischer rings in the eyes)

Hepatosplenomegaly

Causes:
    Myeloproliferative disease
    Lymphoproliferative disease
    Liver cirrhosis and portal hypertension
    Infection (viral hepatitis, cytomegalovirus, malaria, leishmaniasis, schistosomiasis, tuberculosis)

Hepatomegaly

Causes:
    Cirrhosis (secondary to alcohol, drugs, autoimmune or deposition disorders)
    (Note: the liver is not always enlarged in cirrhosis)
    Infections (viral hepatitis, infectious mononucleosis, Lyme disease)
    Malignancy (in which the liver may be hard and irregular)
    Congestive cardiac failure

Splenomegaly

Causes:
Myeloproliferative disease
Lymphoproliferative disease
Liver cirrhosis and portal hypertension
Infection (viral hepatitis, cytomegalovirus, malaria, leishmaniasis, schistosomiasis, tuberculosis and infectious mononucleosis)
Chronic myeloid leukaemia, lymphoma, myelofibrosis, malaria and leishmaniasis are the most likely causes of extreme splenomegaly

Transplanted kidney

Clinical signs: On inspection the patient may have signs of previous dialysis (an arteriovenous fistula on their forearm or scars from vascular access around their neck). They will also have an abdominal scar with an associated palpable mass or fullness normally in an iliac fossa

Causes: Common reasons for a renal transplant are diabetes mellitus, hypertension, polycystic kidney disease and glomerulonephritis. The patient may display additional signs suggesting which of these is most likely

Scenario

Mr Simmons has attended with worsening abdominal pain. Examine his abdomen and describe your findings and diagnosis to the examiner.

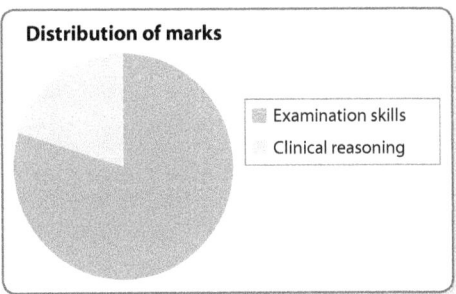

Distribution of marks
- Examination skills
- Clinical reasoning

Mark sheet	Achieved	Not achieved
Introduces self to patient appropriately		
Confirms patient identity		
Explains reason for examination and obtains consent		
Enquires regarding presence of pain and offers analgesia if needed		
Cleans hands appropriately		
Positions and exposes patient correctly		
Performs initial inspection from end of bed		
Inspects hands and fingernails		
Inspect eyes and mouth		
Checks for presence of lymphadenopathy		

Cont'd...

Cont'd...

Mark sheet	Achieved	Not achieved
Inspects for signs of chronic liver disease		
Performs light and deep palpation		
Palpates for the liver		
Palpates for the spleen		
Palpates bimanually for the kidneys		
Correct use of percussion		
Examines for ascites appropriately		
Correct use of auscultation		
Comments on hernia orifices, rectal examination, urine dip		
Thanks patient and offers to help patient redress		
Correctly identifies clinical signs		
Correctly states diagnosis		
Describes appropriate management plan		
Global mark from patient		
Global mark from examiner		

3.4 Upper limb neurology examination

Begin by introducing yourself, washing your hands, confirming the name of the patient and asking for permission to examine them.

Ask if the patient has any pain and offer analgesia if appropriate.

The patient should be positioned sitting upright with both of their arms exposed up to and including the shoulders.

General inspection

Stand at the end of the bed and perform a general inspection. The main features to note are:
- Scars or deformity
- Muscle wasting
- Fasciculation

A peripheral nervous system examination requires an assessment of tone, power, reflexes, sensation and coordination. Each is performed in turn as outlined below with both limbs being compared to each other.

Tone

To assess tone hold the patient's hand. Pronate and supinate the forearm and also flex and extend the elbow. Assess the amount of resistance to movement encountered.

Decreased tone generally occurs due to a lower motor neurone lesion. An increase in tone can be divided into certain subtypes:
- Lead pipe rigidity implies tone is consistently increased during movement and is commonly associated with Parkinson's disease
- Cogwheel rigidity implies a rise and fall in tone as if turning a large wheel or handle, and is said to represent the tremor of Parkinson's superimposed on lead pipe rigidity

Power

Tests for limb power aim to isolate individual muscle groups with specific nerve innervations. Each muscle group is tested by asking the patient to perform a specific movement against resistance applied by the doctor performing the examination.

The power is then graded from 0 to 5 based on the Medical Research Council grading system.

0. No movement
1. Flicker of movement visible in muscle
2. Movement but not against gravity
3. Movement against gravity but not against resistance
4. Decreased power against resistance
5. Normal power against resistance

Box 3.4.1 Myotomes of the upper limbs

Movement	Muscle	Root	Nerve
Shoulder abduction	Deltoid	C5	Axillary
Elbow flexion	Biceps	C6	Musculocutaneous
Elbow extension	Triceps	C7	Radial
Wrist flexion	Flexor carpi radialis and ulnaris	C8	Median and ulnar
Wrist extension	Extensor carpi radialis and ulnaris	C7	Radial
Finger abduction	Dorsal interossei	T1	Ulnar
Thumb abduction	Abductor pollicis brevis	C8	Median

Reflexes

Proceed to test the patient's reflexes using a tendon hammer. While eliciting the reflex ensure adequate exposure to observe the respective muscle for contraction. If you are unable to elicit the reflex after two attempts, try once more while asking the patient to clench their teeth at the moment you use the tendon hammer (this is called reinforcement). The reflexes to test are:

Biceps   C5-6
Brachioradialis C6-7
Triceps   C7-8

Sensation

Sensation should ideally be tested in all modalities: pain (pinprick), light touch, vibration, temperature and proprioception. It is not normally expected to test temperature sensation during an examination.

Before beginning ensure the upper limbs are in the anatomical position. This will avoid confusion when assessing each of the dermatomes in turn (**Figure 3.4.1**):
- Check light touch with cotton wool. The skin should be touched but not stroked
- Pain (pinprick) should be tested with a neuro tip

For both light touch and pain the patient should be shown what sensation to expect on a neutral part of their body before starting the examination. The easiest way to do this is to touch their face or upper chest with the cotton wool or neuro tip beforehand so they are aware of what the normal sensation should feel like.

Vibration is tested using a 128 Hz tuning fork. Ask the patient to say whether the tuning fork is vibrating or not. Place it over a distal bony prominence (distal interphalangeal joint) and move proximally until they can correctly identify vibration.

Finally proprioception is tested by assessing joint position sense. This is achieved by flexing or extending a distal joint while the patient has their eyes closed and asking them if the distal part is moving up or down. If the patient cannot correctly identify this movement move to a more proximal joint until they can do so.

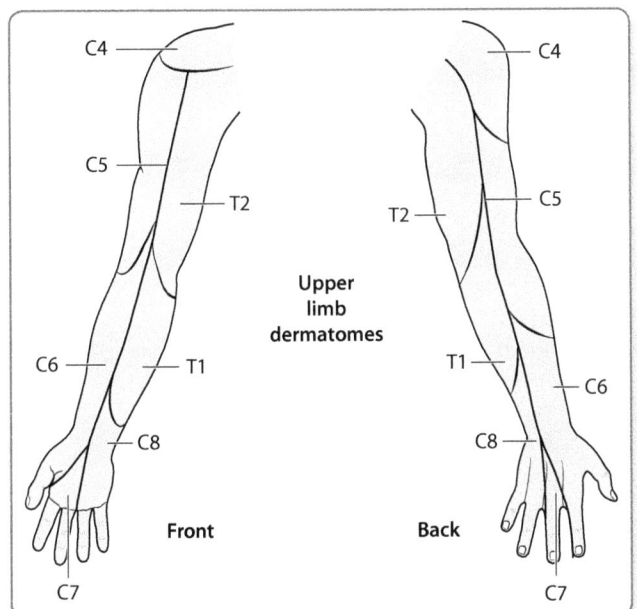

Figure 3.4.1 Upper limb dermatomes.

Coordination

Ask the patient to touch their nose and then your index finger, which should be positioned at a distance such that their arm must extend fully to reach it. Ask them to do this 3 or 4 times. Check both limbs. Note any ataxia or intention tremor.

Ending the examination

Thank the patient, help them redress and ensure they are comfortable.
Tell the examiner you would like to:
- Examine the remainder of the peripheral nervous system

Scenario

Miss Price is a 39-year-old office worker. She is complaining of weakness and altered sensation in one of her arms. Perform a peripheral nervous system examination of her upper limbs and explain your findings and a management plan to her.

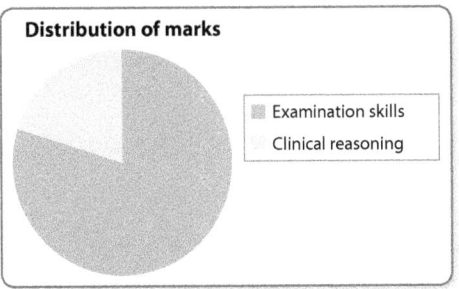

Mark sheet	Achieved	Not achieved
Introduces self to patient appropriately		
Confirms patient identity		
Explains reason for examination and obtains consent		
Enquires regarding presence of pain and offers analgesia if needed		
Cleans hands appropriately		
Positions and exposes patient correctly		
Performs initial inspection from end of bed		
Inspects upper limbs for scars, wasting, fasciculation		
Assesses tone in upper limbs		
Assesses power in upper limbs		
Assesses reflexes in upper limbs		
Assesses sensation in upper limbs		
Assesses coordination in upper limbs		
Thanks patient and offers to help patient redress		
Correctly identifies clinical signs		
Correctly states diagnosis		
Describes appropriate management plan		
Global mark from patient		
Global mark from examiner		

Suggested reading

Michael O'Brien. Aids to the examination of the peripheral nervous system (5th edn). Philadelphia: Saunders Ltd; 2010.

3.5 Lower limb neurology examination

Begin by introducing yourself, washing your hands, confirming the name of the patient and asking for permission to examine them. A peripheral nervous system examination of the lower limbs requires an assessment of gait, tone, power, reflexes, sensation and coordination. Each is performed in turn as outlined below with each limb being compared to the other.

Ask if the patient has any pain and offer analgesia if appropriate.

Gait

Always start by assessing the patient's gait. Ask the patient to walk a few steps away from you then turn around and come back. While they are standing also ask to inspect their lower back for any deformity or scars suggesting previous surgery.
Signs that may be present include:
- Loss of arm swing and festinant gait (small, shuffling steps and difficulty stopping) – suggestive of Parkinson's disease
- Foot drop – a lower motor neurone lesion of L4-5 (common peroneal nerve)
- A scissoring gait – suggesting spasticity caused by an upper motor neurone lesion

Inspection

They should then be positioned so they are sitting up on a trolley or couch with both of their legs exposed.
Stand at the end of the bed and perform a general inspection. The main features to note are:
- Scars or deformity
- Muscle wasting
- Fasciculation

Tone

To assess tone roll the patient's legs (one at a time) from side to side. Then having ensured there is no pain, flick the patient's knee upwards off the bed and observe whether or not the whole of the distal leg rises off the bed, which would demonstrate hypertonicity. Finally gently roll the patient's ankle and briskly dorsiflex their foot. More than five beats of clonus is considered abnormal.

Power

Tests for limb power aim to isolate individual muscle groups with specific nerve innervations. Each muscle group is tested by asking the patient to perform a specific movement against resistance applied by the doctor performing the examination.

Box 3.5.1 Myotomes of the lower limbs

Movement	Muscle	Root	Nerve
Hip flexion	Iliopsoas	L1-2	Femoral
Hip extension	Gluteus maximus	L5-S1	Inferior gluteal
Knee extension	Quadriceps	L3-4	Femoral
Knee flexion	Hamstrings	S1	Sciatic
Ankle dorsiflexion	Tibialis anterior	L4	Deep peroneal
Ankle plantarflexion	Gastrocnemius	S1-2	Tibial
Big toe extension	Extensor hallucis longus	L5	Deep peroneal

The power is then graded from 0 to 5 based on the Medical Research Council grading system.
0. No movement
1. Flicker of movement visible in muscle
2. Movement but not against gravity
3. Movement against gravity but not against resistance
4. Decreased power against resistance
5. Normal power against resistance

Reflexes

Proceed to test the patient's reflexes using a tendon hammer. While eliciting the reflex ensure adequate exposure to observe the respective muscle for contraction. If you are unable to elicit the reflex after two attempts, try once more while asking the patient to clench their teeth at the moment you use the tendon hammer (this is called reinforcement). The reflexes to test are:

Knee	L3-4
Ankle	S1-2
Plantar	If toes extend this is Babinski's sign indicating an upper motor neurone lesion.

Sensation

Sensation should ideally be tested in all modalities: pain (pinprick), light touch, vibration, temperature and proprioception. Assess each dermatome in turn (**Figure 3.5.1**). It is not normally expected to test temperature sensation during an examination:
- Check light touch with cotton wool. The skin should be touched but not stroked
- Pain (pinprick) should be tested with a neuro tip

For both light touch and pain the patient should be shown what sensation to expect on a neutral part of their body before starting the examination. The easiest way to do this is to touch their face or upper chest with the cotton wool or neuro tip beforehand so they are aware of what the normal sensation should feel like.

Figure 3.5.1 Lower limb dermatomes.

Vibration is tested using a 128 Hz tuning fork. Ask the patient to say whether the tuning fork is vibrating or not. Place it over a distal bony prominence (e.g. Great toe interphalangeal joint) and move proximally until they can correctly identify vibration.

Finally proprioception is tested by assessing joint position sense. This is achieved by flexing or extending a distal joint while the patient has their eyes closed and asking them if the distal part is moving up or down. If the patient cannot correctly identify this movement move to a more proximal joint until they can do so.

Coordination

Ask the patient to lift one of their feet and hold it in the air above the contralateral knee. Then ask them to slide it down the front of the shin as far as the ankle and keep repeating the process. Then ask them to do the same with the other foot.

Ending the examination

Thank the patient, help them redress and ensure they are comfortable.
Tell the examiner you would like to:
- Examine the remainder of the peripheral nervous system

Scenario

Mr Carlisle is a 68-year-old retired man complaining of difficulty walking. Perform a neurological examination of his legs and explain your findings and a management plan to him.

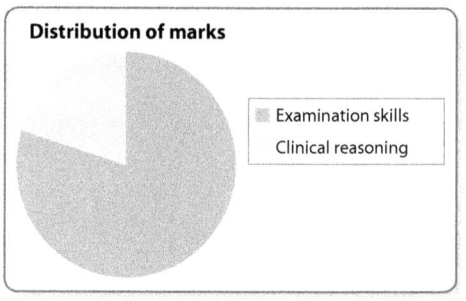

Distribution of marks
- Examination skills
- Clinical reasoning

Mark sheet	Achieved	Not achieved
Introduces self to patient appropriately		
Confirms patient identity		
Explains reason for examination and obtains consent		
Enquires regarding presence of pain and offers analgesia if needed		
Cleans hands appropriately		
Positions and exposes patient correctly		
Performs initial inspection from end of bed		
Inspects lower limbs for scars, wasting, fasciculation		
Assesses tone in lower limbs		
Assesses power in lower limbs		
Assesses reflexes in lower limbs		
Assesses sensation in lower limbs		
Assesses coordination in lower limbs		
Asks patients to walk, assesses gait		
Thanks patient and offers to help patient redress		
Correctly identifies clinical signs		
Correctly states diagnosis		
Describes appropriate management plan		
Global mark from patient		
Global mark from examiner		

Suggested reading

Michael O'Brien. Aids to the examination of the peripheral nervous system (5th edn). Philadelphia: Saunders Ltd; 2010.

3.6 Cranial nerve examination

Begin by introducing yourself, washing your hands, confirming the name of the patient and asking for permission to examine them.

Ask if the patient has any pain and offer analgesia if appropriate.

You should position yourself directly opposite the patient. This is particularly important for the examination of visual fields when the patient's visual fields are compared to your own.

General inspection

Begin by performing a general inspection of the patient's face. Possible findings are:
- Ptosis
- Unequal pupils
- Facial asymmetry/weakness
- Scars

Where possible examine each cranial nerve in turn. By using a clear and reproducible pattern it is less likely any steps will be forgotten.

Cranial nerve 1 (olfactory)

It is unlikely you will be expected to examine this nerve. However ask the patient if they have noticed any problems with their sense of smell.

Cranial nerve 2 (optic)

Visual acuity

Ask the patient to cover each eye in turn and read the letters on a Snellen chart. A near vision Snellen chart is read at 30 cm, whereas a normal Snellen chart is read at 6 m. If they are unable to read letters assess their ability to count fingers, and if not possible their ability to see movement. If neither of these is possible assess their ability to see light using a torch.

Decreased visual acuity may be due to refractive errors (which will be corrected using a pinhole), anterior eye disease, retinal disease or pathology of the optic nerve.

Colour impairment is assessed using Ishihara charts and comparing one eye with the other, or by comparing the intensity between eyes of the colour of a bright red object such as a child's toy. Although this can be mentioned it is not normally expected in examinations.

Visual fields

Position yourself directly opposite the patient, approximately one arm's length away from them. Ask them to look at you and cover one of their eyes. Cover your corresponding eye opposite the one they have covered. Move your free hand with one outstretched finger (or a white hatpin) in from the corner of the upper and lower quadrant of the visual field and ask the patient to say when they first see your finger. This assesses the temporal (lateral) quadrants. To assess the nasal (medial) you will need to swap the hand covering your eye and then using your free hand repeat the process. Then repeat these steps for the opposite eye.

Pupils

Begin by checking the pupils are equal in size. A small pupil may suggest Horner's syndrome while a large pupil and ptosis suggest a third nerve palsy. Check the direct and consensual light reflexes and swing the light from one eye to the other to assess for a relative afferent pupillary defect. To check accommodation, ask the patient to look at an object behind you over your shoulder. Then hold a finger or object in front of their nose and ask them to look at it. As the pupils converge they should constrict.

Fundoscopy

Be prepared to perform fundoscopy though due to time constraints it may not be expected as part of this examination.

Cranial nerves 3 (oculomotor), 4 (trochlear) and 6 (abducens)

These nerves are responsible for eye movement and are examined together. Ask the patient to keep their head still but keep looking at your index finger. In the air in front of the patient slowly write a letter H in the air with your finger and ask them to tell you if they experience any double vision. Also while doing this watch their eyes for nystagmus or ptosis.
- A third cranial nerve lesion results in ptosis (levator palpebrae weakness), an unresponsive dilated pupil (due to disruption of parasympathetic fibres) and the eye being held in a down and out position
- A fourth cranial nerve lesion results in weakness of the superior oblique muscle and causes double vision when the patient looks down and in
- A sixth cranial nerve lesion results in weakness of the lateral rectus muscle and causes double vision on lateral gaze to the side of the lesion

Cranial nerve 5 (trigeminal)

This nerve provides motor innervations to the muscles of mastication, and sensation to the face.
- To assess the motor component of this nerve ask the patient to clench their teeth together. Palpate the temporal and masseter muscles assessing for equal contraction and any wasting
- To assess the sensory component of this nerve assess light touch and pin prick sensation in the distribution of the nerve's three branches (ophthalmic, maxillary and mandibular)
- Comment on the need to check the corneal reflex and jaw jerk though to maintain patient comfort these are rarely performed. The corneal reflex is tested by touching the cornea with a piece of cotton wool

Cranial nerve 7 (facial)

This nerve supplies the motor component of the muscles associated with facial expression.

Note any facial asymmetry with particular attention to forehead wrinkling and the nasolabial folds. Ask the patient to raise both their eyebrows, close both their eyes, show you their teeth, smile and then puff out their cheeks. Paralysis of the whole side of the face is caused by a lower motor neurone lesion. If the forehead is spared this is an upper motor neurone lesion as the forehead is innervated bilaterally by the upper motor neurones.

This nerve also supplies the stapedius muscle and a lesion results in hyperacusis. It also supplies taste sensation to the anterior two-thirds of the tongue.

Cranial nerve 8 (auditory)

Rinne's test compares air versus bone conduction. Strike a 256-Hz or 512-Hz tuning fork and place it next to the external auditory meatus. Then place the base of the tuning fork on the mastoid process and ask the patient which sounds loudest. If bone conduction is better this suggests conductive deafness which is often due to middle ear disease or ear wax.

Weber's test requires the tuning fork to be struck and then placed in the middle of the forehead or vertex of the skull. In conductive deafness sound is louder in the affected ear while with sensorineural deafness it is louder in the unaffected ear.

Cranial nerves 9 (glossopharyngeal), 10 (vagus) and 12 (hypoglossal)

The ninth cranial nerve mainly provides sensation to the posterior third of the tongue while the tenth is a motor nerve supplying the muscles of the palate, larynx and pharynx. Together they respectively form the afferent and efferent limbs of the gag reflex.

Assess for symmetry of the palate and uvula when the patient says 'aah'. Also comment on the need to test the gag reflex.

The twelfth nerve is a motor nerve supplying the tongue. Inspect the tongue and look for any fasciculation. Then ask the patient to protrude it. It will deviate towards the side of a lesion.

Cranial nerve 11 (accessory)

Assess power in the trapezius by asking the patient to shrug their shoulders against resistance. Then assess power in each sternocleidomastoid by asking the patient to turn their head to each side against resistance.

Ending the examination

Finally thank the patient and ensure they are comfortable. If relevant offer to examine the peripheral nervous system.

Common cases

Seventh nerve palsy

This leads to a side of the face being paralysed. Patients are unable to close their affected eye or raise their eyebrow. The nasolabial fold is absent and the mouth droops. If the weakness is caused by an upper motor neurone lesion such as a stroke the forehead is spared as it receives bilateral upper motor neurone innervations. If however the problem is a lower motor neurone lesion the forehead will also be weak.

Causes include:
- Bell's palsy
- Ramsay Hunt syndrome
- Pontine tumours
- Acoustic neuroma
- Cholesteatoma
- Parotid tumours or infection

Third nerve palsy

A third nerve palsy results in a dilated pupil, ptosis and a pupil pointing down and outwards. Parasympathetic fibres run on the outside of the third cranial nerve. Thus compression of the nerve leading to interruption of these fibres, by an intracerebral aneurysm or tumour causes a dilated pupil.

Horner's syndrome

This condition is caused by interruption of the sympathetic chain. It has four features:
1. Ptosis
2. Miosis
3. Anhydrosis
4. Enophthalmos

A lesion can occur anywhere along the sympathetic chain and it's easiest to divide causes anatomically:

- Brainstem — Stroke, tumour, demyelination
- Spinal cord — Syringomyelia, trauma
- Thoracic outlet — Pancoast's tumour, cervical rib
- Carotid artery — Aneurysm, dissection

Cerebellopontine angle syndrome

This condition manifests as a mixture of signs affecting the fifth, seventh and eighth cranial nerves. Loss of facial sensation, the corneal reflex and sensorineural hearing loss should alert you to this possible diagnosis. Signs may vary considerably. Common causes are an acoustic neuroma or meningioma at the cerebellopontine angle.

Scenario

Mrs Smith has not been feeling well with a headache for a few days. She is now saying something 'is not right' with her face. Examine her cranial nerves and explain the likely diagnosis and a management plan to her.

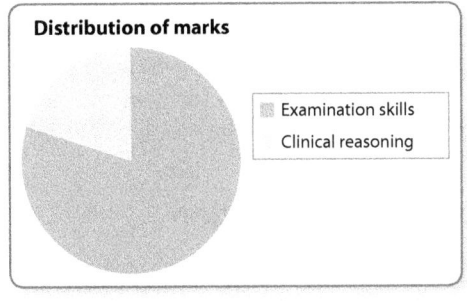

Distribution of marks
- Examination skills
- Clinical reasoning

Mark sheet	Achieved	Not achieved
Introduces self to patient appropriately		
Confirms patient identity		
Explains reason for examination and obtains consent		
Enquires regarding presence of pain and offers analgesia if needed		
Cleans hands appropriately		
Positions self directly opposite patient		
Performs initial inspection for scars and facial asymmetry		
Comments on the need to test sense of smell		
Assesses visual acuity of each eye		
Assesses visual fields in each eye		
Assesses pupillary reflexes		
Comments on the need to perform fundoscopy		
Assesses for ptosis		
Assesses eye movement and asks regarding diplopia		
Assesses power in masseter and temporalis muscles		
Assesses sensation in all three zones of face, comparing both sides		
Comments on need to check corneal and jaw jerk reflexes		
Assesses facial movements/power		
Asks about altered taste		
Assesses hearing in each ear using the Weber and Rinne tests		
Examines uvula and comments on checking the gag reflex		
Assess power of the trapezius muscles		
Asks patient to protrude tongue and check for wasting and deviation		
Correctly identifies clinical signs		
Correctly states diagnosis		
Describes appropriate management plan		
Global mark from patient		
Global mark from examiner		

3.7 Respiratory examination

Begin by introducing yourself, washing your hands, confirming the name of the patient and asking for permission to examine them.
   Ask if the patient has any pain and offer analgesia if appropriate.
   The patient should be positioned at 45° with their chest and neck exposed.

General inspection

Stand at the end of the bed and perform a general inspection. The main features to note are:
- The patient's general appearance and level of comfort
- The presence of any chest wall deformities
- Is the patient breathless? Are they using accessory muscles?
- The respiratory rate should be counted at this point, also make a note of the breathing pattern and chest wall movement
- Are there any scars indicating previous interventions (surgery, chest drains, pleural aspiration)?
- The presence of any medical equipment or medication (sputum pot, inhaler, nebuliser, oxygen)

Hand inspection

The next step is to inspect the hands for:
- Clubbing (present in lung malignancy, fibrosing alveolitis, mesothelioma and chronic suppurative lung diseases such as bronchiectasis and cystic fibrosis)
- Peripheral cyanosis as indicated by a bluish discolouration of the fingers
- Tar staining indicating a significant smoking history
- Wasting of the hand may indicate a Pancoast's tumour (with brachial plexus invasion)

Pulses

Ask the patient to hold their arms out with wrists extended and check for a flap from CO_2 retention.
   Palpate the radial pulse to assess the heart rate and whether or not the pulse is bounding in nature.

Head and neck examination

Move up to the patient's face and inspect for:
- Horner's syndrome which may suggest a Pancoast's tumour
- Central cyanosis as indicated by a bluish discolouration of the tongue
- Pursed lip breathing which may suggest chronic obstructive pulmonary disease

Move to the patient's neck:
- Assess the jugular venous pressure (JVP). If elevated and pulsatile it may suggest cor pulmonale. If elevated and non-pulsatile this may be a sign of superior vena cava obstruction
- Palpate the trachea to assess its position in the suprasternal notch

- Palpate for cervical lymphadenopathy. This is best done with the patient sat forward while standing behind them

Chest examination

The chest should be examined next. Having just sat the patient forward, it is likely to be easier to start with the posterior chest wall. Remember to inspect again for any scars that may be on the patient's back and not visible anteriorly (there may be valuable information to gain from this further inspection and for this reason also it may be wise to start by examining the posterior chest). This minimises the number of times the patient is required to move. Whether you start with the anterior or posterior chest wall completely examine the chosen chest wall before moving on, thus again minimising the number of times the patient moves forwards and backwards. The main steps when examining the chest are:
- **Palpation (chest expansion):** place your hands onto each side of the chest with fingers parallel to the ribs and thumbs just off the skin in the midline. As the patient inhales make a note of the distance your thumbs move away from each other. Unilaterally decreased chest expansion indicates abnormal pathology on the affected side
- **Percussion:** as with each step of the chest examination compare the right and left side at the same level. Percuss anteriorly over the clavicles, the right and left upper and lower chest and then in the axillae. Posteriorly percuss both sides at three separate levels. Make note of whether the percussion note sounds dull, resonant or hyper-resonant
- **Auscultation:** as for percussion compare left and right at each level (**Figure 3.7.1**). This is traditionally performed using the diaphragm of the stethoscope though in the supraclavicular fossa when listening to the lung apices the bell may fit better

To assess vocal resonance listen to each area again while asking the patient to say 'ninety nine'. Areas of consolidation increase the audible sound while an effusion leads to diminished vocal resonance.

Figure 3.7.1 Positions for chest auscultation.

Finally ensure you have assessed for signs of cor pulmonale. To do this you should check for sacral oedema while examining the back and at the end of your examination check for pedal oedema.

Ending the examination

Thank the patient, help them redress and ensure they are comfortable.
Tell the examiner you would like to:
- Check pulse oximetry
- Check the patient's peak flow if relevant
- See a sputum sample if relevant

Common cases

As with all systems examinations the key to reaching the correct diagnosis is identifying the clinical signs and then using clinical reasoning or pattern recognition to come to a final diagnosis. **Figure 3.7.2** below explains the main clinical findings of several common respiratory conditions.

Pathology	Image	Tracheal deviation	Percussion note	Breath sounds	Vocal resonance
Lung fibrosis		Central	Dull	Bronchial breathing Inspiratory crackles	
Consolidation		Central	Dull	Bronchial breathing Coarse crackles	Increased
Collapse, Lobectomy or Pneumonectomy		Towards side of collapse	Dull	Decreased	Decreased

Cont'd...

Cont'd...

Pathology	Image	Tracheal deviation	Percussion note	Breath sounds	Vocal resonance
Pleural effusion		Central or away from side of effusion	Stony dull	Decreased	Decreased
Pneumothorax		Central or away in tension pneumothorax	Hyper-resonant	Decreased	Decreased

Figure 3.7.2 Common clinical patterns on respiratory examination.

Scenario

Mrs Jones is complaining of increased breathlessness for the past 3 weeks. Examine her respiratory system.

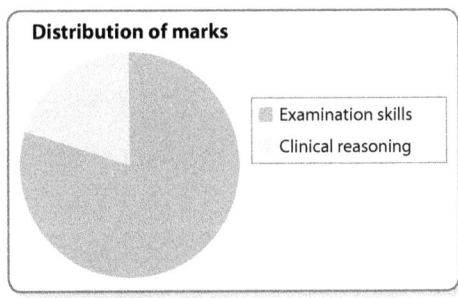

Distribution of marks
- Examination skills
- Clinical reasoning

Mark sheet	Achieved	Not achieved
Introduces self to patient appropriately		
Confirms patient identity		
Explains reason for examination and obtains consent		
Enquires regarding presence of pain and offers analgesia if needed		
Cleans hands appropriately		
Positions and exposes patient correctly		
Performs initial inspection from end of bed		
Inspects hands and fingernails		
Inspects for flap or tremor		

Cont'd...

Cont'd...

Mark sheet	Achieved	Not achieved
Inspects eyes and mouth		
Palpates for lymphadenopathy		
Palpates trachea		
Palpates the apex beat		
Anteriorly – Examines chest expansion		
Anteriorly – Percusses correctly		
Anteriorly – Auscultates correctly		
Anteriorly – Assesses vocal resonance or tactile vocal fremitus correctly		
Posteriorly – Examines chest expansion		
Posteriorly – Percusses correctly		
Posteriorly – Auscultates correctly		
Posteriorly – Assesses vocal resonance or tactile vocal fremitus correctly		
Examines for signs of cor pulmonale		
Comments on need for pulse oximetry, peak flow, arterial blood gas as appropriate		
Thanks patient and offers to help patient redress		
Correctly identifies clinical signs		
Correctly states diagnosis		
Describes appropriate management plan		
Global mark from patient		
Global mark from examiner		

3.8 Thyroid examination

As well as examining the thyroid gland this examination normally includes an assessment of thyroid status, i.e. deciding if the patient is hypo-, eu- or hyperthyroid.

Begin by introducing yourself, washing your hands, confirming the name of the patient and asking for permission to examine them.

Ask if the patient has any pain and offer analgesia if appropriate.

General inspection

The patient should be positioned so they are sat upright with their neck exposed. Position yourself opposite the patient and perform a general inspection. The main features to note are:
- The patient's general appearance, e.g. flushing might indicate hyperthyroidism, whereas an obese, hirsute patient might be hypothyroid
- Any visible neck swelling
- The presence of any scars on the neck suggesting previous surgery

Hand inspection

The next step is to inspect the hands for:
- Thyroid acropachy (similar to clubbing)
- Onycholysis, palmar erythema or clamminess suggesting hyperthyroidism
- A resting tremor when the hands are held outstretched. This can be made easier to see by placing a piece of paper over the hands. A tremor again suggests hyperthyroidism

Pulses

Palpate the radial pulse to assess the rate and rhythm. In hyperthyroidism there may be sinus tachycardia or atrial fibrillation.

Head and neck examination

Examine the patient's eyes for:
- Loss of the outer third of the eyebrow which can occur in hypothyroidism
- Exophthalmos – where the sclera is visible between the iris and lower eye lid (caused by autoimmune thyroid disease)
- Proptosis – where the eyeball is seen to protrude from the orbit when standing behind the patient and looking from above (the distinction between proptosis and exophthalmos is often unclear – some suggest it signifies the amount of displacement of the eyeball while others use exophthalmos when the cause is an endocrinopathy)
- Lid retraction – where the sclera is visible between the iris and upper eye lid
- Lid lag – where the eyelid 'lags' behind the globe on downward gaze (lid lag and lid retraction are a result of increased sympathetic activity, which in this context may be caused by hyperthyroidism)
- Eye movements – ophthalmoplegia resulting in diplopia occurs in Graves' disease due to infiltration and inflammation of the ocular muscles

Next, stand behind the patient and palpate the thyroid gland. Try to ascertain the gland's size and texture. Also note if it is smooth or nodular.

Ask the patient to take a sip of water and hold it in their mouth. Then palpate the swelling again and ask the patient to swallow. A thyroid mass will rise on swallowing. Then ask the patient to protrude their tongue and if the mass rises it may be a thyroglossal cyst.

Palpate for any cervical lymphadenopathy and if present clarify whether the nodes are tender, soft and mobile or hard and fixed. Depending on their nature they may represent an inflammatory process or malignancy.

Next palpate the trachea to check if it is central or deviated to one side.

Percuss down the sternum to assess whether any thyroid swelling extends retrosternally.

Auscultate over the swelling for a bruit which can occur in Graves' disease.

Inspect the patient's lower limbs for pretibial myxoedema. This occurs in Graves' disease and causes waxy indurated plaques over the shins, though they can also occur on other areas of the body. They are normally painless.

Finally offer to elicit peripheral reflexes which may be brisk in hyperthyroidism or slow relaxing in hypothyroidism.

Ending the examination

Thank the patient, help them redress as necessary and ensure they are comfortable.
Tell the examiner you would like to arrange:
(This will vary depending on the history provided and the clinical findings elicited)
- Electrocardiography
- Blood tests (full blood count, electrolytes, liver function tests, erythrocyte sedimentation rate, thyroid function tests)
- A review by an endocrinologist
- Imaging of the thyroid which may be an ultrasound, CT scan or MRI

Common cases

Hyperthyroidism

If provided, a history may describe restlessness, feeling shaky, palpitations, sweating, heat intolerance, and weight loss. Clinical signs may be agitation, a tremor, palmar erythema and clamminess, tachycardia and/or atrial fibrillation, lid lag and lid retraction. A goitre may be present. Causes include:
- Toxic multinodular goitre
- Toxic adenoma
- Graves' disease
- Thyroiditis
- Excess thyroxine

Hypothyroidism

If provided, a history may describe lethargy, weight gain, cold intolerance, muscular aches and constipation. Clinical signs may include dry skin and hair with a coarse appearance, peripheral oedema, signs of heart failure and slow relaxing reflexes. Again, a goitre may be present. Causes may be:

- Autoimmune
- Thyroiditis
- Iodine deficiency
- Following treatment for hyperthyroidism

Graves' disease

This is an autoimmune disease in which there are antibodies that stimulate TSH receptors. The antibodies also cross react with orbital tissue causing multiple eye signs. The patient's thyroid status may vary but there are some signs specific to this disease process:
- Proptosis and ophthalmoplegia
- A bruit over the thyroid
- Pretibial myxoedema

Thyroid mass

Based on their characteristics thyroid masses can be divided into:
Diffuse goitres
- Graves' disease
- Thyroiditis (Hashimoto's or subacute)
- Physiological (non-toxic) goitre
- Lymphoma

Nodular
- Toxic multinodular goitre
- Carcinoma
- Cyst
- Adenoma

Scenario

Miss Carla Sadek, a 28-year-old receptionist has attended the ED feeling clammy and experiencing palpitations for a few days. Examine her thyroid gland and explain your diagnosis and a management plan to her.

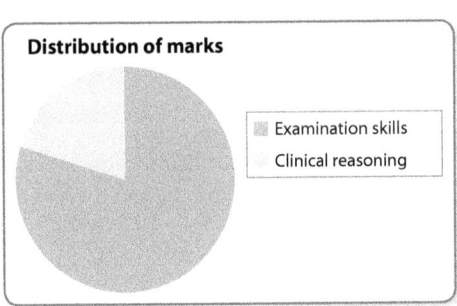

Distribution of marks

- Examination skills
- Clinical reasoning

Mark sheet	Achieved	Not achieved
Introduces self to patient appropriately		
Confirms patient identity		
Explains reason for examination and obtains consent		
Enquires regarding presence of pain and offers analgesia if needed		
Cleans hands appropriately		
Positions and exposes patient correctly		

Cont'd...

Cont'd...

Mark sheet	Achieved	Not achieved
Performs initial inspection from end of bed		
Assesses thyroid status:		
– inspects fingers for signs of thyroid acropachy		
– assesses hands for resting tremor and clamminess		
– palpates radial pulse to assess rate and rhythm		
– examines eyes for proptosis/exophthalmos		
– examines eye movements and checks for lid lag/retraction		
– inspects lower limbs for pretibial myxoedema		
– examines reflexes		
Assesses thyroid gland:		
– inspects neck swelling from in front of patient		
– palpates for tracheal deviation		
– palpates neck swelling from behind patient		
– assesses swelling's mobility on swallowing (with water), and when protruding tongue		
– auscultates swelling for bruit		
– examines for retrosternal extension of swelling by percussion		
Thanks patient and offers to help patient redress		
Correctly identifies clinical signs		
Correctly states diagnosis		
Describes appropriate management plan		
Global mark from patient		
Global mark from examiner		

3.9 Eye examination

Common eye emergencies include an acute red eye, sudden painful or painless loss of vision, and eye trauma. In all of these a systematic assessment is essential. Although a full ophthalmological examination is not possible in the ED setting, the brief but thorough examination practiced by most emergency physicians should be carried out. Slit lamp examination, tonometry and direct ophthalmoscopy are extensions of the eye examination and should be carried out when appropriate. For the purpose of this OSCE, a scheme of eye examination without these is outlined.

Begin by introducing yourself, washing your hands, confirming the name of the patient and asking for permission to perform the examination. Ask if the patient has any pain and offer analgesia if appropriate. Briefly confirm the patient's presenting symptoms and history. Outline your examination before you start. You may have to apply local anaesthetic eye drops if there is a lot of pain or blepharospasm.

General inspection

As with all facial examinations it is best to perform this by direct confrontation, i.e. position yourself so you are directly facing the patient and ideally at the same height. Make note of:

- **External appearance** – is there any asymmetry? Check for ptosis, proptosis or head positioning as compensation. Is the patient photophobic? Is there any obvious squint?
- **Lids, lacrimation and lashes** – is there any eye lid swelling? Is it localised or is it diffuse? Is there excessive lacrimation or are the eyes dry? Is there any blepharitis with swollen lid margin? Are the lids properly positioned or is there any ectropion? Look at the conjunctiva for any follicles or granulomas as signs of allergy or infection
- **Cornea, conjunctiva and sclera** – is the cornea hazy or clear? Are there any foreign bodies visible? Does the sclera look white or icteric? Are the blood vessels normal or dilated? Is there any subconjunctival haemorrhage? Is there any conjunctival oedema? Always evert the eyelids (**Figure 3.9.1**) and check the fornices for foreign bodies or pustular discharge. Corneal ulceration and abrasions can be highlighted with fluorescein. Are the changes unilateral or bilateral?

Visual acuity

Check both far and near vision.
- **Far vision** – check this by using a Snellen chart. The patient stands at 6 metres from it (or 3 metres from a mirror, reading a reflection of the chart). Test one eye at a time while occluding the other without pressing on it. Check the vision with glasses (if the patient wears them) and with pinhole correction. Visual acuity is recorded as distance from the chart (i.e. 6) as the numerator over the number of the lowest line read as the denominator
- **Near vision** – check each eye individually using a near-vision Snellen chart or ask the patient to read a newspaper at reading distance. If necessary patients should use their reading glasses for presbyopia correction

Figure 3.9.1 Everting the eyelid.

Visual fields

- **Confrontation method (Figure 3.9.2)** – position yourself directly opposite the patient, approximately one arm's length away from them. Ask the patient to look at you and cover one of their eyes. Cover your eye opposite the one they have covered. Move your free hand with one outstretched finger (or a white hatpin) inwards from the corner of the upper and lower quadrant of the visual field and ask the patient to say when they first see the finger or pin. This assesses the temporal (lateral) quadrants. To assess the nasal (medial) quadrants, swap the hand covering your eye and then using your free hand repeat the process. Then repeat these steps for the opposite eye
- **Neglect** – check if the patient is neglecting one side relative to the other. While in the same position as before, ask patient to look at your nose. Hold both your hands in the upper outer visual fields and move the fingers of either one or both. Ask the patient which one is moving. When moving both hands if the patient only recognises movement on one side, they may be neglecting the other side. This can be a sign of stroke or trauma

Pupils

An implanted intraocular lens appears as a shimmering light in the pupil when the eye moves. Check for shape, size and symmetry of the pupil. Previous surgery may make it look irregular, dilated and fixed. Check pupillary reflexes:
- **Direct reflex** – pupil constricts in response to light shone in the eye
- **Consensual reflex** – pupil constricts in response to light shone in the contralateral eye

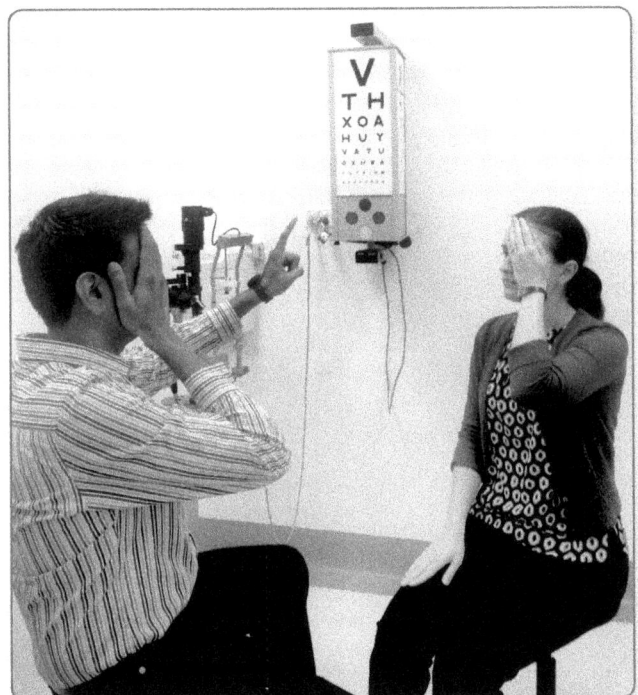

Figure 3.9.2 Confrontation method to check visual fields.

- **Accommodation** – pupils constrict when focusing from far to near objects. To check accommodation, ask the patient to look at an object on the facing wall. Then hold a finger or object in front of their nose and ask them to look at it. As the pupils converge they should constrict
- **Swinging light reflex** – when a light is shone in one eye and then moved to shine in the other eye, both pupils should stay constricted due to the direct and consensual pathways. In a relative afferent pupillary defect (RAPD), when the light is shone in the affected eye the pupillary constriction is notably subtler and may give the impression that the pupils have in fact dilated

Fundoscopy

Check the red reflex from approximately 30 cm. Check systematically the retina, optic disc and macula. Details of this examination are in described in section 6.17.

Eye movements

Ask the patient to keep their head still but to keep looking at your index finger. In the air in front of the patient write a letter H with your finger and ask them to tell you if they experience any double vision. Normally eyes pursue the finger smoothly. Observe the eyes for nystagmus or ptosis.

Ending the examination

Thank the patient and ensure they are comfortable. Comment on the need to complete the examination by examining the eyes with a slit lamp and checking the intraocular pressure using tonometry. Mention that colour vision should also be tested using Ishihara charts.

Scenario

Mrs Galloway is a 32-year-old woman who presents with red eyes. Examine her eyes, give a differential diagnosis and explain a management plan to her.

Distribution of marks
- Communication skills
- Examination skills
- Clinical reasoning

Mark sheet	Achieved	Not achieved
Introduces self to patient appropriately		
Confirms patient identity		
Explains reason for examination and obtains consent		
Cleans hands appropriately		
Confirms history – red eyes		
Positions self directly opposite patient		
Performs initial inspection		
Checks visual acuity – far vision		
Checks visual acuity – near vision		
Checks visual fields		
Checks pupillary reflexes		
Performs fundoscopy – checks red reflex		
Performs fundoscopy – checks each eye systematically		
Checks eye movements		
Comments on need to evert eyelids		
Comments on need for slit lamp examination		
Describes appropriate differential diagnosis and management plan		
Global marks from patient		
Global marks from examiner		

Chapter 4

Joint examination

4.1 Introduction
4.2 Ankle and foot examination
4.3 Back examination
4.4 Elbow examination
4.5 Hand examination
4.6 Hip examination
4.7 Knee examination
4.8 Neck examination
4.9 Shoulder examination

4.1 Introduction

When approaching a joint examination objective structured clinical examination (OSCE), begin as always by introducing yourself to the patient, clarifying the purpose of the meeting, offering analgesia and cleaning your hands. It may be appropriate to take a brief focused history to confirm certain points:
- The information in the scenario brief
- The mechanism of injury, if any
- Occupation
- Hand dominance (in the case of upper limbs)

However, if the purpose of the OSCE is to perform an examination, you must not spend too much time taking a history as this will earn few marks and consume valuable time. A useful format for limb and joint examinations is:
- Inspection
- Palpation
- Movement:
  - Active movement
  - Passive movement
  - Grading muscular power
- Special tests
- Neurovascular assessment

Inspection

- **General resting posture and/or gait:** general attitude of the limb (limb positioning)—this provides clues to tendon injury, disc prolapse, fracture, muscle weakness
- **Skin:** scars, sinuses, swellings, contractures, erythema/colour change, atrophy, loss of hair or nail, ulceration
- **Subcutaneous tissue:** oedema, contractures, haematoma, swellings
- **Muscle and tendons:** atrophy, hypertrophy, contractures, bulge (Popeye sign of biceps rupture), tendon ruptures, muscle haematoma
- **Bone:** deformity, swelling, shortening
- **Joint:** deformity, shortening, contractures, effusion

Ideally expose the entire limb that is being examined and the opposite limb to compare the findings. Ask for a chaperone as appropriate. It is advisable to expose the limb above the elbows for a hand examination and above the knees for an ankle and foot examination.

A deformity is described by the position of the part distal to the deformity. Therefore, if the tibia is more medially angulated than normal at the knee, then it is a genu varum deformity (**Figure 4.1.1**). If the apex of the deformity is in the tibia, then it is tibia vara. This can be decided with the patient in the standing or supine position. In this case, if the medial malleoli are approximated, the knees cannot touch each other. The opposite is genu valgum.

Positioning limbs correctly before comparing them is essential not to miss subtle abnormalities. Deformities at the elbow can easily be missed if the forearm remains in a mid-prone position. They become more apparent when the forearm is placed in full supination.

Figure 4.1.1 Genu varum.

For this reason, a limb should be placed in as close to anatomical position as possible when inspecting it.

For the lower limb examination, if the patient can walk, inspection of gait gives valuable clues to the site of any pathology. Common gait abnormalities are an antalgic gait, Trendelenburg gait, and a high-stepping gait (these are discussed further in section 4.6). Some deformities are dynamic and watching the patient walk will expose the extent of the deformity and any compensation that the patient offers to accommodate the deficit.

Changes in the limb can be due to pathology anywhere in the skin (burns), subcutaneous tissue (oedema), muscle (haematomas), tendon (tenosynovitis or tendon rupture), bones (fracture, osteosarcoma), joints (arthritis, joint effusion), blood vessels (venous and ischaemic ulceration) or nerves (diabetic neuropathy). For example, a swollen leg could be due to deep vein thrombosis, gastrocnemius haematoma or cellulitis, or foot drop can be because of common peroneal nerve injury, ankle sprain or an Achilles tendon injury. Careful consideration of any abnormality is important and a systematic inspection focusing on skin, muscle, bone and joint changes will help to localise the pathological process.

Palpation

Most joints are directly palpable (apart from the hip) and palpation gives valuable information about the nature of any pathology by assessing for the presence of tenderness, warmth or swelling.

Warn the patient you are going to touch them and enquire about the presence of pain. Begin with general palpation of the area in question using the palmar (to check for tenderness) and dorsal (to assess for warmth) aspect of the examining hand. This helps to confirm any inspection findings and gain patient confidence as long as caution is taken not to hurt them.

After this initial step, palpate the joint more systematically. Palpate bony landmarks, muscle and tendon groups and any major nerves, focussing on one point at a time when eliciting tenderness. Localised tenderness usually suggests an injury or inflammation of a particular structure, whereas diffuse tenderness is usually seen when there is a more general process like cellulitis or arthritis. Also palpate for a joint effusion if it is appropriate.

Movement

- **Active movement**: the patient should be systematically directed to move the joint themselves. The range of movement can be compared with the normal side to measure the extent of any limitation. Checking active movements first also helps to localise any areas of concern which the clinician can then focus on while checking movements passively
- **Assisted movement**: this is where the patient moves the limb but some assistance may be provided by the examiner to take the joint through its full range of motion. This is especially relevant in shoulder examination when demonstrating a painful arc or a ruptured rotator cuff
- **Passive movement**: after checking active movement, passive movement can then be checked by the examiner moving the limb/joint in question. This is useful as sometimes the patient may not be able to move a limb due to muscle/tendon injury or paralysis. However, the presence of a full passive range of movement indicates the absence of any injury to the joint itself. With passive movement, one should also be able to feel for any crepitus by resting a hand on the joint during movement
- **Power**: finally the power of muscle groups should be tested and graded as per the medical research council scale (see section 3.4). It should be clear as to whether power is reduced because of true neurological weakness or due to pain

Special tests

These tests vary for different joints and assess specific structures around the joint. Regarding the shoulder, special tests assess the rotator cuff, signs of impingement and instability. At the knee, they assess the extensor mechanism, the collateral and cruciate ligaments, and menisci and look for signs of patella-femoral dysfunction. At the hip, they test for fixed deformities, particularly Thomas test for fixed flexion. Similarly, in a hand examination, a detailed assessment of the deep and superficial flexor and extensor tendons and small muscles of the hand are important.

Neurovascular assessment

Finally, an assessment of the neurovascular status of the limb should be performed. Indeed the focus of the OSCE may be on the neurovascular status itself. If this is the case, palpation of pulses and detailed examination of each nerve and its sensory and motor component, should be completed. In case of injuries where there may be underlying nerve or blood vessel injury, this is particularly important, e.g. traumatic knee dislocations have a very high incidence of popliteal artery injury and it would be negligent not to examine the foot pulses.

A quick screening examination of the joint above and below should also be performed if time permits. These can be the source of referred pain especially in children.

Closing the examination

Remember to make sure you leave the patient comfortable, help them redress if necessary and thank them. Demonstrating this respect for the patient is fundamental in clinical practice and in the exam will translate to making a good impression and will contribute to a higher global score.

The above format for joint examinations provides a framework with which the following examinations will be discussed.

4.2 Ankle and foot examination

Begin by introducing yourself, confirming the name of the patient, asking for permission to examine them and cleaning your hands. Ask if the patient has any pain and offer analgesia if appropriate.

Inspection

Inspect for any obvious deformity. A foot that is positioned at a 90° angle to the tibia with both the heel and toes touching the floor is described as plantigrade. Feet can present with many deformities, the commonest of which are equinovarus (ankle in plantar flexion and foot in adduction), pes cavus (high-arched foot), pes planus (flat foot), hallux valgus (lateral deviation of the big toe), hammer toe (fixed flexion of a single IP joint) or claw toes (fixed flexion of all the toes).

Ask the patient to walk. Some deformities are dynamic and become obvious when the patient walks, e.g. foot drop. Foot drop is associated with a high-stepping gait (in order to clear the ground) and a 'slap' of the foot on the floor when it returns to the ground.

Palpation

Begin by palpating the ankle and continue distally to the foot and toes. Important bony and soft tissue landmarks should be palpated. Around the ankle these are the medial and lateral malleoli, anterior talofibular ligament (injured in most ankle sprains), the deltoid ligament, the peroneal, tibialis and Achilles tendons, and the dorsalis pedis and posterior tibial pulses (**Figures 4.2.1 to 4.2.3**).

Proceed to holding the heel square in the palm of your nondominant hand to palpate the foot and toes with the other hand. Important landmarks in the foot are the calcaneum and navicular bones, the base of the fifth metatarsal, head of first and fifth metatarsals, and the individual toes.

Presence of localised tenderness and swelling correlates well with these underlying structures and therefore it is important to relate the signs to them accordingly.

Movement

The ankle and foot comprise a series of joints that should be individually assessed.

The ankle joint is a hinge joint responsible for dorsi and plantar flexion of the foot. The subtalar joint or the talocalcaneal joint is responsible for eversion or inversion of the heel and with it the foot. The midfoot joint (or Lisfranc joint) is the tarsometatarsal joint.

To examine these, with the heel held in the nondominant hand, the examining hand moves the foot in dorsi and plantar flexion to assess the ankle joint. Keep the foot plantigrade and ankle fixed with the nondominant hand, move the heel and foot together in inversion and eversion to assess the subtalar joint. Finally to check the midfoot, keep the heel fixed with the nondominant hand and move the forefoot up and down and side to side. Compare the range of movements to the other side. Then the individual toes can be assessed separately.

Figures 4.2.1 and 4.2.2 Ankle and foot anatomical landmarks (medial and lateral views).

Figure 4.2.3 Ankle and foot anatomical landmarks (anterior view).

Special tests

- **Calf squeeze test**: with the patient in the prone position, squeeze the calf noticing any movement of the foot. If the Achilles tendon is intact, the foot will move in plantar flexion
- **Morton's neuroma**: pain in the metatarsal head while walking is termed as metatarsalgia. One of the causes of this pain is a digital nerve neuroma usually in the 3rd or 4th web space. There can be sharp localised pain on the plantar aspect. Occasionally, the neuroma can be felt to move up and down between the metatarsal heads on compressing the forefoot sideways with one hand and feeling for the neuroma with the other

Diagnoses to consider

- **Traumatic diagnoses include**: ankle sprain, fractured base of fifth metatarsal bone, ankle fracture, midfoot fracture, dislocation or fracture of toes, and an Achilles tendon injury
- **Non-traumatic diagnoses include**: osteoarthritis, rheumatoid arthritis, septic arthritis, cellulitis, diabetic foot, acute or chronic ischaemia, tenosynovitis, compartment syndrome, DVT, stroke, spinal cord compression and spina bifida

Scenario

Miss Perkins has come to the ED with a right ankle injury. She was playing football and when she went for a run, she heard a snap and had a shooting pain in the back of her heel. Examine her ankle and explain your diagnosis and a management plan to her.

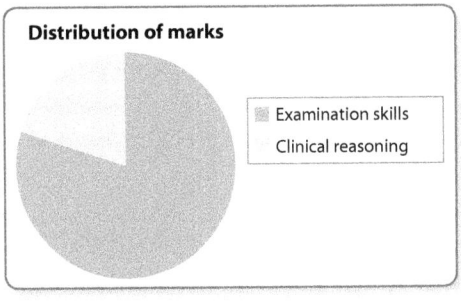

Distribution of marks
- Examination skills
- Clinical reasoning

Mark sheet	Achieved	Not achieved
Introduces self to the patient appropriately		
Confirms the patient identity		
Explains reason for examination and obtains consent		
Enquires regarding presence of pain and offers analgesia if needed		
Confirms the history and asks about mechanism of injury		
Cleans hands appropriately		
Adequate exposure of both legs up to the knee		
Assessment with patient standing:		
– looks from front, back and side for skin changes, deformity, localised or generalised swelling		
– assesses posture on tip toe and heel standing		
– inspects gait and comments on any asymmetry or posture changes		
Assessment with patient sitting:		
– confirm any inspection findings from before		
– palpates in logical manner		
– checks active movement		
– checks passive movements		
– checks power in ankle muscle groups		
– checks integrity of Achilles tendon, performs calf squeeze		
– feels dorsalis pedis and posterior tibial pulse		
Thanks the patient and offers to help the patient redress		
Comments on need to examine joint above and below		
Correctly identifies clinical signs		
Correctly states diagnosis		
Describes appropriate management plan		
Asks if the patient has any questions		
Global mark from the patient		
Global mark from the examiner		

4.3 Back examination

Begin by introducing yourself, confirming the name of the patient, asking for permission to examine them and cleaning your hands. Ask if the patient has any pain and offer analgesia if appropriate.

Inspection

Expose the patient from the waist up. Inspect their back from the side and from behind. Look for any changes suggesting underlying pathology such as scars, redness, or deformities. Spinal deformities may be fixed (due to primary vertebral pathology) or mobile. Mobile deformities can be postural or due to compensating for pain or perispinal problems. For example, a short leg on one side can cause scoliosis and fixed flexion at the hip will cause an exaggerated lumbar lordosis. Mobile deformities disappear with sitting or forward flexion unlike fixed deformities (**Figure 4.3.1**).

- **Scoliosis:** this is lateral curvature of the spine, best seen from the posterior aspect. Mobile scoliosis is commonest due to postural problems. Fixed scoliosis on the other hand is associated with a rib hump that does not disappear with any manoeuvres
- **Kyphosis:** this is anteroposterior curvature of the spine with anterior concavity. It is normal in the thoracic spine. It can be exaggerated in elderly patients (senile kyphosis) with osteoporosis, in teenagers with Scheuermann's disease or in young patients with ankylosing spondylitis. A localised prominent angular kyphosis is usually due to an underlying vertebral fracture

Figure 4.3.1 Back anatomical landmarks.

- **Lordosis**: this is anteroposterior curvature with posterior concavity. It is normal in cervical and lumbar spine and can be obliterated by the presence of pain. Exaggerated lumbar lordosis with a step in the lumbosacral area can indicate underlying spondylolisthesis

Palpation

Palpate from the cervical spinous processes to the base of the spine noting any tenderness warmth, step or deformity.

Movement

Assess flexion by asking the patient to bend forwards as far as they can. Lateral flexion can be assessed by asking the patient to slide their hand down the outside of their leg as far as they can. To assess the degree of rotation, ask them to keep their legs and hips still and turn to each side.

Special tests

Straight leg raising (Lasègue's test)

This test can be done both actively and passively. With the patient supine, the knee is kept extended and the leg is slowly raised with flexion at the hip. Presence of radiating pain in the gluteal region, posterior thigh and calf signifies a positive test. Normally, it should be possible to raise the leg from 80° to 90° flexion without causing any pain. The test is positive if the pain starts below 30° flexion. Forced dorsiflexion of the foot just below the angle where pain starts, may reproduce the pain.

Bowstring test

The examiner lifts the patient's leg as for the straight leg raising test. At the point where the patient feels pain, the knee is flexed without lowering the leg. This should result in relief from pain as tension in the sciatic nerve is reduced. Pressure just behind the lateral femoral condyle on the common peroneal nerve, to stretch it like a bowstring, may reproduce the sharp stabbing pain in the leg. This is more specific for sciatic root entrapment.

Well-leg-raising test

Straight leg raising on the unaffected side reproduces radicular pain in the affected leg. This is highly specific for nerve root irritation and a large central disc prolapse.

Femoral stretch test (reverse Lasègue's test)

The test aims to identify nerve root irritation of high lumbar roots (L2, 3, 4). With the patient in prone position, the knee is passively flexed. If this produces radicular pain and paraesthesia in the anterior thigh, it is suggestive of irritation of the femoral nerve roots. Extension of the hip will further enhance the pain. On full flexion of the knee if the patient has pain and paraesthesia in the ipsilateral gluteal region, this may indicate a more distal disc prolapse.

Joint examination

Neurological examination of the lower limbs is essential to complete any examination of the back. This is discussed in more detail in section 3.5.

Diagnoses to consider

These include musculoskeletal back pain, ankylosing spondylitis, prolapsed vertebral disc, compression fractures, cauda equina syndrome, spinal infections, pyelonephritis, psoas abscess, retroperitoneal haematoma.

Scenario

Mr Singh is a 23-year-old student who has come to the ED with pain and stiffness in his back. Examine his back and explain your diagnosis and a management plan to him.

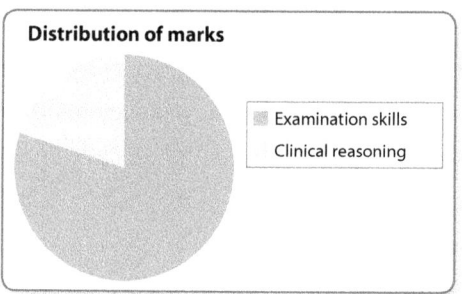

Distribution of marks
- Examination skills
- Clinical reasoning

Mark sheet	Achieved	Not achieved
Introduces self to patient appropriately		
Confirms patient identity		
Explains reason for examination and obtains consent		
Enquires regarding presence of pain and offers analgesia if needed		
Confirms the history and asks about any injury		
Cleans hands appropriately		
Adequate exposure of back		
Assessment with patient standing:		
– inspects from the behind patient		
– inspects from the side of the patient		
– palpates back systematically		
– assesses forward flexion, extension, lateral flexion		
– screens power in legs with standing on heel and toe		
Assessment with patient supine:		
– tests for nerve root tension		
Neurological examination:		
– tone and power		
– reflexes		

Cont'd...

Cont'd...

Mark sheet	Achieved	Not achieved
– sensory examination		
– mentions need for examination of anal tone		
Thanks patient and offers to help patient redress		
Correctly identifies clinical signs		
Correctly states diagnosis		
Describes appropriate management plan		
Asks if patient has any questions		
Global mark from patient		
Global mark from examiner		

4.4 Elbow examination

Begin by introducing yourself, confirming the name of the patient, asking for permission to examine them and cleaning your hands. Ask if the patient has any pain and offer analgesia if appropriate.

Inspection

Ensure the patient's upper limbs are exposed up to their shoulders. Ensure full inspection from the front and behind. It is easy to miss a posterior scar (**Figure 4.4.1**).

Normally there is a slight valgus position at the elbow joint called the carrying angle. This is most pronounced with the elbow in extension and forearm fully supinated. It is approximately 11° in men and 13° in women. Any increase in carrying angle is called cubitus valgus and a decrease is called cubitus varus (**Figure 4.4.2**). The commonest cause of cubitus varus is a non-united supracondylar fracture and of cubitus valgus is a non-united lateral condyle fracture.

Slight hyperextension at the elbow up to 15° is common, especially in women; however if more than that, consider hypermobility syndrome. Hypermobility syndrome is diagnosed by a total score above five in the following scoring system:
- Touch thumb to volar forearm   2
- Dorsiflex little finger >90°   2

Figure 4.4.1 Elbow exposure.

Figure 4.4.2 Cubitus valgus.

- Hyperextension at elbows   2
- Hyperextension at knees   2
- Touch the ground with palms   1
- Maximum total score   9

Palpation

Aim to palpate the bony and soft tissue structures around the elbow. Start from the medial epicondyle, ulnar nerve just behind the medial condyle and olecranon. Move laterally to the lateral condyle, radial head, lateral epicondyle and radial nerve, carefully looking for localised tenderness or swelling. The anterior structures are the biceps tendon, median nerve and brachial artery which are medial to the biceps tendon.

Confirm the relationship of the three prominent bony points namely the medial and lateral epicondyle and the olecranon which should roughly form an isosceles triangle when the elbow is positioned in 90° flexion. These structures lie in a straight line with the elbow extended. A disturbed relationship is seen in a dislocated elbow or elbow fractures. However, it is maintained in supracondylar fractures.

The radial head can be palpated just under the lateral condyle. With the elbow flexed, gentle rotation of the forearm with the examiner's thumb on the radial head, helps to localise and palpate any tenderness. Effusion of the elbow joint can be felt as a fluctuant swelling in the lateral aspect between olecranon, capitellum and the radial head.

Movement

Assess the degree of flexion and extension in the joint actively and passively. Do the same for pronation and supination. Always remember to examine both sides and be attentive to the patient's level of comfort.

Special tests

- **Lateral epicondylitis (tennis elbow):** this is inflammation in the common extensor origin due to movements that involve strong gripping and wrist extension. There is usually tenderness at the lateral epicondyle that increases on full flexion of the elbow, pronation of the forearm and forced dorsiflexion of the wrist
- **Medial epicondylitis (golfer's elbow):** there is tenderness on the medial epicondyle at the common flexor origin. Pain increases with forced extension of wrist with the forearm supinated and elbow flexed. This is less common than lateral epicondylitis

Diagnoses to consider

- Traumatic conditions to consider are fractures or dislocation of elbow, radial head injury or a pulled elbow
- Non-traumatic conditions to consider are golfer's elbow, tennis elbow, olecranon bursitis, osteoarthritis and septic arthritis

Joint examination

Scenario

Miss Reardon is an 18-year-old gymnast who has come to the ED after a fall onto her elbow which has been painful since then. Examine her elbow and discuss your diagnosis and management plan with her.

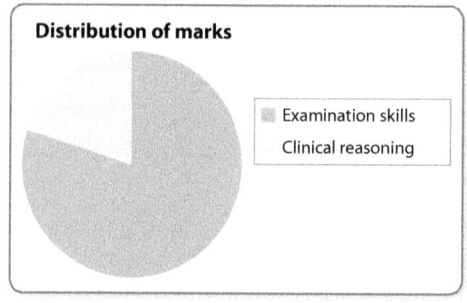

Distribution of marks
- Examination skills
- Clinical reasoning

Mark sheet	Achieved	Not achieved
Introduces self to patient appropriately		
Confirms patient identity		
Explains reason for examination and obtains consent		
Enquires regarding presence of pain and offers analgesia if needed		
Confirms the history of injury		
Cleans hands appropriately		
Exposes both upper limbs		
Inspects arms appropriately		
Checks carrying angle and hyperextension		
Palpates systematically		
Checks active flexion		
Checks active extension		
Checks supination and pronation with elbows flexed at 90°		
Checks for passive range movements		
Checks power of muscle groups		
Performs tests for medial or lateral epicondylitis if relevant		
Palpates brachial and radial pulse		
Screens for ulnar, median and radial nerve motor and sensory functions		
Compares both sides		
Comments on need to examine joint above and below		
Thanks patient and offers to help patient redress		
Correctly identifies clinical signs		
Correctly states diagnosis		
Describes appropriate management plan		
Asks if patient has any questions		
Global mark from patient		
Global mark from examiner		

4.5 Hand examination

Begin by introducing yourself, confirming the name of the patient, asking for permission to examine them and cleaning your hands. Ask if the patient has any pain and offer analgesia if appropriate.

Inspection

Expose both upper limbs to above the elbows and ask the patient to place the hands on a pillow or examination table as appropriate (**Figures 4.5.1** and **4.5.2**).

It is important to notice whether there is a localised or generalised pattern of disease. Rheumatoid hand deformities will involve multiple joints, especially metacarpophalangeal joint (MCPJ) or proximal interphalangeal joints (PIPJ), whereas osteoarthritis will involve distal interphalangeal joints (DIPJ). Skin and nail changes suggest psoriasis (remember psoriatic plaques may be present over the extensor surfaces of the elbow). Clawing suggests ulnar nerve entrapment. Inspect up to the elbows as there may be scars suggestive of nerve injury or evidence of rheumatoid nodule suggesting rheumatoid arthritis.

Localised deformity or swelling could indicate localised trauma, e.g. Boutonniere deformity in a single joint with rest of the hand normal. This could be due to localised

Figures 4.5.1 and 4.5.2 Positions for hand examination.

Figure 4.5.3 Normal finger cascade.

rupture of the extensor tendon due to infection, e.g. septic arthritic, or trauma, e.g. penetrating wound.

Inspection of the neutral position of the fingers (cascade) gives clues to underlying tendon or nerve injury. Normally with the wrists extended, the fingers should gently flex with the MCPJs at approximately 30° flexion at the index finger and 70° flexion at little finger. When the fingers are flexed they should all point towards the same point, normally around the scaphoid bone (**Figure 4.5.3**). Similarly with the wrist flexed, there should be some degree of additional extension at the fingers, maximum in the index and least in little finger. Any change in the cascade can point to an underlying tendon injury.

Next ask the patient to make a fist. The fingers should all curl up, with MCPJs flexed at 90° to the palm. Any tendency of the finger to rotate or trigger can be easily noticed.

Palpation

By light touch compare the temperature of the hands to identify localised areas of warmth. Then systematically palpate the bones and joints. The order is not vital as long as it is clearly systematic, e.g. metacarpals, then each digit, then each joint.

Movement

Testing long flexor tendons

It is important to appreciate certain facts to understand these clinical tests:
1. Flexor digitorum profundus (FDP) flexes the DIPJ and flexor digitorum superficialis (FDS) flexes the PIPJ. Flexion at the MCPJ is affected by the intrinsic muscles of the hand
2. FDP or the deep flexor tendons share a common muscle belly unlike the FDS or the superficial flexor tendons, which have a single muscle belly for each tendon
3. There is sometimes no superficial flexor for the little finger or a separate deep flexor of the index finger
    a. **Testing FDP:** hold the individual finger PIPJ in extension and ask the patient to flex the tip of the finger
    b. **Testing FDS:** since the FDP crosses the PIPJ it needs to be inactivated so the movement at PIPJ is purely by the FDS. By holding the remaining fingers firmly in extension, the FDP is inactivated (all tendons share a common muscle belly, as per number 2 above, and if the rest of the fingers are held in extension, the other can't

work independently). Any flexion at the PIPJ now is due to FDS. There may be a false positive in the little finger as some people do not have a separate FDS tendon to their little finger

In the index finger there is a separate FDP, so holding other fingers in extension won't immobilise the FDP for this finger. Asking the patient to perform a firm pinch keeping the DIPJ in extension confirms that FDS is intact.

Flexor pollicis longus or the long flexor to the thumb is tested by holding the thumb MCPJ in extension and asking the patient to flex the interphalangeal joint.

Testing long extensor tendons

These insert at the base of the proximal phalanx and extend the MCPJs. They continue on the dorsum of the fingers and opposite the PIPJ gives off a central slip and two lateral bands. The central slip helps to extend the PIPJ and lateral bands the DIPJ. They act principally via the intrinsic muscles (therefore, one can still flex the IPJs with the MCPJ in extension). Injury at the MCPJ leads to a characteristic drop finger deformity and the patient will not be able to extend the MCPJ.

- **Elson's test**: the central slip gets injured in small wounds to the back of the PIPJ and if not detected, can lead to a swan neck deformity. To test it, stabilise the finger across the edge of the table, with the PIPJ flexed and ask the patient to extend it. If the slip is functioning, the finger will extend and the DIPJ will be flail. However, if the central slip is ruptured, attempts at extension will cause the DIPJ to extend (via lateral bands)

Injury at the DIPJ leads to a mallet finger deformity with inability to extend the flexed tip of the finger.

Testing the ulnar collateral ligament of the thumb

Gamekeeper's or skier's thumb is excluded by stabilising the metacarpal and stressing the ligament using the examiner's thumb as the fulcrum. Compare both sides and test the normal side first. Any exaggerated laxity suggests injury. This can be difficult to identify when the patient is in pain.

Special tests

- **Kanavel's signs** are seen in infective tenosynovitis with the presence of:
  - Passive flexion posture of finger
  - Fusiform swelling of the finger
  - Intense pain on passive extension
  - Tenderness on palpation
- **Finkelstein's test** for De Quervain's tenosynovitis (inflammation of abductor pollicis longus and extensor pollicis brevis): there is tenderness on the radial styloid and involved tendon sheaths. There might be crepitus. Holding the patient's thumb in their palm in full flexion, followed by adduction of the wrist elicits pain in the radial aspect of the forearm
- **Allen's test**: occlude the radial and ulnar artery and ask the patient to open and close their fist a few times. The hand and fingers should now be pale as all the venous blood will be drained. On releasing the pressure on the ulnar side, the hand should immediately pink up confirming an intact ulnar arterial supply. If it does not pink up in 5–6 seconds, the test is positive and indicates no ulna arterial flow

Any complaints of loss of sensation or weakness should be followed by a detailed neurological assessment. This is discussed in detail in section 3.4.

Functional assessment of the hand

An assessment of what the patient cannot do is informative in terms of impairment. All of these tests are not necessary but may be appropriate.
- Tip pinch – ask the patient to hold a pin firmly between the tip of index finger and thumb
- Side (key) pinch – ask the patient to hold a key between the side of the index finger and thumb
- Power grip – ask the patient to firmly grip a pen in the hand and attempt to take it out
- Hook – assess this by hooking the patient's flexed fingers with your own and attempting to straighten them
- Grasp – ask the patient to pick up a cup or a ball

Simple tasks to assess function are to ask a patient to write with a pen or to undo buttons on their clothing.

Diagnoses to consider

- Traumatic diagnoses include flexor or extensor tendon rupture, ulnar, median or digital nerve injury and thumb ulnar collateral ligament injury
- Nontraumatic diagnoses include tenosynovitis, cellulitis, palmar space infections, septic arthritis, osteo/rheumatoid arthritis, carpal tunnel syndrome, stroke, brachial artery embolism and subclavian thrombosis

Scenario

Miss Monks is a 24-year-old musician. She presents to the ED with a swollen hand and no history of trauma. Examine her hands and explain your differential diagnosis and management plan to her.

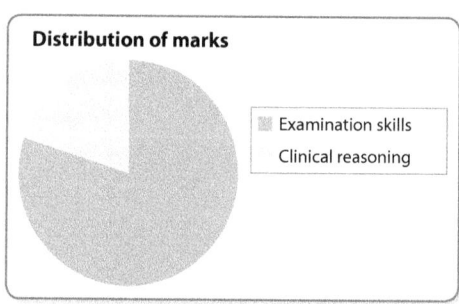

Distribution of marks
- Examination skills
- Clinical reasoning

Mark sheet	Achieved	Not achieved
Introduces self to patient appropriately		
Confirms patient identity		
Explains reason for examination and obtains consent		
Enquires regarding presence of pain and offers analgesia if needed		
Confirms brief history		
Cleans hands appropriately		

Cont'd...

Cont'd...

Mark sheet	Achieved	Not achieved
Exposes both limbs		
Appropriately positions the hands for inspection		
Inspects joints appropriately		
Palpates systematically		
Checks active movements at fingers and thumb		
Checks passive movements at individual joints		
Checks power of superficial and deep tendons appropriately		
Checks power of finger extensors		
Checks ulnar, median and radial nerves sensory component		
Checks ulnar and median nerve motor component		
Checks ulnar collateral ligament stability		
Checks radial pulse and performs Allen's test		
Performs a functional assessment		
Comments on need to examine joint above		
Thanks patient and offers to help patient redress		
Correctly identifies clinical signs		
Correctly states diagnosis		
Describes appropriate management plan		
Asks if patient has any questions		
Global mark from patient		
Global mark from examiner		

4.6 Hip examination

It is important to be able to examine this large joint in an efficient and systematic way eliciting important signs specific to the clinical situation.

Begin by introducing yourself, confirming the name of the patient, asking for permission to examine them and cleaning your hands. Ask if the patient has any pain and offer analgesia if appropriate.

Inspection

It is useful to begin the hip examination by asking the patient to walk and observing their gait for any abnormalities. Before the patient starts to walk, look at both hips and limbs for visible abnormalities, which include scars and muscle wasting. The common gait abnormalities are antalgic and Trendelenburg gaits.

- An antalgic gait is when the patient spends very little time weight-bearing on the affected joint and quickly shifts their weight on the opposite limb
- **Trendelenburg gait**: this occurs due to weakness of hip abductors. When weight-bearing on the joint in question, the patient cannot keep the pelvis stable and has to move their body across the midline to the same side (Trendelenburg lurch) in order to prevent the pelvis from falling to the opposite side. The Trendelenburg test aims to detect this weakness and should be performed after watching the patient walk
- **Trendelenburg test (Figure 4.6.1)**: one method of performing this test is with the patient standing and the examiner sitting or kneeling in front of the patient. The examiner then asks the patient to support themselves by placing their hands on the examiner's shoulders. The examiner holds the patient's pelvis at the anterior superior iliac spines (ASIS) and asks the patient to lift their affected leg and stand on the unaffected leg. This process is repeated with the stance on the affected leg. If the pelvis dips on the unaffected side when standing on the affected side, the test is positive. There can be a false positive if the patient is in pain or cannot weight-bear

Figure 4.6.1 The Trendelenburg test.

Next ask the patient to lie down supine and complete a general inspection of their legs. Then assess leg length:
- Apparent length is measured with the patient lying supine and the legs parallel to each other in the midline. Measure from a fixed point in the midline, which can be the umbilicus (xiphisternum is a long way away and you may not have a tape measure that long) to the medial malleolus (**Figure 4.6.2**)
- True length is measured by correcting any pelvic tilt. Therefore before measuring the true length, one makes sure that the line joining two ASIS is perpendicular to the midline, or the pelvis is squared. One may have to move the affected limb away or towards the midline in order to square the pelvis and then leave the limb in that new position to measure limb length. This is measured from the ipsilateral ASIS to the medial malleolus. This manoeuvre also unmasks any deformity at the hip (abduction or adduction) that is being compensated for with pelvic tilt (**Figure 4.6.3**)

True limb length discrepancy exists when there is an actual difference in the limb length due to loss or gain of bone height. This can be at the level of any joint or bone but most commonly it is the hip that is affected.

Apparent discrepancy exists when there is no actual difference in the length of the bony skeleton but the limb appears short (or long) due to pelvic tilt altering the functional length of the limb. An adduction deformity at the hip causes apparent shortening and an abduction deformity causes apparent lengthening. In these cases when the patient tries to

Figure 4.6.2 Measuring apparent leg length.

Figure 4.6.3 Measuring true leg length.

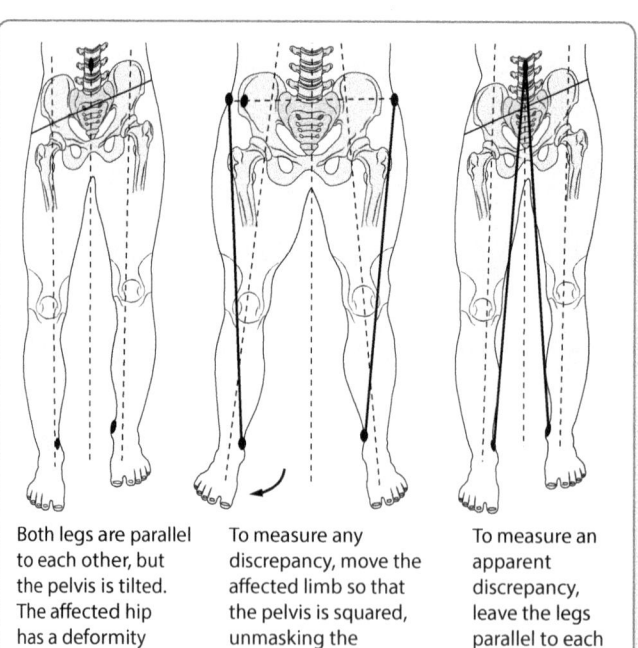

Figure 4.6.4 Measuring leg length discrepancy.

Both legs are parallel to each other, but the pelvis is tilted. The affected hip has a deformity causing apparent lengthening.

To measure any discrepancy, move the affected limb so that the pelvis is squared, unmasking the deformity at the hip.

To measure an apparent discrepancy, leave the legs parallel to each other.

walk, in order to bring the leg to the midline, they compensate by tilting the pelvis causing apparent discrepancy of the limb length (**Figure 4.6.4**).

Palpation

The hip is too deep to palpate reliably. It is however worth palpating the greater trochanter to assess for trochanteric bursitis.

Movement

Assess flexion, extension, internal and external rotation. Passive flexion is tested with the knee at approximately 90° and pushing the knee towards the chest. Extension is best tested by placing your hand under the respective thigh and asking the patient to push it into the bed. Internal and external rotation are also tested with the knee at 90° and by rotating the hip while keeping the knee fixed (**Figure 4.6.5**).

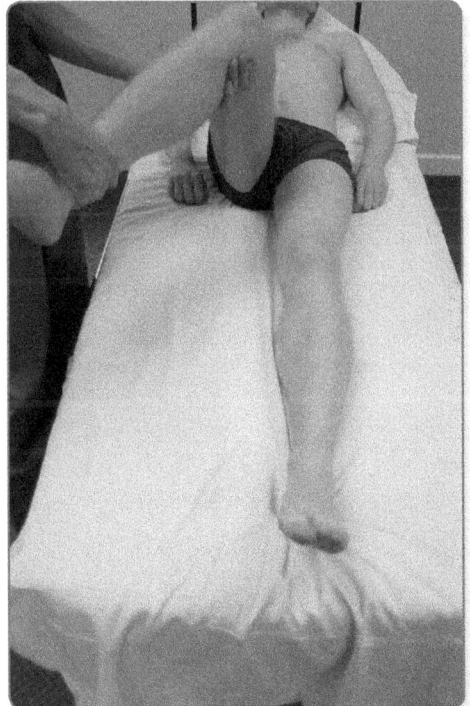

Figure 4.6.5 Assessing internal hip rotation.

Special tests

- **Thomas test**: just like pelvic tilt compensates for abduction or adduction deformity, lumbar lordosis compensates for a flexion deformity at the hip. The aim of the Thomas test is to eliminate this compensation and identify any fixed flexion deformity (**Figures 4.6.6** and **4.6.7**)

While supine, the leg may appear flat on the examination table. Putting a hand under the lumbar spine checks whether the lumbar lordosis is exaggerated or not. This can be further eliminated by flexing the opposite hip. If the affected limb then moves into a flexed position, that means a fixed flexion deformity exists. This can be measured as an angle between the long axes of the thigh to the horizontal plane.

Figure 4.6.6 Thomas test.

Figure 4.6.7 Performing Thomas test.

Diagnoses to consider

Diagnoses to consider during hip examination are listed in **Table 4.6.1**.

Table 4.6.1 Hip examination diagnoses to consider

	Look	Feel	Move	Special tests
Simple groin strain	Antalgic gait No shortening	Tender in the adductor insertion	Pain on abduction, normal range of movements	No fixed deformity
Transient synovitis	Antalgic gait Flexed, abducted, externally rotated leg Apparent lengthening	Tender around the hip joint	Global reduction in all the movements	Thomas test positive
Osteoarthritis	Antalgic gait Flexed and adducted position Apparent shortening	Tender globally	Crepitus Fixed flexion and adduction deformity	Thomas test positive
Slipped capital femoral epiphysis	Antalgic gait Adducted and externally rotated leg True shortening	Tender globally	Limitation of abduction and internal rotation	Thomas test positive
Coxa vara	Trendelenburg gait Muscle wasting in the thigh True shortening	Non-tender unless arthritic	Limited abduction Limited external rotation	

Scenario

Mr Smith is a 39-year-old recreational runner. He presents with left hip pain after his last running session. He is otherwise well and not on any medications. Examine his hip and make a management plan with him.

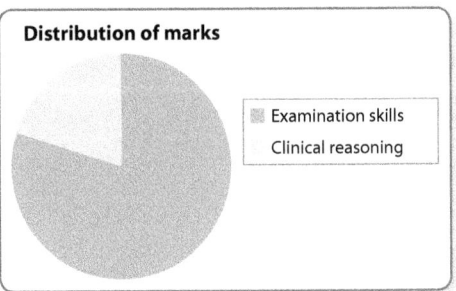

Distribution of marks
- Examination skills
- Clinical reasoning

Mark sheet	Achieved	Not achieved
Introduces self to patient appropriately		
Confirms patient identity		
Explains reason for examination and obtains consent		
Enquires regarding presence of pain and offers analgesia if needed		
Confirms the history briefly		

Cont'd...

Cont'd...

Mark sheet	Achieved	Not achieved
Cleans hands appropriately		
Exposes both lower limbs and lower back		
Assessment with patient standing:		
– looks at the hips from front, side and back		
– inspects the gait		
– performs Trendelenburg test		
Assessment with patient supine:		
– inspects the hips and lower limbs		
– performs palpation		
– measures true and apparent limb length		
– checks active movements at hip		
– checks passive movements systematically		
– performs Thomas test correctly		
– checks the neurovascular status of the limb		
Comments on need to examine the joint above and below		
Thanks patient and offers to help patient redress		
Correctly identifies clinical signs		
Correctly states diagnosis		
Describes appropriate management plan		
Asks if patient has any questions		
Global mark from patient		
Global mark from examiner		

4.7 Knee examination

Begin by introducing yourself, confirming the name of the patient. Ask if the patient has any pain and offer analgesia if appropriate.

Inspection

Inspect both knees with the patient standing. Look for any skin change, swelling or varus (bow legged)/valgus (knock-knee) deformity (**Figures 4.7.1** and **4.7.2**). Inspect from behind the knee to assess the popliteal fossa for any swelling, e.g. Baker's cyst.

Ask the patient to walk and observe their gait. Then ask them to lie down. Again inspect the knees for any visible signs. Then move on to feeling the joint.

Figure 4.7.1 Varus deformity.

Figure 4.7.2 Valgus deformity.

Palpation

Begin by feeling the temperature of the knee with the back of your hand and compare it with the other knee and parts of the leg (**Figure 4.7.3**).

Aim to palpate bony and soft tissue structures and identify areas of localised tenderness. These findings usually relate to underlying anatomy and thus indicate the structures affected. Start medially on the tibial and femoral condyles, tibial collateral ligament and the medial quadriceps. Move on to the quadriceps, patella, patellar tendon and the tibial tuberosity. Finally move to the lateral aspect palpating the lateral femoral condyle, lateral tibial condyle and the head of the fibula.

The joint line is best palpated with the knee in flexion. Keeping the knee in approximately 90° of flexion, identify the hollow on either side of the patellar tendon. The joint line is either

Figure 4.7.3 Palpating the joint for warmth.

side of it, and can be palpated. Move gradually from front to back feeling the tibial plateau and the femoral condyles above. Tenderness on the joint line is usually present in meniscal injuries or ligament sprains. Swellings on the joint line can be from a meniscal cyst which is commoner on the lateral aspect.

Knee effusion

Examine for an effusion of the knee. This is suggested by swelling that fills the juxtapatellar hollows and is likely to be intra-articular. It can extend above the patella and present as suprapatellar swelling (**Figure 4.7.4**).

A small sized effusion will fill up the fossa around the patella, most prominent on the medial side. Firmly squeeze the thigh milking down the fluid in the suprapatellar pouch and maintain the hand in this position. Gently apply pressure to the medial side of the knee and then the lateral side watching for any bulging on the opposite side.

If a larger effusion is suspected, perform a patellar tap. Empty the suprapatellar pouch as described above. With the thumb and fingers of the other hand push the patella sharply down.

Figure 4.7.4 'Milking' a knee effusion out of the suprapatellar pouch.

One can feel it, tap the femoral condyle and then bounce back, indicating fluid in the joint. This is positive for a moderate-size effusion and may be negative in a very tense effusion. During this manoeuvre be attentive to the patient's level of comfort.

Movement

The knee's main movements, flexion and extension should be examined, both actively and passively with attention paid to the range of movement achieved and the presence of any crepitus. To test the extensor apparatus of the knee, ask the patient to perform a straight leg raise. Ask the patient to raise the leg keeping the knee in full extension and look for any lag in extension. This could be due to quadriceps weakness or rupture, a patellar fracture, a patellar tendon injury or avulsion of the tibial tuberosity. Tenderness on any of these structures (or possibly the presence of a palpable gap) can help to confirm a diagnosis.

Special tests

- **Medial and lateral collateral ligaments:** apply varus and valgus stress with the knee in full extension and in 20° of flexion (this relaxes the cruciate ligaments and the knee capsule). It is easier to perform with the lower leg held in the examiner's axilla and the hands on either side of the knee. From this position, the examiner can provide varus or valgus strain feeling for any abnormal mobility. There is some movement when the knee is flexed as the rest of the knee ligaments are relaxed and purely collaterals are tested, whereas any movement in full extension is abnormal (**Figure 4.7.5**)

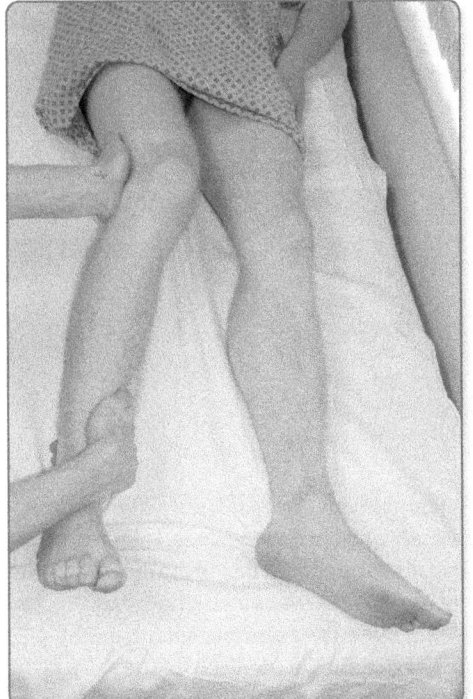

Figure 4.7.5 Stressing the medial collateral ligament.

- **Cruciate ligaments drawer test**: keep the knees flexed at approximately 90° and the feet pointing forwards. Note any sagging of the tibial condyle as compared with the other side (**Figure 4.7.6**). This could mean a ruptured posterior cruciate ligament (PCL). Next the examiner stabilises the patient's legs by sitting close to, or gently on top of, the patient's feet (this manoeuvre braces the feet against the examiner so the following step can be performed). If both the tibial condyles are at the same level, grasp the leg firmly with fingers in the popliteal fossa and thumbs on the tibial tubercle. Check that the hamstrings are relaxed and attempt to move the leg forwards with a firm jerk (**Figure 4.7.7**). Any excessive movement suggests a ruptured anterior cruciate ligament (ACL)

Figure 4.7.6 Assessing for sagging of a tibial condyle and posterior cruciate ligament rupture.

Figure 4.7.7 Assessing for anterior cruciate ligament rupture.

- **Lachman's test**: this is more specific for ACL integrity. With one hand, grasp the femur just above the knee, and with the other, grasp the tibia just below the knee, keeping the knee in 20° flexion. Attempt lifting the tibia forwards. One should be able to feel a definite end to movement indicating an intact ACL. Any excessive movement is abnormal
- **McMurray's test**: start with the knee in full flexion. Place the examiner's hand on the patella with the fingers palpating the joint line. For the medial meniscus, externally rotate the foot and apply valgus strain to the knee. Now gently extend the knee feeling

for any clicks or noting pain as the knee is extended. For the lateral meniscus, internally rotate the foot and apply varus strain to the knee extending it at the same time
- **Patellar apprehension test**: hold the leg with the knee in full extension. Gently flex the knee applying pressure on the medial aspect of the patella attempting to displace it laterally. The patient will feel the sensation of dislocation and will stop the examiner progressing with the test

Diagnoses to consider

- Traumatic diagnoses include collateral or cruciate ligament injuries, fractures and meniscus tears
- Non-traumatic diagnoses include osteoarthritis, septic arthritis, internal derangement of the knee, Baker's cyst and referred hip pain

Scenario

Mr Nevitt is a 35-year-old surf instructor who has come to the ED with left knee pain. While playing football this evening he was involved in a tackle. He was helped off the ground and now has pain on the inside of his knee. Examine his knee and make a management plan.

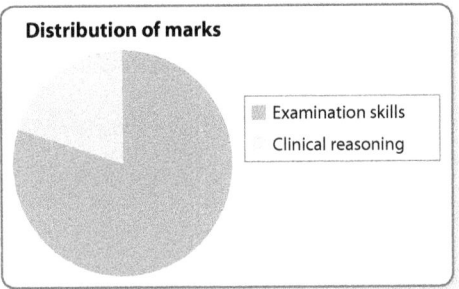

Distribution of marks
- Examination skills
- Clinical reasoning

Mark sheet	Achieved	Not achieved
Introduces self to patient appropriately		
Confirms patient identity		
Explains reason for examination and obtains consent		
Enquires regarding presence of pain and offers analgesia if needed		
Confirms the history		
Cleans hands appropriately		
Adequate exposure of both knees		
Assessment with patient standing:		
– inspects knees from the front, side and in the popliteal fossa		
– inspects the gait		
Assessment with patient supine:		
– Inspects the legs appropriately		
– palpates in a logical manner		
– palpates for knee effusion		
– checks active movements		
– checks passive movements		

Cont'd...

Cont'd...

Mark sheet	Achieved	Not achieved
– checks power of muscle groups		
– performs patellar apprehension test		
– tests collateral ligaments integrity		
– tests anterior and posterior cruciate ligament integrity		
– performs Lachman's test		
– performs McMurray's test		
– completes neurovascular assessment of distal limb		
Comments on need to examine joint above and below		
Thanks patient and offers to help patient redress		
Correctly identifies clinical signs		
Correctly states diagnosis		
Describes appropriate management plan		
Asks if patient has any questions		
Global mark from patient		
Global mark from examiner		

4.8 Neck examination

Begin by introducing yourself, confirming the name of the patient, asking for permission to examine them and cleaning your hands. Ask if the patient has any pain and offer analgesia if appropriate.

Inspection

This should be performed from the front, sides and back looking for skin changes, swelling, deformity and scars. From the front also look at the patients face for signs of Horner's syndrome and note any abnormality in their voice or breathing.

Horner's syndrome consists of drooping of the eyelid (ptosis), pupillary constriction (miosis) and reduced sweating (anhidrosis), all on the ipsilateral side due to loss of sympathetic tone to the superior tarsal muscle, pupillary constrictor and facial sweat glands. This may reflect interruption of the sympathetic chain in the neck. In the context of neck pain, potential causes are an abscess, malignancy, goitre, carotid artery or aortic dissection though there are many others.

Palpation

Palpation is best done with the clinician standing behind and to the side of the patient. Systematically palpate the vertebrae starting at the occipital part of the cervical spine to the thoracic region and moving from midline laterally (**Figure 4.8.1**). Focus on any localised areas of tenderness or swelling and assess fully. Also, while standing behind the patient, palpate the neck anteriorly and the supraclavicular fossae (**Figure 4.8.2**).

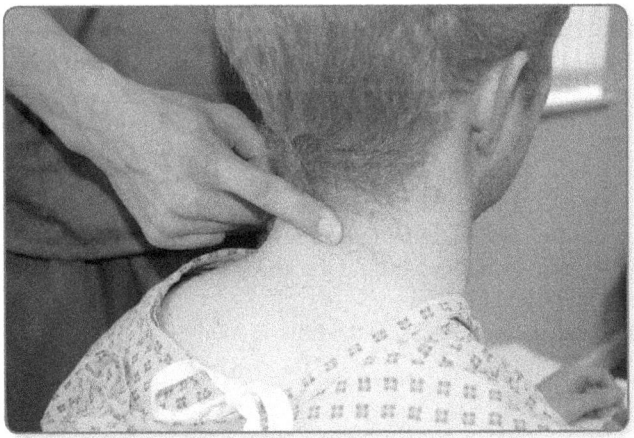

Figure 4.8.1 Palpating for bony tenderness of the cervical spine.

Figure 4.8.2 Palpating the anterior neck.

Movement

Movements to be examined are forward, right and left flexion, extension and rotation to each side. In the case of trauma, consider whether or not it is safe to assess movements of the neck. This will depend on the scenario provided.

Special tests

Signs of spinal cord compression

- **Hoffman's test**: this test elicits a pathological reflex present in spinal cord compression. Hold the middle finger at the middle phalanx between the index and middle finger of the examiner's hand. Flick the distal phalanx at the pulp with the examiner's free thumb. The test is positive if the patient's index finger and thumb flex
- **Lhermitte's test**: also called barber's chair phenomenon, flexion or extension of the neck produces electric shock-like sensation in the legs. This sign is mostly associated with multiple sclerosis

Signs of meningism

- **Kernig's test**: this test can be performed with the patient supine or in a chair. The hip and knee are flexed to 90° and attempt is made to extend the knee. The test is positive if the manoeuvre causes pain in the neck or back
- **Brudzinski's test**: flexion of the neck causes flexion of the hips and knees

Signs of thoracic outlet obstruction

- **Adson's test**: palpate the radial pulse and, while keeping the elbow extended, abduct (to 30°), externally rotate and extend the shoulder. Then ask the patient to take a deep breath and hold in inspiration and turn the head to the ipsilateral side. The test is positive if there is a loss of the radial pulse. Always compare with the other side

Neurovascular examination

Neurological evaluation is both for the spinal cord and for peripheral nerves as they exit the neck via the brachial plexus. Therefore, the patient can have weakness and a sensory deficit in a spinal cord injury pattern or a peripheral nerve injury pattern. Spinal cord involvement usually has bilateral features with clinical signs in lower limbs as well, whereas peripheral nerve injury (e.g. a traction injury of the brachial plexus) is usually unilateral and confined to the injured limb. Knowledge of both segmental distribution and nerve distribution is therefore essential (**Figure 4.8.3** and **Table 4.8.1**).

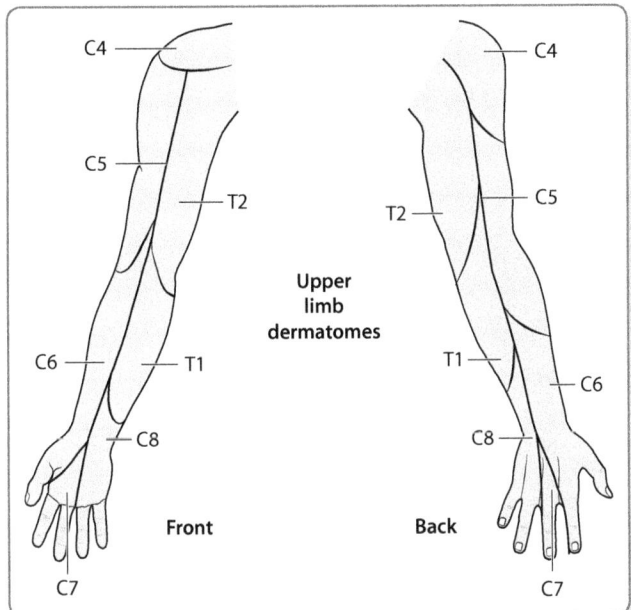

Figure 4.8.3 Upper limb dermatomes.

Table 4.8.1 Myotomes of the upper limbs

Movement	Muscle	Root	Nerve
Shoulder abduction	Deltoid	C5	Axillary
Elbow flexion	Biceps	C5–6	Musculocutaneous
Elbow extension	Triceps	C7	Radial
Wrist flexion	Flexor carpi radialis and ulnaris	C8	Median and ulnar
Wrist extension	Extensor carpi radialis and ulnaris	C7	Radial
Finger abduction	Dorsal interossei	T1	Ulnar
Thumb abduction	Abductor pollicis brevis	C8	Median

Upper limb reflexes are:
- Biceps — C5–6
- Brachioradialis — C6–7
- Triceps — C7–8

Diagnoses to consider

- Traumatic diagnoses include arthritic neck pain, post-traumatic neck pain and carotid artery dissection (not always traumatic)
- Non-traumatic diagnoses include retropharyngeal abscess, lymphadenopathy, goitre, meningitis and thoracic outlet obstruction

Scenario

Dr Goodman is a 48-year-old maths professor. He has come to the ED with sudden severe pain in his neck. Examine his neck and explain your differential diagnosis and management plan to him.

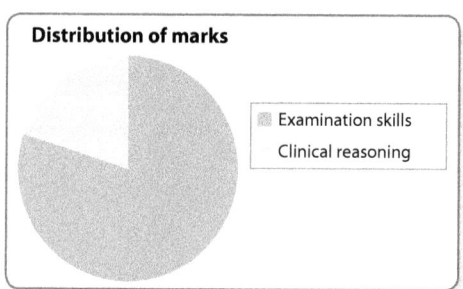

Distribution of marks
- Examination skills
- Clinical reasoning

Mark sheet	Achieved	Not achieved
Introduces self to patient appropriately		
Confirms patient identity		
Explains reason for examination and obtains consent		
Enquires regarding presence of pain and offers analgesia if needed		
Confirms the history and asks about mechanism of injury		
Cleans hands appropriately		
Performs adequate inspection		
Palpates the cervical spine methodically		
Assesses movements		
Neurological examination:		
– tone and power in shoulder, elbow, wrist and hand		
– deep tendon reflexes – biceps, triceps and supinator reflexes		
– sensory examination for light touch		
– tests for spinal cord involvement		
– assesses signs of meningism		
Performs or describes Adson's test		
Palpates carotid pulses		
Comments on need to examine shoulders and thoracic spine		
Thanks patient and offers to help patient redress		
Correctly identifies clinical signs		
Correctly states diagnosis		
Describes appropriate management plan		
Asks if patient has any questions		
Global mark from patient		
Global mark from examiner		

4.9 Shoulder examination

Begin by introducing yourself, confirming the name of the patient, asking for permission to examine them and cleaning your hands. Ask if the patient has any pain and offer analgesia if appropriate.

Inspection

Look at the shoulders from the front, the sides and the back for any changes suggestive of pathology. Do not forget to examine the axilla (**Figure 4.9.1**).

Figure 4.9.1 Shoulder inspection.

Palpation

With the dorsum of your hand feel both shoulders to assess for any difference in warmth between them.

Palpation of the shoulder starts anteriorly and proceeds through the following structures; the sternoclavicular joint and the clavicle (**Figure 4.9.2**) proceeding to the

Figure 4.9.2 Palpating the clavicle.

acromioclavicular joint, coracoid process and biceps tendon, greater tuberosity of humerus and posteriorly to the acromion, spine of the scapula, suprascapular and infrascapular muscles. Aim to elicit any areas of localised tenderness, which usually correspond to an underlying structure.

Movement

Asking the patient to put their hands behind their head and then behind their back, is a quick screening manoeuvre that detects any changes in shoulder movement.

Test forward flexion, abduction, extension, internal and external rotation actively and then passively.

Abduction is tested in the coronal plane and flexion and extension in the sagittal plane. Shoulder abduction is a complex movement involving glenohumeral and scapulothoracic movements. There is normally a gradual transition from pure glenohumeral to pure scapulothoracic movement as the patient abducts. This gradual transition is lost in joint disruption or damage to the tendons that stabilise the joint. The patient will not be able to initiate the movement in the case of a supraspinatus tear. Once initiated, there may be pain on continuing abduction which is a sign of impingement. If the pain is towards the end of abduction, this may be due to acromioclavicular joint arthritis.

Rotation should be checked with the shoulder in neutral position and with the elbow in 90° flexion. Patients with recurrent dislocations will find it difficult to externally rotate as it can cause dislocation.

Ask the patient to push against a wall while inspecting their back. This forces the serratus anterior to stabilise the scapula. Therefore if the scapula lifts up or 'wings' during this manoeuvre, it indicates weakness of serratus anterior and possible damage to long thoracic nerve.

Assessment of the rotator cuff

The rotator cuff is made up of infraspinatus and teres minor (principle external rotators), supraspinatus (principle abductor) and subscapularis (principle internal rotator) of the shoulder. Their tendons combine to form a single unit which acts to stabilise the humeral head in the glenoid cavity during active movements.

Rotator cuff pathology is a spectrum from tendonitis, to impingement to a full tear of the tendon leading to weakness of the respective muscle. The aim of the clinical examination is to distinguish which structure is affected and to what degree.

Special tests

The tests aim to identify any weakness in the various rotator cuff muscles by isolating and testing them individually. All the tests are done with the examiner standing behind the patient.
- **Jobe's (Empty can) test**: this aims to test for pathology in supraspinatus tendon. Ask the patient to flex both shoulders by 90° and place them in 30° of abduction with their thumbs pointing down. Weakness to downward force applied to the arm in this posture points to a supraspinatus tear (**Figure 4.9.3**).

Figure 4.9.3 Testing supraspinatus.

- **Resisted external rotation:** this test is for pathology of the infraspinatus muscle. The patient is asked to keep their arms parallel to the body, elbows at 90° flexion and forearm in mid-prone position. Keeping the elbows tucked in, the patient is asked to externally rotate the shoulder against resistance. Weakness indicates a tear and pain indicates possible impingement of the infraspinatus (**Figure 4.9.4**)

Figure 4.9.4 Testing infraspinatous.

- **Gerber's lift off test:** this aims to isolate the subscapularis. The patient is asked to internally rotate the shoulder and rest the dorsum of the hand against the mid or lumbar spine. The examiner then applies resistance to the palm and asks the patient to lift their hand off their back. Weakness during this manoeuvre may indicate a subscapularis tear (**Figure 4.9.5**)
- **Drop test:** the patient's arm is passively abducted with their hand above the head and then they are asked to lower it down gradually. If there is a rotator cuff tear, the arm drops in mid range or the patient has to support the arm to bring it down. It usually indicates a tear of supraspinatus

Figure 4.9.5 Testing subscapularis.

- **Neer's test for impingement**: performed from behind the patient, the examiner passively flexes, abducts and then internally rotates the shoulder by 90°. The aim is to bring the greater tuberosity under the acromion and therefore elicit pain due to impingement. If the patient complains of pain in the anterior or lateral shoulder, the test is positive. It is not very specific to impingement and can be positive in osteoarthritis and capsular tears

Tests for instability

- **Sulcus test**: downward traction by the examiner on the arm produces a depression below the acromion indicating inferior dislocation
- **Apprehension test**: this can be done with the patient sitting or lying. The examiner moves the shoulder to 90° abduction and gently starts external rotation while applying anterior pressure on the humeral head from behind. The patient will sense when the shoulder may dislocate and shows signs of apprehension (**Figure 4.9.6**)

Figure 4.9.6 The apprehension test.

Diagnoses to consider

- **Tendonitis**: it is usually the supraspinatus that gets inflamed and oedematous because of persistent friction as it moves under the acromion arch. Tenderness on the anterior edge of the acromion with the shoulder extended indicates inflamed supraspinatus tendon
- **Painful arc syndrome**: ask the patient to abduct. Pain starts at about 60° and continues to about 120° and during this range, the examiner may have to assist in moving the shoulder. Pain eases towards the end of abduction. Ask the patient to bring the arm back to neutral and then perform abduction with full external rotation of the arm. This is relatively painless as the structures move away from the subacromial region
- Traumatic diagnoses include muscle sprains, shoulder dislocation, clavicle fracture, acromioclavicular joint dislocation and ruptured rotator cuff
- Nontraumatic diagnoses include osteoarthritis, impingement syndrome, chronic instability, frozen shoulder, acute calcific tendonitis, septic arthritis or referred pain from peritoneal inflammation

Scenario

Miss Ali is a 28-year-old netball player. She has come to the ED with pain in her right shoulder after a match. Examine her shoulder and explain your diagnosis and a management plan to her.

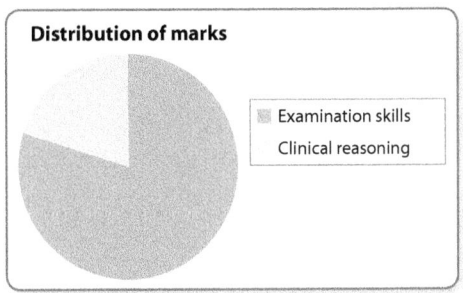

Distribution of marks
- Examination skills
- Clinical reasoning

Mark sheet	Achieved	Not achieved
Introduces self to patient appropriately		
Confirms patient identity		
Explains reason for examination and obtains consent		
Enquires regarding presence of pain and offers analgesia if needed		
Confirms the history		
Cleans hands appropriately		
Adequate exposure of both shoulders		
Performs adequate inspection		
Examines for winging of scapulae		
Palpates systematically		
Checks active movements		
Checks scapulothoracic coordination from back		
Checks internal and external rotation		
Stabilises scapula and checks passive movements of the glenohumeral joint		
Assesses power of flexors, extensors and abductors		
Assesses power of all rotator cuff muscles specifically		

Cont'd...

Cont'd...

Mark sheet	Achieved	Not achieved
Checks for impingement		
Checks for instability		
Examines neurovascular status of limb		
Comments on need to examine the joint above and below		
Thanks patient and offers to help patient redress		
Correctly identifies clinical signs		
Correctly states diagnosis		
Describes appropriate management plan		
Asks if patient has any questions		
Global mark from patient		
Global mark from examiner		

Chapter 5

Psychiatry

5.1 Introduction
5.2 Depression
5.3 Assessing the risk of self-harm
5.4 Mania
5.5 Schizophrenia/psychoses
5.6 Mini-mental state examination
5.7 Substance abuse history – alcohol
5.8 Assessing mental capacity

5.1 Introduction

The assessment of psychiatric patients is a common undertaking in the ED and the ability to do so is assessed frequently. Core skills relate to performing a mental state examination, completing a mini-mental state examination (MMSE), assessing risk of self-harm and taking a substance abuse history.

A good level of communication skills is imperative as due to their presentation patients may have several barriers to developing a rapport. An initial introduction with an explanation of what you are trying to achieve during the meeting is always a good way to begin. Good use of open questions before more focused closed questioning is helpful as is appropriate use of silence.

Taking a basic history follows the standard format but additional areas to enquire about specifically are past psychiatric history, forensic history (any criminal records or illegal activities) and substance abuse. Some patients may be quiet or impossible to engage (psychotic patients) and others may display challenging behaviour (manic patients who are sexually inappropriate) that candidates will have to manage while performing their assessment. Even if answers are not forthcoming or patients exhibit difficult behaviour a good candidate will cover all areas in their questioning, remain professional and display good communication skills.

There is a lot to cover and good time-keeping is essential not to run out of time during these objectively structured clinical examination (OSCE) stations.

The mental state examination

This examination is a structured approach to assessing an individual's state of mind at a given time. It is a challenging task in exam conditions as there is a lot to cover and you may be faced with patients who are not forthcoming with information. By adhering to a relatively structured approach you can demonstrate your awareness of all the areas that are to be covered. The examination can be divided into several areas some of which require close observation while others require direct questioning. Together, once the following areas have been covered, the information gained can be unified to suggest a likely diagnosis:

Appearance
- Clothing – in terms of appropriateness, colours, style, personal hygiene – hair, facial hair, cleanliness

Behaviour
- Posture/position – standing, sitting, pacing around and fidgeting
- Eye contact
- Nature of any gestures made – aggressive, irritable

Speech
From the time of introductions speech can be assessed. Some open questions about what has been happening to the patient are a good starting point.
- The rate, tone, volume and quality should always be considered
- Presence of pressure of speech, flight of ideas, knight's move thinking or neologism (made up words that make little sense) will all indicate certain diagnoses
- The content of speech is also important. Examples are delusions, depressive or suicidal ideas being expressed

Mood
After forming an impression based on the above it is appropriate to ask some general questions to assess mood. The patient can be asked how they feel about their current situation and about any relevant symptoms they are experiencing.

It is also vital to directly assess whether or not the patient has any suicidal ideation. Depending on their response and presentation a more thorough risk assessment may need to be undertaken.

Thoughts
At this point, the patient should be asked if there are any thoughts they are preoccupied by. There may be ideas of persecution or paranoia, hopelessness, delusions of grandeur or flight of ideas.

In the case of schizophrenia thought may be particularly delusional with the presence of thought insertion, withdrawal or broadcasting. Somatic passivity where the individual feels controlled by external forces is another feature. Auditory hallucinations, particularly in the third person are frequently experienced. However, bear in mind other patients may experience visual, olfactory and tactile hallucinations also.

Thus, this area of the examination should involve asking about recurring thoughts, obsessions, phobias, abnormal beliefs and abnormal experiences.

Cognition
Ideally cognition would be assessed with the abbreviated mini-mental state examination; however, in the exam time is limited. It is acceptable to ask basic questions to ascertain whether or not the patient is orientated in terms of time, place and person. Furthermore, a judgement can be made of whether their memory and concentration skills are impaired.

Insight
Again a simple question such as 'What do you think is wrong with you?' or 'Do you think you need any treatment?' will help establish whether or not the patient recognises themselves to be unwell and to what degree.

Performing a mental state examination

Like any examination the routine of performing a mental state examination should be well rehearsed so it can be done smoothly in an exam setting. Though the areas to be assessed do not vary the specific symptoms and signs that are sought will vary considerably with each type of presentation. As well as performing a mental state examination the marks in each area will be given to candidates who demonstrate an awareness and understanding of specific psychiatric disease patterns during their history taking and assessment. For this to be possible candidates must have an awareness of the common presentations.

Ultimately, the above information should be assimilated and summarised with a view to establishing the possible diagnosis and its severity. A referral or management plan can then be formulated.

Suggested reading

Royal College of Emergency Medicine (RCEM). Mental Health in Emergency Departments. A Toolkit for Improving Care. RCEM. London: RCEM; 2017.

Dick T. Mental Health in the ED. RCEM Learning. London: RCEM Learning; 2018.

5.2 Depression

Depression generally presents with persistent low mood, decreased energy levels and an inability to enjoy things one previously did. Causes are commonly multi-factorial but acute presentations can follow significant life-events (reactive depression) and anniversaries of such events, or be the result of more chronic processes.

Patients may be observed to display signs of apathy and self-neglect in terms of personal hygiene and clothing. Their actions may be slow and require effort (psychomotor retardation). Eye contact can be poor due to reduced self-esteem.

Their mood is likely to be apathetic and pessimistic with nothing to look forward to. Also activities that were enjoyed are not any longer (anhedonia). Specific questions in this area should ask about sleep and eating patterns as patients often sleep poorly, experiencing early morning waking and poor appetite. Risk of self-harm and suicide must always be addressed by sensitive but direct questioning. The SAD PERSONS score can be used to attempt to quantify the risk of self-harm (**Box 5.3.1**).

Thoughts may include recurrent negative ideas relating to self-worth and guilt, or relate to life-events that have precipitated the acute episode. In severe cases psychotic symptoms corresponding to this pattern of thought may also develop.

Subsequently cognition may be impaired due to decreased concentration and also poor short-term memory. A degree of insight is normally retained in all but the most severe cases though this can be limited due to the influence of the patient's mood and thoughts.

Depending on the severity of the presentation and the patient's level of risk, management will vary. In those who are felt to require early assessment or admission discussion with psychiatry services is advisable.

Scenario

Mr Jackson is a 58-year-old man who has been brought to the ED by a friend who is worried about him. Mr Jackson had not been answering his phone until his friend visited and banged on the door for 15 minutes. Take a brief history, perform a mental state examination and explain your findings to the examiner.

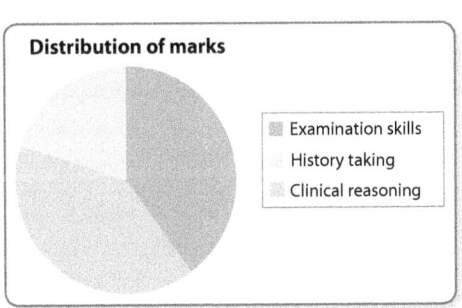

Distribution of marks
- Examination skills
- History taking
- Clinical reasoning

Mark sheet	Achieved	Not achieved
Introduces self to patient		
Confirms identity of patient		
Explains purpose of meeting		
Takes history of:		
– presenting complaint		
– past psychiatric history		
– past medical history		
– medications, drugs and substance use		

Cont'd...

Cont'd...

Mark sheet	Achieved	Not achieved
– family history		
– social history		
– forensic history		
Comments on mental state examination findings regarding:		
– appearance		
– behavior		
– speech		
– mood		
– thoughts		
– hallucinations/delusions		
– cognition		
– insight		
Presents mental state examination findings to examiner appropriately		
Suggests likely diagnosis and management plan		
Global mark from patient		
Global mark from examiner		

Instructions for actor

You are Howard Jackson a 58-year-old engineer for a telephone and broadband company. Your friend and work colleague has made you come to the ED today. He is worried by your recent behaviour. In the past 3 weeks you are regularly late for work or calling in sick. You have not been physically unwell but feel you have no energy. You saw your general practitioner 2 weeks ago and had some blood tests including checking your thyroid and they were all normal. You were meant to go back but couldn't be bothered.

You feel exhausted, don't have much appetite and are finding it hard to sleep for more than a couple of hours as you always wake up in the early hours and feel restless. During the day you often feel like crying. You have no medical problems or medications. You smoke 30 cigarettes a day but don't drink alcohol or take other drugs at all. You've never had problems with the police. You're divorced and have no family but a few good friends at work who you have not talked to about your mood.

You know you are low in mood and at risk of losing your job. You have not considered harming/killing yourself. You find it hard to make eye contact with the doctor as you feel like it may make you burst into tears. You are concerned about taking antidepressants as you've heard they have lots of side-effects (but do not know what they are) and feel embarrassed to talk to a counsellor or psychiatrist. However, you do want help and are prepared to take advice from the doctor.

Suggested reading

Depression in adults. Clinical guideline 90. National Institute for Health and Care Excellence, London, 2009.

5.3 Assessing the risk of self-harm

Assessing a patient's risk of serious self-harm or suicide is a challenging but important task. It is unrealistic to refer all attendances of deliberate self-harm for a formal psychiatric assessment. Thus, it is the emergency physician's role to make as thorough a risk assessment of each individual case as possible, and having done so decide which cases require a referral and which cases can be safely discharged.

The final decision to self-harm is multi-factorial. The National Institute for Health and Care Excellence (NICE) recommends that several issues are taken into account when assessing risk including the patient's:
- Previous methods and frequency of current and past self-harm
- Current and past suicidal intent
- Depressive symptoms or psychiatric illnesses and their impact on self-harm
- Personal and social precipitants for self-harm
- Specific risk factors or protective factors that influence the possibility of further self-harm
- Coping strategies
- Presence of other risk-taking behaviour such as unprotected sexual activity, drug or alcohol misuse

Certain factors constituting a 'serious attempt' are associated with a significant suicidal intent. These generally reflect that the attempt was premeditated and organised over a period of time. The individual may have:
- Taken time to obtain the means to commit suicide
- Taken care of all of their personal affairs (e.g. paid bills, made a will)
- Gone to efforts not to be found/discovered.

Several demographic factors are also associated with a high risk of self-harm including:
- Extremes of adult age
- Being male
- Social isolation – living alone, being unemployed/retired, being separated, divorced or widowed
- Chronic illness
- Substance abuse
- Access to violent means for self-harm

Several risk assessment scales have been developed to assist in decision making. Though they offer well-defined methods of assigning a numeric risk score to assess individuals, it is agreed that these scores should be used with caution to predict ongoing risk, as they oversimplify very complicated and unpredictable issues. These scales are, however, useful in screening risk in the ED and focus the mind on areas that need consideration. Below as an example is the SAD PERSONS scale which offers a useful mnemonic (**Box 5.3.1**).

It may be helpful to remember that the examiner has a checklist-style mark sheet, and it is likely to have been constructed with a risk assessment scale (such as SAD PERSONS) in mind. Consequently, following such a screening checklist in your OSCE makes it easier for the examiner to follow your progress and award marks.

Psychiatry

Box 5.3.1 SAD PERSONS scale

Factor	Score
• Sex (male)	1
• Age (below 45 years or over 65 years)	1
• Depression	1
• Previous suicide attempt	1
• Ethanol use	1
• Rational thought loss	1
• Social isolation	1
• Organised plan for suicide	1
• No spouse	1
• Sickness	1
Total score	Recommended action (as a guide only)
0–4 lower risk	Can be discharged
5–6 moderate risk	Consider admission
7–10 high risk	Admit

Scenario

Anna Peters was brought to the ED by her parents. Her investigations are all normal (including paracetamol/salicylate levels). Take a history from the patient and explain what is going to happen next.

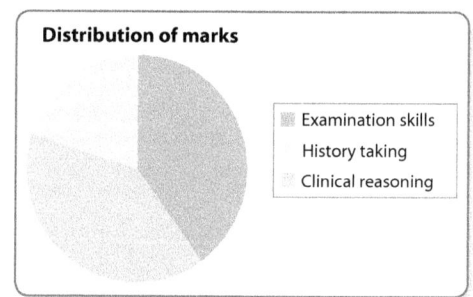

Distribution of marks
- Examination skills
- History taking
- Clinical reasoning

Mark sheet	Achieved	Not achieved
Introduces self to patient appropriately		
Explains reason for reviewing patient		
Confirms patient identity		
Uses open and closed questions appropriately		
History of presenting complaint		
Previous psychiatric history		
Previous medical history		
Drug history (must include recreational drugs)		
Family history		
Social history (must include school, bullying and friends)		

Cont'd...

Cont'd...

Mark sheet	Achieved	Not achieved
SAD PERSONS score		
– sex		
– age		
– depression		
– previous suicide attempts		
– excessive alcohol or drug use		
– rational thought loss		
– separated/widowed/divorced		
– organised attempt		
– no social support		
– stated future intent		
Uses information obtained to draw appropriate conclusion		
Explains plan to patient involving parents and mental health services		
Talks to patient sensitively using silence where appropriate		
Global mark from patient		
Global mark from examiner		

Instructions for actor

You are Anna Peters. You are 14 years old and study at school. After thinking about it for a couple of weeks you took an overdose yesterday. You do not want to talk to the doctor but if they talk to you in a kind and sensitive manner you slowly start answering their questions.

You stayed home from school after pretending to feel ill. From the family medicine cupboard you took a strip of paracetamol and another strip of ibuprofen (ten tablets of each). You did not take anything else. You took the overdose in the morning as you thought you would be dead before your parents came home from work. You wanted to die and only called 999 because you got such bad stomach cramps. You did leave a letter.

You live at home with your parents who are both accountants in the city. They are not at home very much as they work long hours. Your family have just moved to the area for your parent's jobs. You have no friends at school but have started getting messages on social media making fun of your hair and your teeth. You've tried contacting friends from your old school but since the school holidays they have stopped replying to you. You do not like the teachers as they aren't very enthusiastic or motivating. You've been shouted at a couple of times for being late to class but you didn't want to go in early because you thought you would be bullied before the teacher arrived.

You are normally well. You take no medications and do not smoke, drink or take any drugs. You have never taken an overdose before.

You are uncomfortable when talking to the doctor but do answer questions except when asked why you took the overdose. You do not really know the answer to this and just become tearful. You also do not know if you would do the same thing again but still feel like things may be better for your parents if you weren't around.

Suggested reading

Self-harm. Clinical guideline 16. National Institute for Health and Care Excellence, London, 2004.

5.4 Mania

The presenting problem for these patients may vary but can usually be described as 'behaving strangely'. In simple terms the underlying problem relates to a pathological over-stimulation of mood with a subsequent impact on several areas of behaviour. The cause varies and mania can develop after depression, stress, medications or arise spontaneously.

Patients typically appear to be dressed in inappropriately flamboyant and bright clothing with perhaps excessive make-up and jewellery. Their level of elation is not congruent with the situation as they are excessively cheerful and over-familiar as well as having increased energy levels.

Speech may be loud with an excess of thoughts that they may try to express. This can result in pressure of speech and flight of ideas. Correspondingly their mood is euphoric.

Thoughts are normally unrealistic and demonstrate a lack of insight. Patients commonly exhibit delusions of grandeur and have unrealistic ideas as to how they will spend their time and indeed their money. This disinhibition can also result in irritability and anger when confronted and patients may also be violent. Hallucinations and delusions do occur but unlike those in schizophrenia they are normally consistent with the patient's mood.

There is an impaired level of cognition with impaired concentration and poor judgement. Clearly patients have poor insight into their behaviour and engage in risk-taking activities with higher levels of gambling, promiscuity and excessive spending.

These patients commonly need admission for assessment and treatment.

Scenario

Mr Jones is a 38-year-old business man. He has been found walking down the middle of the street asking passers-by to join him in a bar for drinks to celebrate. When stopped by the police he began singing to them and insisted they should keep his house keys as he was moving to a bigger, better mansion after winning the lottery later today.

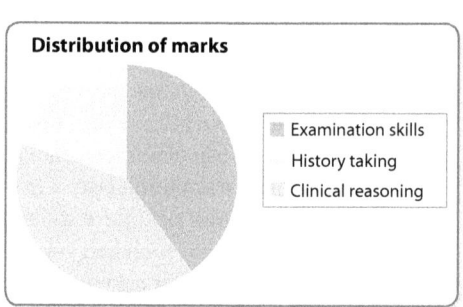

Distribution of marks
- Examination skills
- History taking
- Clinical reasoning

Mark sheet	Achieved	Not achieved
Introduces self to patient		
Confirms identity of patient		
Explains purpose of meeting		
Takes history of:		
– presenting complaint		
– past psychiatric history		
– past medical history		
– medications, drugs and substance use		
– family history		

Cont'd...

Cont'd...

Mark sheet	Achieved	Not achieved
– social history		
– forensic history		
Comments on mental state examination findings regarding:		
– appearance		
– behaviour		
– speech		
– mood		
– thoughts		
– hallucinations/delusions		
– cognition		
– insight		
Presents mental state examination findings to examiner appropriately		
Suggests likely diagnosis and management plan		
Global mark from patient		
Global mark from examiner		

Instructions for actor

Your name is William Jones. You work as an estate agent selling 'luxury homes'. Today you realised that it's finally your turn to get a luxury house of your own. You have bought one thousand lottery tickets and are certain you are going to win. Instead of going to work you put on your most colourful suit and wanted to celebrate. All your friends are busy so you thought you'd go for a walk and see if you could make any new friends to help you celebrate.

When the doctor arrives you are very excited at the opportunity to see them. You give them a hug and start telling them about your good fortune. If they interrupt you or ask you to sit down you get a little irritated and try to tell them everything is fine and it's a great day. You will not agree to sit down but do not mind if they do so. You want to tell them all about the house you intend to buy. You have already chosen it. It has lots bedrooms for when friends visit, lots of staff to help you out, a swimming pool and space for all the cars you will buy. You refuse to give the address or location as it's your special secret.

You make good eye contact but are very excited and can't stay still. You do get irritated with the serious questions but are not aggressive or rude.

You evade any questions about your past medical problems and personal life. If asked, the only information you provide is that your girlfriend has moved out and your general practitioner does prescribe you a tablet but you can't remember what for and have decided you do not need it. The rest of the questions and their answers are not important as your fortune is going to change.

5.5 Schizophrenia/psychoses

Though a formal diagnosis of schizophrenia cannot be made in the ED, features suggesting it can be sought. Clearly, in those who previously have a formal diagnosis, an acute exacerbation is likely, but in first presentations thorough assessment and follow-up will be necessary to distinguish schizophrenia from other acute psychoses. Presentations can vary and influence all elements of the mental state examination.

Patients may present in inappropriate clothing with elements of self-neglect. Their behaviour and mood can be influenced by hallucinations and disordered thought leading to agitation or aggression.

Schneider's first rank symptoms were previously considered diagnostic of schizophrenia:
- Thoughts are commonly affected by thought insertion, removal or broadcasting
- Auditory hallucinations are also common and typically they are voices discussing the patient in the third person
- Delusional ideas often relate to everyday happenings being given special significance. Often this relates to paranoia and feelings of persecution
- Somatic passivity is a process whereby a patient feels their body and actions are controlled by external powers

These features are now recognised to occur in other disease processes though they are common in schizophrenia and should actively be sought during an assessment.

Cognition and insight can both be significantly impaired.

These patients can be challenging to assess because there are often more barriers to developing a rapport and effective communication. It is not uncommon in the exam to be confronted by an agitated patient who will not sit down or answer any questions they are asked.

Scenario

A woman calling herself Jackie has been brought to the ED by ambulance. She was found hiding behind a van in a car park. She told the paramedics she was hiding from the devil who is trying to kill her. She is refusing to sit down or talk to anyone. She continually paces across the room repeating 'the devil is going to kill me'. Take a history and perform a mental state examination. Explain your findings to the examiner.

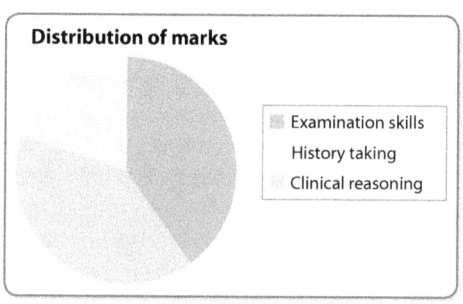

Distribution of marks
- Examination skills
- History taking
- Clinical reasoning

Mark sheet	Achieved	Not achieved
Introduces self to patient		
Confirms identity of patient		
Explains purpose of meeting		

Cont'd...

Cont'd...

Mark sheet	Achieved	Not achieved
Attempts to take history of:		
– presenting complaint		
– past psychiatric history		
– past medical history		
– medications, drugs and substance use		
– family history		
– social history		
– forensic history		
Comment on mental state examination findings regarding:		
– appearance		
– behaviour		
– speech		
– mood		
– thoughts		
– hallucinations/delusions		
– cognition		
– insight		
Presents mental state examination findings to examiner appropriately		
Suggests likely diagnosis and management plan		
Global mark from patient		
Global mark from examiner		

Instructions for actor

You are extremely anxious and scared as you believe the devil is trying to kill you. You are restless and pacing around the room. When the doctor speaks to you, stop and listen. Then you tell them the devil is trying to kill you. Occasionally, you make eye contact with the doctor and repeat the same statement trying to convince them that what you believe is true. The rest of the time you pace around the room repeating the same phrase again and again. You say nothing else and will not sit down for more than a few seconds when offered a chair. If the doctor tries to restrain you, begin repeating the same phrase louder and louder.

5.6 Mini-mental state examination

This is a validated test which provides a score that quantifies cognitive ability and helps to identify impairment in several areas. Over a period of time it can also be used to monitor changes in cognitive ability. It is often used as a screening test to assist in the diagnosis of dementia. In the emergency setting there is an ever-ageing population and recognising signs of dementia will allow for early investigation and follow-up in a group that may not otherwise receive help until the disease has progressed significantly.

The mini-mental state examination (MMSE) assesses orientation, registration (immediate learning), short-term memory and language functioning. The total score is 30. Scores over 25 are considered normal. The National Institute for Health and Care Excellence (NICE) consider scores of 21–24 as mild impairment, 10–20 as moderate and less than 10 severe. Caution should be used in certain cases depending on the patient's education level, grasp of the English language, and presence of learning or communication related disabilities.

There are several alternative tests which perform a similar function or allow for screening of cognitive impairment. These include abbreviated mental tests (with AMT-4 or AMT-10) or the Montreal Cognitive Assessment (MoCA).

The MMSE is structured as follows:
- Orientation in time – five points are given for asking increasingly specific questions regarding the time (e.g. one point for each of: year, season, month, day and time)
- Orientation in place – five points are given for increasingly specific questions regarding location (e.g. one point for each of: country, county, city, hospital, ward)
- Registration – three points are given for being able to repeat the names of three simple objects – one point each
- Attention – five points are given for being able to spell WORLD backwards or subtract increments of 7 from 100 (one point each time)
- Recall – three points are given for remembering the same three objects from earlier
- Language – two points are given for naming two everyday objects
- Language – one point for repeating 'No ifs, ands or buts'
- Language – three points for following a three-stage command (e.g. take this paper in your hand, fold it in half, place it on the table)
- Language – one point for reading and following an instruction (e.g. close your eyes)
- Language – one point for writing a sentence (must contain a subject and a verb but poor spelling shouldn't lose marks)
- Ask the patient to copy a drawing which is typically two intersecting pentagons – one point (**Figure 5.6.1**)

Patients with cognitive impairment require investigations to exclude an organic cause for their condition. Depending on the severity and nature of the impairment they may be managed in the community or require admission. This decision lies with the assessing doctor who must take into account the severity and nature of the problem as well as the patient's social circumstances.

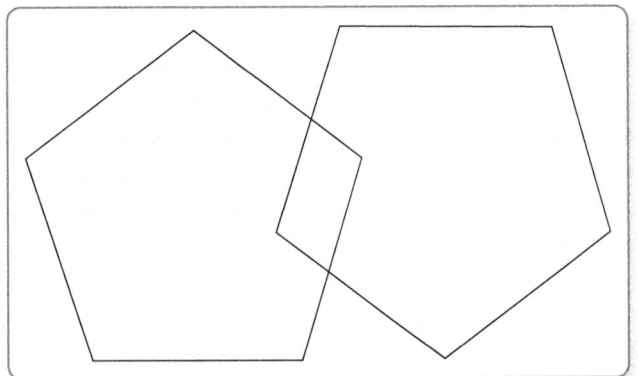

Figure 5.6.1 Intersecting pentagons.

Scenario

Mr Herbert is a 79-year-old man who presented after a minor fall. He has no injuries. He lives alone and has been brought to the ED by his anxious daughter who says he has begun to seem quite muddled in recent months and is struggling with living alone since his wife died. Perform a mini-mental state examination and feedback your findings to the examiner.

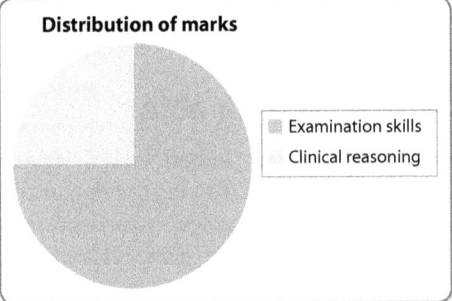

Mark sheet	Achieved	Not achieved
Introduces self to patient appropriately		
Confirms patient identity		
Explains reason for examination and obtains consent		
Assesses orientation in time (asks five questions)		
Assesses orientation in place (asks five questions)		
Assesses registration (asks to repeat three objects)		
Assesses concentration (asks to spell world backwards or subtract 7 from 100 again and again)		
Assesses short-term memory (asks to recall three previous objects: watch, shoe, car)		

Cont'd...

Cont'd...

Mark sheet	Achieved	Not achieved
Assesses language (asks to identify/name two objects) (asks to repeat phrase) (asks to follow a three stage instruction) (asks to read an instruction and follow it) (asks to write a full sentence) (asks to copy a diagram)		
Adds up score out of 30 points		
Aware that scores less than 25 are significant		
Talks to patient reassuringly during examination		
Ends examination appropriately		
Global mark from patient		
Global mark from examiner		

Instructions for actor

Your name is James Herbert. Your daughter has brought you to the ED because she says you are always confused. You tell the doctor you are fine and they are wasting their time. You are a retired history professor and lecturer at the local university and can manage fine in the house alone. You are proud of the fact that you have no medical problems and take no medication at all.

You agree to perform the tasks the doctor asks you to but insist they are wasting their time. During the task you cannot remember the month, year or season. If asked to count or spell backwards you are unable to do this. When asked to copy a diagram you fail to do this correctly.

You complete the remainder of tasks correctly.

Suggested reading

Royal College of Emergency Medicine (RCEM). Clinical Standards for Emergency Departments. RCEM. London: RCEM; 2014.

5.7 Substance abuse history – alcohol

Alcohol related presentations are an everyday part of the ED workload. An awareness of how to take a relevant history to screen for alcohol dependence and the ability to recognise and manage alcohol withdrawal are fundamental.

Many patients are reluctant to admit to their alcohol use and sensitive but direct questions are required. Particular presentations are more commonly associated with alcohol. These commonly include falls, collapses, seizures, head injury and assaults.

The candidate should demonstrate awareness that alcohol related questions may be considered very personal and make the patient feel defensive. It is always advisable to explain that the questions being asked are routine and not intended as criticism of the individual patient.

There are several screening tools available to assess risk of harmful alcohol intake. The **CAGE** questions indicate likely alcohol dependence if three answers are positive:
- Have you ever felt you should **C**ut down on your drinking?
- Do you get **A**ngry if people mention your drinking?
- Do you feel **G**uilty about your drinking?
- Do you ever have an '**E**ye-opener' when you wake up to settle your nerves?

The Paddington alcohol test (PAT) is another quick screening tool that is updated annually. It is intended to help with early identification of individuals who are at increased risk of alcohol misuse. Patients who are 'PAT positive' are offered written information about alcohol misuse and where to seek further help including talking to an alcohol specialist worker. The PAT 2011 test is formed of three questions:

1. **How often do you drink alcohol?**
   For those who never drink alcohol the next questions are not relevant. For those who drink every day the following questions should also be asked.
2. **What is the most you will drink in any one day (in units)?**
   If more than 8 units/day for men or 6 units/day for women the test is considered positive. These amounts are double the recommended daily limit and indicate a group that may benefit from provision of advice and information regarding alcohol (**Table 5.7.1**).
3. **Do you feel your attendance in ED is related to alcohol?**
   If the answer is yes the test is considered positive.

The amount of alcohol consumed is also not as significant as the impact on an individual's life. For this reason enquiries should be made into work, finances, criminal activity, relationships and any other substance use.

The remaining history must be taken adequately with due attention to other medical problems, medication and allergies.

Table 5.7.1 Alcohol units by type		
Beer/lager/cider	2 units/pint	1.5 units/can
Strong beer/lager/cider	5 units/pint	4 units/can
Wine	1.5 unit/glass	9 units/bottle
Spirits	1 unit/25 mL measure	30 units/750 mL bottle

Alcohol dependence is suggested by compulsion to drink alcohol and signs of acute withdrawal. Signs such as tremors, sweats, anxiety, nausea and vomiting are common. The nature of these patients and their presentations also means they often require a short stay on a clinical decisions unit/observation ward. It is not uncommon for such patients to develop acute withdrawal.

There is an increasing move to identify alcohol misuse in the ED setting so it can be addressed directly. The main goals relate to helping patient's recognise the risks associated with alcohol misuse and then motivating and empowering them to modify their drinking habits. Many EDs have access to alcohol specialist workers who can assist with thorough assessments and management plans in the ED and in the community.

Scenario

Mr Jones is a 38-year-old man who has spent the night on the ED observation ward after a fall with a minor head injury. He was examined, assessed appropriately and considered medically fit. He did not originally admit to drinking alcohol. The nurse in charge has asked you to see him as he has become increasingly shaky and agitated this morning. He told her, he needs a 'shot of vodka and will be fine'. Take a relevant history from him.

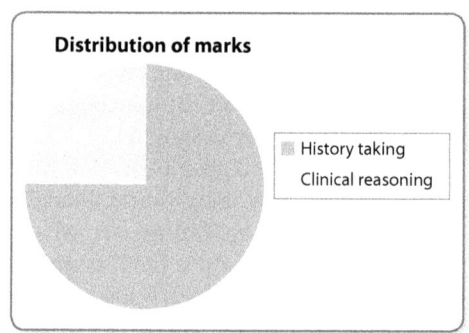

Distribution of marks
- History taking
- Clinical reasoning

Mark sheet	Achieved	Not achieved
Introduces self to patient appropriately		
Confirms patient identity		
Explains reason for concern and further discussion		
Asks screening questions for alcohol misuse (e.g. CAGE questions)		
Enquires about:		
– daily alcohol intake		
– choice of alcohol (narrowing of repertoire)		
– physiological symptoms relating to dependence		
– home circumstances		
– family/social support		
– employment/finances		
– other substance use		
– mood/risk of self-harm		
– forensic history – problems with the police		
– past medical history		

Cont'd...

Cont'd...

Mark sheet	Achieved	Not achieved
– medication/allergies		
– family history		
– patient's thoughts/insight regarding alcohol use		
Explains risks associated with excess alcohol intake		
Accepts patient's refusal to be admitted		
Acknowledges patient's wish to seek further help		
Advises referral to drug and alcohol services		
Closes discussion appropriately		
Global mark from patient		
Global mark from examiner		

Instructions for actor

Your name is Dylan Jones and you are a 38-year-old man who is currently working as a gardener. You don't really remember but have been told you came to the ED by ambulance after being found on a park bench. You had gone out with a friend last night to the pub but when they went home you continued drinking on your own as you had today off. You have become very shaky and clammy and the nurse was worried. You are not worried by this as it happens most days and settles after you have a drink of either vodka or cider, the two drinks you like. Each day you have around ten alcoholic drinks at home or while working.

You do not see this as a problem as you manage financially but you have lost a few days of work because you didn't get up in time. You have drunk this heavily for the last year and feel it's just a habit you have got into. You have no medical problems and medications and do not smoke or take other drugs. You live alone and are self-employed. You have had no problems with your mood as far as you are concerned. You have never been in trouble with the police but have been to the ED two or three times after incidents like last night, once when you got beaten up in a pub.

You do feel guilty about your drinking and are regretful that you've ended up in the ED again. You have considered reducing the amount of alcohol you drink but admit you've found it hard to do so. You are keen to get help.

Suggested reading

Paddington alcohol test. Imperial Healthcare NHS Trust, 2009.
Alcohol dependence and harmful alcohol use. Clinical guideline 115. National Institute for Health and Care Excellence, London, 2011.

5.8 Assessing mental capacity

Mental capacity assessment is an important task that should be understood and rehearsed well in advance of the exam. Different countries, including those making up the UK, have their own legislation to define mental capacity, its assessment and the procedures to follow. While a full discussion of specific legislation is outside the scope of this book, the following discussion aims to help the working emergency doctor apply the general principles and processes in day-to-day clinical practice.

Mental capacity is the ability to make an informed decision that is task specific. Any person above the age of 16 years is presumed to have mental capacity to make their own decisions about their care and treatment, according to the Mental Capacity Act 2005. In other words, they are capable of make a decision for themselves if provided with sufficient information. Whether their decision seems reasonable is irrelevant; thus, an individual with mental capacity has the right to make a decision which to others may seem unwise or irrational. Mental capacity can be questioned if there is a reason to believe that an impairment of mind or brain exists that limits the ability to make a decision. In such a situation, mental capacity should be formally assessed.

Assessment of mental capacity is a two-stage test (**Figure 5.8.1**):
1. Is there an impairment or disturbance in the functioning of the person's mind or brain?
2. If so, is this impairment or disturbance sufficient that the person is unable to make that particular decision?

Regarding the first part of the test it is important to check that the patient is orientated in time, place and person. Failing stage one is often the result of conditions such as:
- Stroke or head injury
- Mental illness
- Dementia
- Learning disability
- Confusion, drowsiness or unconsciousness due to an illness or its treatment
- Substance misuse, such as alcohol or drug intoxication

This list is not exhaustive. Nor does it mean that the presence of such conditions automatically means that a patient lacks capacity. Remember, mental capacity is task specific and is presumed to be present, and the lack of it may be temporary. A patient with dementia may lack the capacity to consent for surgery, but may be able to make a decision regarding their choice of food. A patient with alcohol intoxication may lack mental capacity now, but may regain mental capacity once sober.

The second stage is the application of a functional test to confirm the presence of mental capacity, or the lack of it. This can be remembered as the mnemonic '**URBI**'. A person is deemed to lack mental capacity if they are unable to do any of the following:
- **U**nderstand the information relevant to the decision
- **R**etain this information
- **B**alance (weigh up) their options
- **I**nform (communicate) others of their decision

Failure of one or more elements discussed will mean the whole test is failed and the individual will not satisfy the test of mental capacity.

All possible means of communication should be used to assist the patient to make a decision. This may include use of communication aids or asking for assistance from relatives, advocates or carers while at the same time-keeping in mind the patient's right to confidentiality.

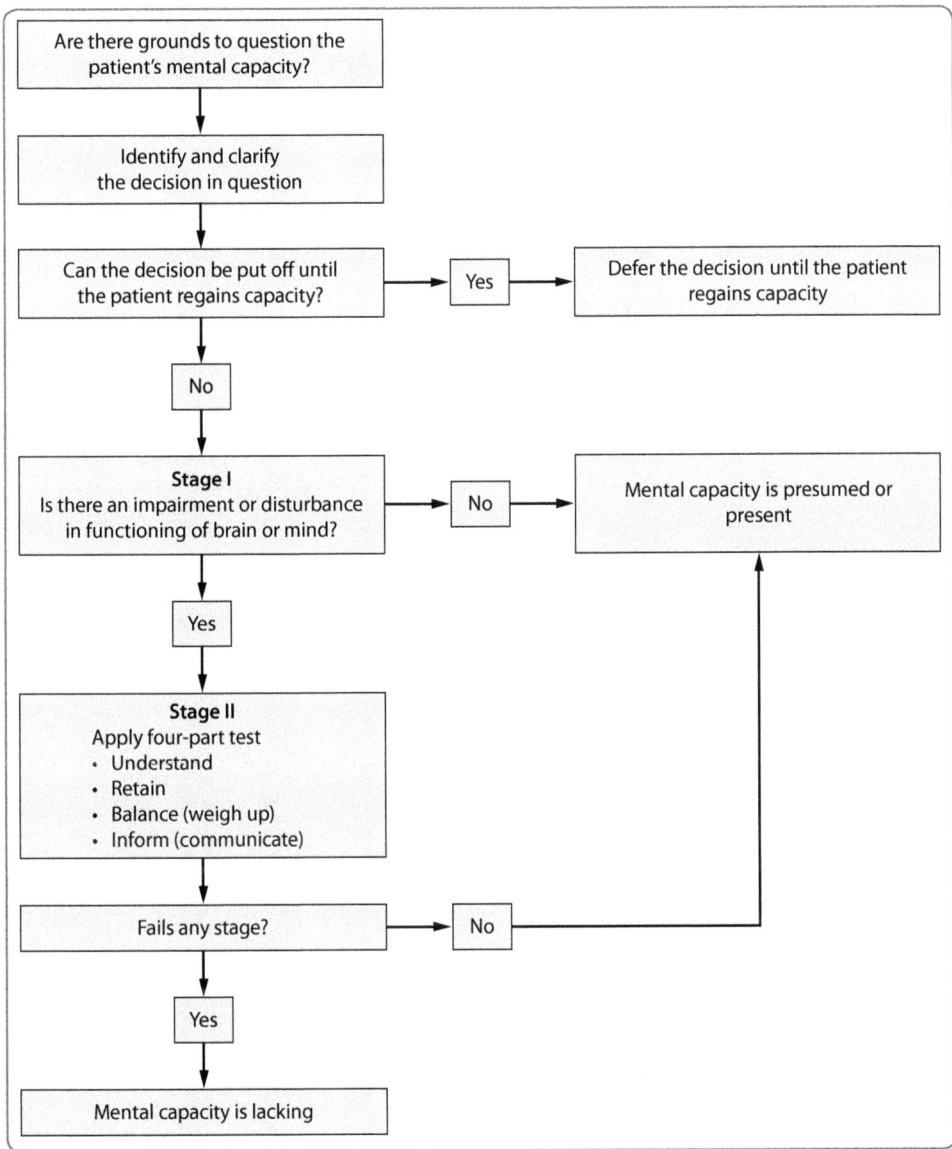

Figure 5.8.1 A simple flowchart for assessing mental capacity.

If the patient is found to lack capacity, subsequent decisions must either be in the patient's best interest or be the least restrictive option available.

Clinically there are two broad situations when one may have to assess mental capacity:
1. A patient who seems to lack capacity (e.g. an elderly patient with delirium),
2. A patient who makes a seemingly unwise decision (e.g. a patient with anaemia who refuses blood transfusion)

In both situations, the assessment remains the same. As stated earlier, an individual with mental capacity has the right to make a decision which to others may seem unwise or irrational.

Scenario

Mr Moore is a 79-year-old man who presented with a red and swollen leg. You have diagnosed cellulitis and admitted him for intravenous antibiotics. You felt that because Mr Moore lives by himself he would not be able to cope. The nurse now informs you that Mr Moore no longer wants to stay in hospital and wants to go home. She feels that Mr Moore now appears confused. Assess Mr Moore and make an appropriate management plan. You have ambulatory care at your hospital.

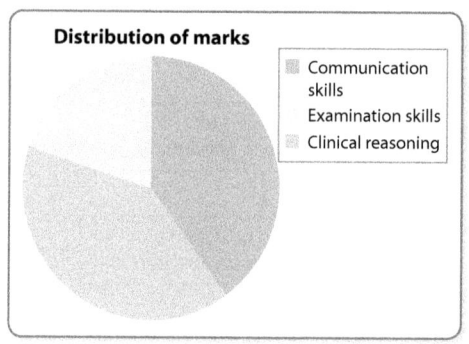

Distribution of marks
- Communication skills
- Examination skills
- Clinical reasoning

Mark sheet	Achieved	Not achieved
Introduces self to the patient		
Explains reason for discussion		
Assesses patients orientation to time		
Assesses patients orientation to place		
Assesses patients orientation to person		
Confirms that the patient is not confused		
Clarifies patient's understanding of his illness so far		
Explains reasons to stay in hospital – benefits		
Explains own concerns if patient goes home – risks		
Explores patient's concerns/reasons for his decision		
Checks patients understanding of situation		
Check patient can retain relevant information		
Check patients is able to balance risks and benefits		
Check patients ability to inform/express his wishes		
Establishes patient has capacity		
Enquires if patient wants to discuss decision with his family		
Respects patient decision to go home		
Agrees an acceptable alternative plan		
Explains about deterioration and provides safety net advice		
Agrees discharge		
Global marks from patient		
Global marks from examiner		

Instructions for actor

You are Frank Moore, a 79-year-old widower. You live by yourself and manage everything on your own. For the last 2 days you have had an increasingly painful and swollen leg.

You have drug-controlled hypertension and type 2 diabetes mellitus. The doctor has a list of your tablets. You don't smoke or drink alcohol.

Your wife died last year in this hospital. You found the experience very upsetting and you would rather be at home than stay here. You understand that the doctors say you have a skin infection and need intravenous antibiotics. You cannot sleep in the hospital but do want help to get better if there are any other options.

You will not agree to a stay in hospital when the doctor asks you to. You are able to explain your reasons to the doctor and are able to understand and repeat back to the doctor the reasons why he/she is concerned and you can repeat the doctor's account of the risks of not staying.

However, you are agreeable to any other options available. You will consider taking tablets and seeing if they work. You would also consider going home and returning daily for antibiotics. You feel well enough to go home; if necessary your son can stay with you or drive you to and from the hospital, or take you to your GP.

Suggested reading

Consent in Adults, Adolescents and Children in Emergency Departments. London: Royal College of Emergency Medicine, 2017.
Church M, Watts S. Assessment of mental capacity: a flow chart guide. Psychiatric bulletin 2007; 31:304–307.
Mental capacity toolkit [England and Wales]. London: British Medical Association, 2016.

Chapter 6

Practical skills and teaching

- 6.1 Introduction
- 6.2 Arterial cannulation
- 6.3 Basic airway management
- 6.4 Ascitic drainage
- 6.5 Central venous cannulation
- 6.6 Inserting a chest drain by blunt dissection
- 6.7 Clearing a cervical spine
- 6.8 Non-invasive ventilation
- 6.9 Direct current cardioversion
- 6.10 Focused assessment with sonography in trauma, aorta and vascular access ultrasound
- 6.11 Hand washing
- 6.12 Intraosseous needle insertion
- 6.13 Knee aspiration
- 6.14 Lumbar puncture
- 6.15 Anterior nasal packing
- 6.16 Femoral and fascia iliaca nerve block
- 6.17 Ophthalmoscopy
- 6.18 Otoscopy
- 6.19 Paediatric asthma – discharge planning and spacer technique
- 6.20 Performing an electrocardiogram
- 6.21 Blood cultures
- 6.22 Backslab application

- 6.23 Pleural aspiration
- 6.24 Rapid sequence induction
- 6.25 Surgical airway
- 6.26 Lateral cervical spine X-ray interpretation
- 6.27 Thomas splint application
- 6.28 Male urethral catheter insertion
- 6.29 Vaginal examination
- 6.30 Fitting a cervical spine collar
- 6.31 Head injury guidelines
- 6.32 Procedural sedation
- 6.33 Slit lamp examination
- 6.34 Wound assessment and management

6.1 Introduction

Practical skills and teaching will feature in the exam and the current exam guidance suggests at least two objective structured clinical examination (OSCE) stations will be based on evaluation of procedural skills. In reality these skills will also arise elsewhere, most likely as part-assessment of teaching technique or resuscitation scenarios. These OSCEs usually involve performing a procedure on your own or completing the procedure while teaching a colleague at the same time. It is often the case that a patient/actor will be present to speak, but the procedure will be performed on an appropriate manikin.

Approach to practical skills OSCEs

Go through the scheme of the procedure in your head while waiting to go in the station. Just like other OSCEs, divide the time appropriately into the introduction, carrying out the task and closing the station.

1. **Introduction – lasting approximately 1 minute**
   Start with introducing yourself, confirming the patient's identity and cleaning your hands. Make sure the patient is comfortable and offer pain relief if appropriate. Take a brief and focused history, confirm the facts already given in the scenario and ask focused questions around the task. This gives an opportunity to 'think out loud' in establishing the indications, necessity of the procedure and considering any complications or contraindications. This also helps you to communicate this thought process to the examiner, thereby demonstrating that you have taken the decision to carry on with the procedure after carefully weighing the risks and benefits.

   The next step is to gain patient consent. Communicate to the patient the indications, contraindications and complications for the procedure in question. Next ask the patient to repeat the information back to you to confirm their understanding and invite any questions they may have.

   It might be stated in the scenario provided that the patient has already been consented for the procedure. In this case, it is safe to proceed directly with the task without seeking consent again.

2. **Procedure – forming the bulk of the station**
   This involves completing the task that the scenario requires in order to pass the station. Therefore, prior to the exam, thinking about and practicing tasks that may arise is vital to appear experienced and efficient in the exam. These are artificial situations; under normal circumstances, you might take much longer to perform the procedure than 5 minutes. However, the focus of the OSCE is to establish that you know the critical steps. It is easy to recognise someone who is slick and experienced with a procedure as compared to someone who is doing the procedure for the first time.
   A quick check of the following points before starting the procedure may be helpful:
   - Position and site
   - Results of relevant investigations, e.g. chest X-ray
   - Drugs (e.g. analgesia and local anaesthetics)
   - Equipment
   - Monitoring
   - Cleaning and preparation (povidone-iodine or chlorhexidine, sterile drapes)
   - Sterile gloves and gown (for invasive procedures)
   - Help needed

During the procedure explain what you are doing (or think out loud) so that the examiner (and patient) knows what is happening. The way to approach this is to keep talking to the actor or the manikin rather than to the examiner, explaining in simple language what is being done.

The time can also be used to invite any questions or explain follow-up plans, e.g. if the patient is going home after a backslab inform them about the potential complications, plaster advice, analgesia, and follow-up while applying the backslab. This saves time and prevents you running out of time during a long procedure.

3. **Closure – final 1 minute**
Thank the patient, invite any questions and ensure equipment has been disposed of correctly, e.g. that sharps have been put in a sharps bin. Highlight any post-procedure steps needed to confirm that the procedure has been done adequately, e.g. swinging of the chest drain, or fluid running without any swelling in the intraosseous needle.

Organise any post-procedure check investigations, e.g. X-ray after manipulation, or chest X-ray after a chest drain.

Finally explain you would like to document the procedure and post-procedure advice in the patient's notes.

Approach to teaching OSCEs

Virtually any type of station can be made into a teaching station. It is easiest to imagine teaching a practical skill, but candidates may also be asked to teach factual information or a communication skill. Regardless of the nature of a teaching station, the same basic principles apply, as outlined below.

In teaching stations, you have to combine the two approaches of performing the task required and teaching at the same time. All of the information in the section above regarding how to approach practical-skills OSCEs therefore still applies.

The poorly prepared candidate in a teaching OSCE will be tempted to simply tell the 'student' everything they know about the procedure/task. This approach will score poorly as many marks are for teaching technique rather than knowledge.

It is vital to begin by clarifying what the individual in question already knows and what they wish to learn. Having identified these learning needs and stating the learning objectives the teaching can begin.

The teaching OSCE can easily drift out of control and, therefore, you need to establish these points early on. For example, an OSCE about otoscopy may easily drift to discussion about causes of perforation or hearing loss and you will lose marks if you do not adequately teach the technique. Therefore establish that the objective is to learn otoscopy and recommend that further learning can be done by other means, e.g. in a tutorial or an online module.

Be non-judgemental; spend time facilitating learning rather than asking the 'student' questions and testing their knowledge.

If each of the below steps are incorporated into your approach to the OSCE, you will be successful (indeed, when the emphasis of the OSCE is teaching, a candidate who follows the below steps may even be successful when they have minimal knowledge of the actual procedure/task, as long as they have 'taught' it well):

- Establish what the 'student' already knows, and what they want to learn
- Set the learning objectives of the encounter based on what they want to learn

- Demonstrate the skill in stages
- Then ask the student to perform the procedure, reinforcing learning
- Correct their technique as necessary and invite questions
- Plan for further learning and development to practice the skill
- Recommend other resources for self-directed learning, e.g. online modules or relevant papers or courses

6.2 Arterial cannulation

Indications

- Monitoring – invasive monitoring of blood pressure
- Diagnostic – repeated blood sampling (specially blood gas measurement)

Contraindications

- Local trauma or infection
- Ischaemic extremity
- Severe bleeding disorder
- Arteriovenous fistula

Complications

- Haematoma
- Embolism or thrombosis leading to ischaemia of the limb
- Accidental arterial drug injection
- Bleeding if it disconnects
- Line sepsis

Common sites for performing the procedure

- Radial artery (most common)
- Ulnar artery
- Dorsalis pedis artery
- Brachial artery
- Femoral artery – during resuscitation and profoundly shocked patients

Allen's test is described in the hand examination OSCE section of this book (see section 4.5). The value of the test is questionable but one needs to be able to perform it in the exam when performing radial or ulnar artery cannulation, to ensure there is collateral circulation to the hand prior to performing the procedure.

Pre-procedure checks

- Drugs – local anaesthetic – 1% lignocaine
- Cleaning and preparation – skin cleaning with chlorhexidine or iodine
- Equipment (**Figure 6.2.1**):
    - Arterial line cannulae (usually 20 or 22 gauge)
    - Extension line, flushed
    - Minor dressings pack
    - Suture, dressing
- Monitoring – pressurised flushing system connected to the monitor
- Sterility – sterile gloves

Figure 6.2.1 Arterial line equipment (a) cleaning swab (b) needle for Seldinger insertion (c) guidewire for Seldinger insertion (d) dressings to secure arterial line (e) alternative arterial line for direct arterial cannulation.

Technique

Start by feeling the arterial pulse and confirm the site for placement.

Position the wrist dorsiflexed about 30–45° on a flat surface. A rolled towel or an inverted kidney dish under the wrist may help. Establish a sterile field and clean the area. Inject 1% lignocaine intradermally to raise a bleb in skin at the proposed site. Holding the cannula in the dominant hand, insert it at a 30–45° angle to the skin guided by the pulse felt with the nondominant hand. The artery is usually deeper than anticipated.

Seldinger technique – the needle is inserted into the artery. Stop when pulsatile blood flows out and insert the wire through the needle into the artery. Once the wire is in, remove the needle and place the catheter over the wire and remove the wire. One hand must always be holding the wire to ensure the wire is not accidentally pushed into the artery, or pulled out of it.

Direct cannulation (with or without transfixing the artery) – the catheter comes 'preloaded' on the needle. Insert the needle in the artery. Upon seeing blood flow in the hub of the needle advance the catheter into the artery and then withdraw the needle.

There are various techniques for this procedure and with experience individuals tend to each develop their own preferred method which may vary with the clinical situation.

Ultrasound-guided cannulation can be a useful skill. When the pulse is difficult to palpate (e.g. hypotension, gross oedema or a larger patient), using an ultrasound probe can help facilitate cannulation. Use a vascular high frequency probe and maintain the sterility by using a sterile sheath and ultrasound gel. Visualise the artery in the longitudinal section (in-line cannulation) and advance the catheter or the needle under direct vision.

Once the catheter is placed in the artery, attach an extension line which has been flushed through with normal saline. Flush the line with saline to keep it open. Secure the line with either a suture placed superficially taking care not to suture the artery underneath or with a clear adherent film dressing. The arterial cannula can then be connected to a pressurised flushing system and allows monitoring of the pulse wave form and blood pressure.

Dispose of all the equipment appropriately and ensure the patient is comfortable.

Scenario

A 52-year-old patient, Mrs Burton, has been diagnosed with community-acquired pneumonia and is in septic shock. Despite fluid resuscitation, she is hypotensive and you need to start invasive blood pressure monitoring. Insert an arterial cannula into Mrs Burton's radial artery. A manikin will be used.

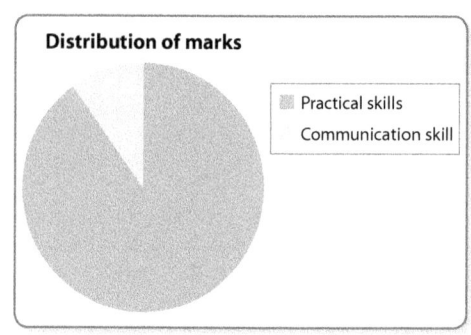

Distribution of marks
- Practical skills
- Communication skill

Mark sheet	Achieved	Not achieved
Introduces self to the patient		
Confirms patient identity		
Asks about presence of pain and offers analgesia		
Briefly asks about medical history, medication and allergies		
Explains procedure to patient		
Obtains patient consent		
Identifies the correct site for radial arterial line		
Correctly performs Allen's test		
Prepares and checks equipment		
Cleans hands and wears gloves		
Correctly positions the wrist		
Establishes a sterile field, uses sterile drapes and gloves		
Adequate skin preparation		
Injects appropriate local anaesthetic		
Use of acceptable technique to cannulate the artery		
Attaches extension line and flushes the cannula		
Secures the cannula in place		
Ensures the site is dressed and line is secured		
Comments on the need for a connection to a pressure transducer		
Disposes of equipment correctly		
Thanks the patient and invites any questions		
Global mark from patient		
Global mark from examiner		

6.3 Basic airway management

Emergency airway management is an essential part of initial assessment. Any problems with the airway should be identified early and dealt with rapidly. It is an everyday scenario that an emergency specialist may have to deal with and therefore could easily be part of any objective structured clinical examination (OSCE). A patient with any degree of airway compromise should be managed in a resuscitation area and appropriate help should be called. Though, this may seem obvious these simple things get forgotten in the heat of the moment and lose marks.

Preparation

- Equipment needed:
  - Pillow
  - Airway trolley containing airway equipment
  - Suction
  - Oxygen supply
  - Nasopharyngeal and oropharyngeal airways
  - Non-rebreathe face mask with reservoir bag
  - Bag valve mask
  - Mapleson-C or Water's circuit – not essential but useful in some circumstances
- Monitoring – end-tidal CO_2, blood pressure, pulse oximetry, ECG
- Drugs (if considering rapid sequence induction and as demanded by the situation)
- Personal protective equipment – gloves, apron, and face mask

Technique

When managing the airway, assessment for airway obstruction and intervention to improve airway patency go hand in hand. However, for the purpose of clarity, they are discussed here separately.

Airway assessment (use the classic look, listen and feel approach)

1. Look at the chest for paradoxical see-saw movements (indrawing with inspiration). Look in the mouth and oropharynx for any secretions/vomitus, blood, foreign bodies, swelling or oedema.
2. Listen for any upper airway sounds. Normal breathing is quiet with gentle flow of air with each respiratory cycle. Stridor, snoring or gurgling sounds may indicate an obstructed airway. Stridor is produced in laryngeal or sub-laryngeal obstruction. It is a harsh sound which can be present during both inspiration and expiration.
   Snoring indicates loose and floppy muscles of the oropharynx. It is usually produced by the tongue falling back leading to airway obstruction.
   Gurgling is produced when there are pooled secretions/fluids at the back of oropharynx.
   Absence of any sounds indicates complete airway obstruction or apnoea.

3. Feel for the air movement across the nares and mouth with your hand or lean forward and use your cheek while listening as described above. Fogging of the face mask with each cycle indicates that patient is moving air with each cycle. If the non-rebreathe mask is held firmly on the face, the reservoir bag will empty with each inspiration again indicating that the patient is 'moving air'.

Airway position

When patients are lying on their back on a flat trolley, the neck tends to extend and head flexes. This happens more commonly in the elderly with osteoarthritis in the neck. Unless there is a risk of neck injury, the head and neck should be positioned with the neck flexed and head extended. This can be done by placing a pillow under the neck and extending the head gently.

In the presence of intact airway reflexes and an otherwise clear airway, a safe airway position can be maintained with the patient in the left lateral position with slight head-down tilt of the trolley. This helps gravitate the secretions out of the mouth and avoids aspiration in the right main bronchus.

Airway suction

If there are secretions/fluids visible in the mouth, they should be suctioned. Use curved tip suction (e.g. Yankauer), and perform suctioning under direct vision (**Figure 6.3.1**). The oropharynx can be suctioned using endotracheal suction catheter introduced through the nose or an airway adjunct if one is in place.

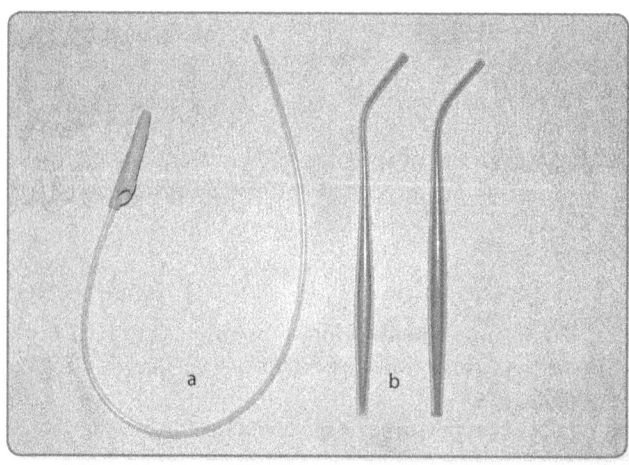

Figure 6.3.1 Suction devices (a) suction catheter (b) Yankauer suction device.

Airway manoeuvres

Once the patient is appropriately positioned, use manoeuvres to open the obstructed airway.
- **Head tilt and chin lift**: place two fingers below the chin and lift it up, extending the head gently at the same time with other hand on the forehead of the patient. This lifts

the tongue and helps to clear the airway. Do not perform a chin lift if the cervical spine requires immobilisation due to concerns of trauma
- **Jaw thrust**: when there are concerns regarding a cervical spine injury, a jaw thrust can be performed while maintaining cervical spine immobilisation. Place the heels of the hands on patient's zygomas and curl the fingers behind the angle of the jaw. Lift the jaw forwards avoiding any neck movements

Airway adjuncts

If the patient cannot maintain an open airway and needs airway manoeuvres to keep it open, use an adjunct to maintain the patency of the airway (**Figure 6.3.2**).
- **Oropharyngeal airway (Guedel airway)**: if the patient is awake and has intact airway reflexes; they can gag on this and will not tolerate the airway. Correct sizing is essential as either a larger or a smaller oropharyngeal airway (OPA) can worsen the airway patency. Size the OPA's length by matching it to the length from the mid-incisors to the angle of the jaw. In adults it is introduced inverted until it reaches the soft palate and is then rotated 180°, this avoids displacing the tongue backwards during insertion
- **Nasopharyngeal airway (NPA)**: this is tolerated better in patients who are more conscious. The NPA's length is measured from the tip of the patient's nose to the tragus of the ear. The correct diameter is the one that will fit in the nares. Lubricate with aqua gel and insert in the direction of the curve perpendicular to the face. If there is obstruction, use the other nostril. These can cause bleeding in the nose and therefore avoid undue force. The NPA should be used with caution in suspected basal skull fractures.

Figure 6.3.2 Airway adjuncts (a) oropharyngeal airways (b) nasopharyngeal airways.

Tracheal intubation

The above procedures can maintain a stable airway but do not represent a definitive airway which is a secured, cuffed tube in the trachea. If there is an indication for a definitive airway, then proceed to rapid sequence induction (this is discussed further in section 6.24).

Surgical airway

A surgical cricothyroidotomy will save an airway in an emergency when other options fail. (This is discussed further in section 6.25).

Post-procedure steps

Connect appropriate monitoring (ECG, blood pressure, pulse oximetry) to the patient and maintain appropriate oxygen saturation. End-tidal CO_2 monitoring is a useful adjunct that gives an accurate respiratory rate. The catheter can be attached to the inside of the face mask (if patient is self-ventilating without any airway device). Keep the patient under observation and look for any signs of deterioration. Consider which investigations must be arranged, ensure help is on its way and begin thinking about a further plan for the patient.

Scenario

A 34-year-old, known epileptic patient named Marcus Dewey has had multiple seizures at home. You are pre-alerted to his arrival in the ED. The paramedics have given him one dose of rectal and another of intravenous diazepam. You have a senior nurse with you. You have 1 minute to prepare your equipment. Teach a junior doctor how to manage the patient's airway with basic airway manoeuvres.

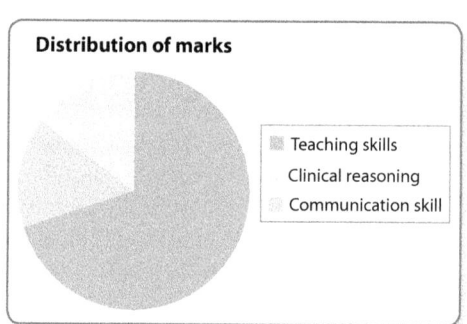

Distribution of marks
- Teaching skills
- Clinical reasoning
- Communication skill

Mark sheet	Achieved	Not achieved
Introduces self to the nurse, informs her about the patient		
Enquires from junior doctor about their previous experience and knowledge		
Sets learning objectives		
Cleans hands and puts on personal protective equipment		
Assembles and checks airway equipment		
Makes a plan and assigns roles – nurse can connect monitoring		
Checks monitoring – pulse oximetry, end-tidal CO_2, blood pressure, ECG		
Calls for help from intensivist/senior staff		
Takes hand over from paramedic		
Looks in the mouth		
Suctions oropharynx with tracheal catheter to clear secretions		
Listens to airway noises – gurgling and snoring		
Feels for air movement and looks for fogging of the mask		
Optimises airway position correctly using a chin lift or jaw thrust		
Confirms need for an airway adjunct-correctly sizes the OPA, inserts it correctly, must remove if patient gags or coughs		

Cont'd...

Cont'd...

Mark sheet	Achieved	Not achieved
Uses NPA if OPA not tolerated. Correctly measures the length and inserts safely		
Uses reservoir bag and high flow oxygen		
Positions patient left lateral position		
Checks observations and continues further assessment of breathing, circulation and disability		
Re-assesses for any obstruction		
Makes further plan for observations and need for further investigations		
Invites questions from junior doctor		
Answers junior doctor's questions appropriately		
Directs to relevant self-learning modules, videos and simulation courses		
Is non-judgemental and facilitates learning		
Global Mark from examiner		
Global Mark from junior doctor		

Suggested reading

Benger J, Nolan J, Clancy M. Emergency Airway Management. Cambridge University Press; 2009.

6.4 Ascitic drainage

Indications

- Diagnostic – investigating a patient with ascites for the cause or when spontaneous bacterial peritonitis is suspected
- Therapeutic – for symptomatic relief in patient with large ascites

Contraindications

- Infection at insertion site
- Acute surgical abdomen
- Distended bowel or bowel obstruction
- Intra-abdominal adhesions
- Too little fluid to tap – this can be confirmed by USS in ED if available
- Uncorrected coagulopathy is a relative contraindication; most patients with liver failure have some degree of coagulopathy and thrombocytopaenia. However, if the coagulopathy is severe or platelets are lower than 40×10^9/L the procedure will normally be deferred until the abnormality is corrected

Complications

- Haematoma at site of procedure
- Introduction of infection
- Hypovolaemia leading to shock and renal failure
- Persistent leakage of ascitic fluid from the drain site
- Haemoperitoneum (uncommon)
- Bowel perforation (uncommon)

Common sites

- Right or left iliac fossa
- Ultrasound guided marking on skin where the collection is closest to the skin

Pre-procedure check

- Drugs – local anaesthetic – 1% lignocaine
- Cleaning and preparation – skin cleaning with chlorhexidine or iodine
- Equipment:
  - Minor dressing pack, with sterile drapes
  - 10 mL syringe and an orange and a green needle
  - 20 mL syringe
  - Bonanno pigtail catheter or other purpose-built paracentesis catheter
  - Drainage bag
  - Dressing and suture to secure the catheter in place
  - Bottles to take samples
- Monitoring – intravenous line connected and running
- Sterility – sterile gloves and field

Technique

Ensure all the equipment is available and easily accessible.

The patient should be lying supine, preferably leaning towards the side where you plan to tap and should have an empty bladder. Percuss the abdomen and confirm dullness to percussion at the chosen site. Hands should be washed and dried before wearing sterile gloves. Clean the selected area with povidone-iodine or chlorhexidine skin solution. Establish sterility and cover the area of the abdomen with a sterile drape leaving a window for the drain insertion.

The site for the procedure is approximately 15 cm lateral and 2-3 cm below the umbilicus. At this point, the rectus and anterior abdominal wall muscles become aponeurotic. This site is also located away from the epigastric arteries. Consider using ultrasound to locate the best site.

Infiltrate an appropriate local anaesthetic at the site, first using an orange 25G needle in the skin and then using a larger 21G green needle in the abdominal wall. On advancing the needle into the peritoneal cavity one can feel a give and aspirate peritoneal fluid.

Attach a 20 mL syringe to the end of the Bonanno catheter. Insert using the so-called Z technique. Pull the skin taught and insert the needle perpendicular to the skin. Release the skin and advance the needle obliquely in the subcutaneous tissue before advancing the needle perpendicular to the abdominal wall in the peritoneal cavity. This ensures that the holes in the skin and the abdominal wall are away from each other and therefore there is less chance of leakage of the fluid after drain removal.

Once in the peritoneal cavity, aspirate the syringe to confirm placement in the ascitic fluid. Once aspirating freely, advance the needle a few millimetres and then advance the catheter further and withdraw the needle from the catheter. If the fluid cannot be aspirated from the catheter when the needle has been withdrawn, do not re-advance the needle in the catheter. This is because the catheter has a 'pig-tail' end which tends to curl up. If the needle is advanced, it may cut through, rather than advance into the catheter.

If necessary take samples for cytology, culture, neutrophil count and albumin as required and connect the catheter to the drainage bag. Secure the catheter in place using a suture.

Clear the sharps and other equipment appropriately. The amount of fluid to be removed and duration for which the catheter is to be left in place will depend on the situation. If the catheter is for therapeutic drainage, it is recommended for it not to remain inserted overnight.

Scenario

Mr Martin Cruise is a 36-year-old man with a history of alcoholic liver disease and cirrhosis. He has attended the ED with a temperature of 38°C. His abdomen is distended and tender. Insert an ascitic drain and to send the fluid for investigation while also relieving some of the discomfort. The patient has had this procedure before.

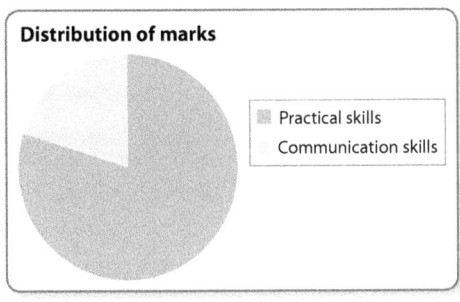

Distribution of marks
- Practical skills
- Communication skills

Mark sheet	Achieved	Not achieved
Introduces self to patient appropriately		
Confirms patient identity		
Asks about presence of pain and offers analgesia		
Briefly asks about medical history, medication and allergies		
Explains procedure to patient		
Performs abdominal examination, demonstrates shifting dullness and localises area of dullness		
Checks any previous surgery on abdomen, enquires about any contraindications		
Obtains patient consent		
Prepares and checks equipment		
Correctly positions the patient and identifies the point of drain placement in lower left or right quadrant		
Cleans hands, wears sterile gloves, establishes a sterile field, uses sterile drapes		
Performs adequate skin preparation		
Correctly infiltrates local anaesthetic		
Correctly inserts the catheter in abdomen, aspirates while inserting the needle		
Secures the catheter in place		
Takes appropriate samples		
Connects the drainage bag		
Disposes of equipment correctly		
Thanks the patient, ensures their comfort and invites any questions		
Global mark from patient		
Global mark from examiner		

6.5 Central venous cannulation

Indications
- Therapeutic – for delivery of drugs, total parenteral nutrition (TPN), temporary pacing wire, dialysis, fluid resuscitation
- Diagnostic – for taking blood samples regularly
- Monitoring – central venous pressure, insertion of pulmonary artery catheter

Contraindications
These are relative contraindications depending on the clinical situation:
- Infection at the chosen site of insertion
- Coagulopathy, low platelet count
- Difficult landmarks, uncooperative patient

Complications
- Early:
  - Arrhythmias
  - Inadvertent arterial puncture
  - Neck haematoma
  - Air or guidewire embolism
  - Pneumothorax – (the risk is highest for subclavian lines insertion), haemothorax
  - Cardiac tamponade, if inserted too far
- Late:
  - Line sepsis
  - Vein thrombosis

Common sites of central line insertion
- Internal jugular vein
- Subclavian vein
- Femoral vein

Ultrasound guidance
The National Institute for Health and Care Excellence (NICE) recommends that 2D ultrasound should be considered in most clinical situations when inserting a central line under elective or emergency conditions to reduce the risk of complications. If ultrasound is available, select a high frequency vascular probe and use a sterile sheath and sterile gel. It is recommended that ultrasound should be used to provide direct visualisation of the vessels during the procedure.

Pre-procedure check
- Drugs – local anaesthetic – 1% lignocaine
- Cleaning and preparation – skin cleaning with chlorhexidine or iodine

Figure 6.5.1 Central line equipment (a) central line (single lumen in photograph) (b) guidewire (c) syringe (d) needle (e) dilator (f) central line clamp/holder.

- Equipment (**Figure 6.5.1**):
  - Central venous catheter – 15 cm for neck and 20 cm for femoral line, all lines flushed
  - 10 mL syringe and saline
  - Extension ports and connectors for each port
  - Minor dressings pack
  - Suture, dressing
- Monitoring:
  - Continuous ECG monitoring
- Sterility – full surgical scrubs, gown, mask, hat, sterile gloves and sterile drapes

Technique for internal jugular vein cannulation

Position the patient supine with trolley tilted head down approximately 10° to 20°. Extend the patient's neck and turn the head slightly to the opposite side from where you intend to insert the central line. Stand at the head-end of the patient with equipment prepared on the trolley next to your dominant hand. Keep the guidewire ready to insert, in front so that you can reach it quickly without much movement. Make sure you can see the ECG trace on the monitor.

Clean and prepare the area with skin disinfectant, and cover the area with a sterile drape, making sure that you can see the landmarks. Inject local anaesthetic in the skin and in the subcutaneous tissue.

The internal jugular vein (IJV) runs vertically downwards from below the mastoid process to just above the clavicle in between the two heads of the sternocleidomastoid (SCM) muscle staying lateral to the internal and then common carotid artery. However, this relationship to the artery is not fixed and in up to 20% of patients the vein may lie anterior to the artery increasing the risk of arterial puncture.

In the low approach, the vein is punctured at the apex between the two heads of SCM, lateral to the pulse and the needle is directed towards the ipsilateral nipple.

Keep the little finger at the cricoid cartilage and palpate the carotid pulse at this level. Insert the needle at a 30° angle to the skin, with the bevel directed upwards, aspirating as you advance the needle. Once the needle enters the IJV venous blood can be aspirated.

Once blood is aspirated, hold the needle with the non-dominant hand maintaining the same position and disconnect the syringe. Any pulsatile flow out of the needle should alert to the possibility of arterial puncture. If there is no pulsatile back flow, pass the guidewire, down the needle. This should pass easily without any obstruction, if resistance is felt resist the temptation to push the guidewire harder. Pass the guidewire beyond the 10 cm mark. Now slide the needle off while holding the guidewire in place. Where the guidewire enters the skin make a small nick in the skin with the blade (blade pointing away from the guide wire to avoid damaging it) to allow for the passage of the dilator.

Pass the dilator over the guidewire, making sure that the other hand holds the wire so that it doesn't get pushed into the vessel. Gently pass the dilator, without undue force in the direction of the wire.

Carefully remove the dilator, keeping the wire in place and press the puncture site with gauze to prevent bleeding. Next pass the catheter over the guidewire and advance it into the vein, it should pass easily. The catheter should be inserted about 12–15 cm so that the tip is positioned just at or above the carina. Finally remove the guidewire.

Aspirate each lumen of the catheter and flush them with normal saline. Place a connector over each lumen port. Secure the catheter with the clamp sutured superficially taking care not to suture the vessel underneath and then cover the insertion site with a clear dressing. Arrange a chest X-ray after IJV or SCV cannulation to confirm catheter position and exclude an iatrogenic pneumothorax.

Distinguishing arterial versus venous puncture

Under certain circumstances there may be doubt as to whether the needle has been advanced into an artery or vein. Dark blood which is not pulsatile is likely to be venous. However, in hypotensive hypoxic patients this may not be the case. If ultrasound is not available to visualise the catheter's placement, alternative methods are to run a blood gas and decide if the results represent arterial or venous blood, or connect a transducer and observe for an arterial or venous wave form.

Technique for subclavian vein cannulation

The patient should be supine with their shoulders relaxed; some prefer to put a small pillow in between the scapulae to facilitate this. The preparation and post-procedure steps for the procedure are the same as for IJV cannulation except the person performing the procedure must be standing to the patient's side at the level of the patient's shoulders.

The subclavian vein is the extension of the axillary vein beyond the first rib. It runs underneath the clavicle, anterior to the subclavian artery to join the IJV, forming the brachiocephalic vein at the sternoclavicular joint.

Keep one finger of the non-dominant hand in the suprasternal notch and other finger at the junction of the lateral and middle third of the clavicle. Insert the needle at this point aiming towards the clavicle. Locate the vein by advancing the needle towards the suprasternal notch running just under the clavicle.

Technique for femoral vein cannulation

Again, prepare for the procedure as described above. Position the patient supine with their hips extended and in neutral rotation. If they can be tilted head up 5° this will assist in filling the vein and thus making it easier to puncture. The preparation and post-procedure steps for the procedure are the same as for IJV cannulation except the person performing the procedure must be standing to the patient's side at the level of the patient's hips.

The femoral vein runs medial to the femoral artery, at the inguinal ligament. The femoral artery is located 2 cm below the midinguinal point, i.e. midway of the anterior superior iliac spine and pubic symphysis.

Palpate the femoral pulse just under the inguinal ligament and insert the needle 1 cm medial to the pulse. Advance the needle at 45° to the skin directed towards the umbilicus until blood is aspirated.

Scenario

Mr Woo is a 54-year-old man who has been diagnosed with septic shock. He has had a 2 L fluid bolus and initial antibiotics; despite this his blood pressure is 74/36 mmHg. He has been catheterised and has passed 15 mL of urine in the last hour. The junior doctor looking after Mr Woo has asked you to teach him how to insert a central line as he has never done it before. Insert a femoral central line while demonstrating the procedure to the junior doctor.

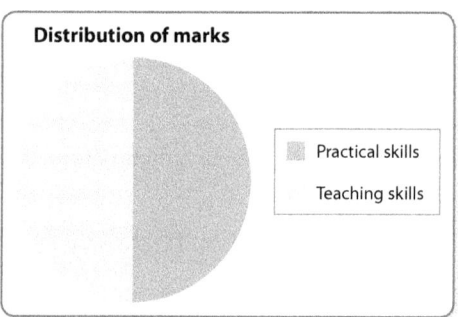

Distribution of marks
- Practical skills
- Teaching skills

Mark sheet	Achieved	Not achieved
Introduces self to the junior doctor and confirms their and the patient's identity		
Clarifies clinical situation and treatment up to now		
Enquires from junior doctor about their previous experience and knowledge		
Sets the learning objectives		
Briefly asks about medical history, medication and allergies		
Explains procedure to patient		
Obtains patient consent		
Explains indications, contraindications and complications		
Checks the equipment		
Flushes the catheter lumens with saline		
Correctly positions the patient and identifies/demonstrates the landmarks in the femoral triangle		
Washes hands and wears sterile gown, gloves and mask		
Performs skin cleaning with povidone-iodine or chlorhexidine		

Cont'd...

Cont'd...

Mark sheet	Achieved	Not achieved
Establishes a sterile field, uses sterile drapes		
Injects appropriate local anaesthetic		
States maximum safe dose of local anaesthetic		
Uses Seldinger technique appropriately, checks for inadvertent arterial puncture while teaching the procedure		
Keeps control of the guidewire at all stages, no undue pressure on the wire		
Secures the catheter in place adequately		
Disposes of equipment correctly		
Thanks the patient and offers to help them redress		
Invites any questions from junior doctor		
Answers junior doctors questions appropriately		
Directs to relevant self-learning modules, videos and simulation courses		
Is non-judgemental and facilitates learning		
Global mark from junior doctor		
Global mark from examiner		

Instructions for actor

Your name is Michael Adekoya. You are a new junior doctor and have not been working in the ED for long. You are aware of central lines but have never seen one put in. Your current patient needs one and you have asked if you can watch the procedure. You are grateful for the opportunity and have some questions.

When the doctors injects local anaesthetic, you ask them what anaesthetic they use and how much.

After the procedure, ask the doctor how to decide which location the central line should be inserted. Also ask how to choose how many lumens the central line should have.

6.6 Inserting a chest drain by blunt dissection

Chest drains are placed in the pleural cavity to drain fluid or air.

Indications

The main reason for placing a drain using blunt dissection in the ED is to drain a haemopneumothorax. Though not all relevant in the ED additional indications for a chest drain which may often be Seldinger drains are:
- A pneumothorax:
  - In any ventilated patient
  - Tension pneumothorax after initial needle decompression
  - Persistent or recurrent pneumothorax after simple aspiration
  - Large secondary spontaneous pneumothorax in patients aged over 50 years
- Malignant pleural effusions
- Empyema and complicated parapneumonic pleural effusion
- Post-surgical
- Haemothorax

Contraindications

- Coagulopathy is a relative contraindication to chest drain insertion

Complications

- Haemorrhage
- Infection at the drain site or in the pleural cavity

Technique

The first step is to confirm the indication for a chest drain to be inserted. This should be done clinically and most circumstances also require checking an up-to-date chest X-ray.

Consent for the procedure should be sought unless the situation renders this inappropriate. Complications to inform the patient of are pain, local or pleural infection, visceral injury or drain blockage.

Chest drain insertion is a painful procedure and a small dose of opiate analgesia with or without sedation should normally be given.

Trauma patients are most likely to be supine but reclining on a bed is also acceptable. The ipsilateral arm needs to be abducted.

The appropriate site of insertion within the safe triangle (**Figure 6.6.1**) and size of chest drain should be confirmed.

Using aseptic technique (drapes/gown/gloves) the area should be cleaned and infiltrated from the skin to the pleura with 1% lignocaine (using up to 3 mg/kg).

A horizontal incision should be made parallel to and above (thus avoiding the

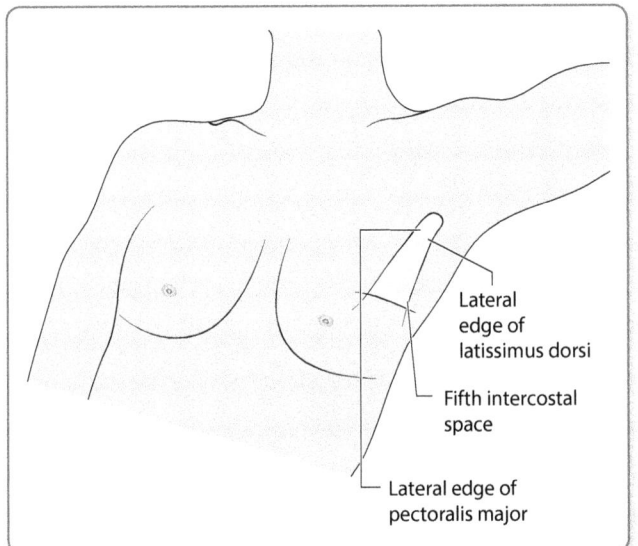

Figure 6.6.1 The safe triangle.

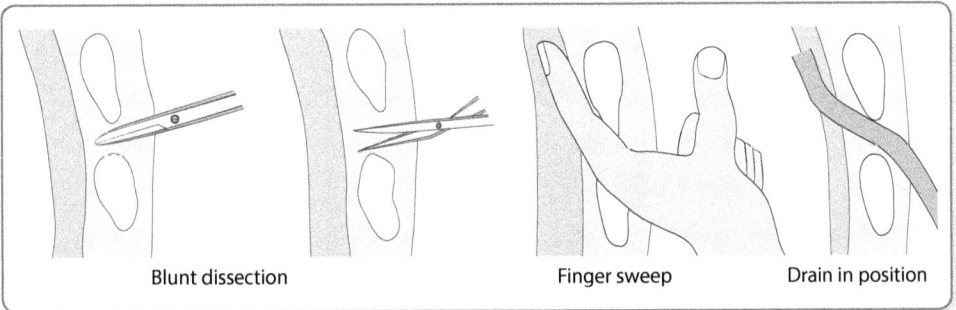

Figure 6.6.2 Inserting the chest drain.

neurovascular bundle) a rib. This should be large enough to accommodate the clinician's finger and the chest drain.

Blunt dissection (**Figure 6.6.2**) is then carried out using forceps until the pleura is breached. Care must be taken not to use excessive force as this may result in the forceps penetrating too deep and causing a visceral injury.

A finger is then inserted into the pleural space to confirm position and ensure no organs are present that may be damaged by the passage of the drain.

The drain is then inserted to an appropriate depth. Due to a high rate of complications trochars should never be used. However, a firm introducer may help guide the drain's insertion (**Figure 6.6.3**).

The drain should be attached to a bottle with an underwater seal (**Figure 6.6.4**). The passage of blood or visible bubbling and swinging of the water in the bottle confirm the drain is working.

The drain should then be sutured in place and the insertion site should then be covered by a clear dressing. The patient should be reassessed and a chest X-ray performed to confirm the drain position.

Figure 6.6.3 Equipment for open chest drain insertion (a) scalpel (b) introducer (c) chest drain (d) suturing equipment (e) gauze and sterile sheet (f) procedure tray (g) suture.

Figure 6.6.4 Chest drain bottle with under water seal.

Scenario

Mr Jones has fallen onto his right side and has a moderate haemopneumothorax. Other injuries have been excluded. You have been asked to insert a chest drain by blunt dissection.

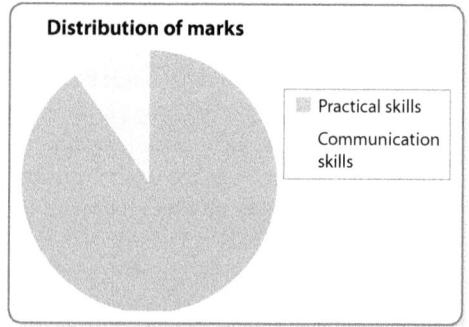

Distribution of marks

- Practical skills
- Communication skills

Mark sheet	Achieved	Not achieved
Introduces self to patient appropriately		
Confirms patient identity		
Enquires regarding presence of pain and offers analgesia		
Briefly asks about medical history, medication and allergies		
States need to listen to lung fields		
Reviews chest X-ray and confirms side to be drained		
Explains procedure to patient		
Obtains patient consent		
Cleans hands and applies sterile gloves and gown		
Prepares and checks equipment		
Prepares and places sterile field/drapes		
Identifies safe triangle for drain placement		
Injects local anaesthetic stating maximum safe dose		
Checks local anaesthetic has worked		
Makes incision correctly stating need to avoid neurovascular bundle		
Uses correct technique for blunt dissection		
Performs finger sweep within pleural space		
Places chest drain without trochar		
Connects drain to bottle with underwater seal		
Confirms drain is bubbling/swinging		
Sutures drain in place		
States need for a chest X-ray to confirm drain position		
Removes drapes and ensures patient comfort		
Correctly disposes of equipment		
Global mark from patient		
Global mark from examiner		

Suggested reading

Havelock T, Teoh R, Laws D, et al. Pleural procedures and thoracic ultrasound: British Thoracic Society pleural disease guideline. Thorax 2010; 65:ii61eii76.

6.7 Clearing a cervical spine

There are two established sets of clinical rules that guide whether imaging is required when assessing a patient with a suspected cervical spine injury. If the rules are satisfied the cervical spine can be cleared based on the clinical information without resorting to X-ray (see Section 6.26).

The National Emergency X-Radiography Utilization Study (NEXUS) published in 2000 attempts to identify five risk factors that indicate a low risk of injury in patients with blunt trauma. They included all patients with blunt neck trauma irrespective of their Glasgow Coma Score (GCS) or clinical condition. Therefore, if a patient satisfies all the NEXUS criteria, the probability of a cervical spine injury is low and hence an X-ray is not required.
- Absence of midline cervical spine tenderness
- Absence of focal neurological deficit
- Normal level of alertness
- No evidence of intoxication
- Absence of any distracting injury causing clinically significant pain

The NEXUS rules have been shown to be 99% sensitive and 12.7% specific for clinically significant cervical spine injuries.

The Canadian C-Spine rules (CCR) were published in 2001 (**Figure 6.7.1**). They included patients >16 years of age, with either neck pain following blunt trauma or no neck pain but injury above the clavicle, not ambulatory or with a dangerous mechanism of injury. In addition, patients had to be alert, i.e. GCS 15 and stable, i.e. systolic blood pressure of >90 mmHg and respiratory rate between 10 and 24 breaths per minute.

They also excluded patients with known vertebral disease, i.e. ankylosing spondylitis, rheumatoid arthritis, spinal stenosis or previous cervical surgery.

These rules have been shown to be 100% sensitive and 42.5% specific for clinically important cervical spine injuries.

In a separate study published in 2003, both these criteria were validated and compared and this showed that the NEXUS criteria are less sensitive and significantly less specific than CCR. The National Institute for Health and Care Excellence (NICE) published guidance regarding cervical spine imaging as part of the guidance for management of head injury patients. The NICE criteria are broadly based on the CCR.

In practice (and the exam), the candidate should take a balanced view and therefore be aware of both the rules. Therefore in this station focus on three main steps:
- History of the mechanism of injury:
  - Dangerous mechanism of injury as described above
  - Whether or not a simple MVC
- Patient factors that preclude clinical assessment – in history and on examination
  - History:
    - Age >65 years
    - Previous neck disease or surgery
    - Limb paraesthesia
  - Examination:
    - Intoxicated patient
    - Glasgow coma score <15
    - Systolic blood pressure <90 mmHg or respiratory rate <10 or >24 breaths per minute

- Distracting injury with clinically significant pain
- Focal neurological deficit
- Range of movement testing if it is safe to do so
  - Check low risk criteria as above

In an OSCE, the candidate will be expected to safely assess the patient and then manage the cervical spine appropriately, including clearing the cervical spine if the criteria are met.

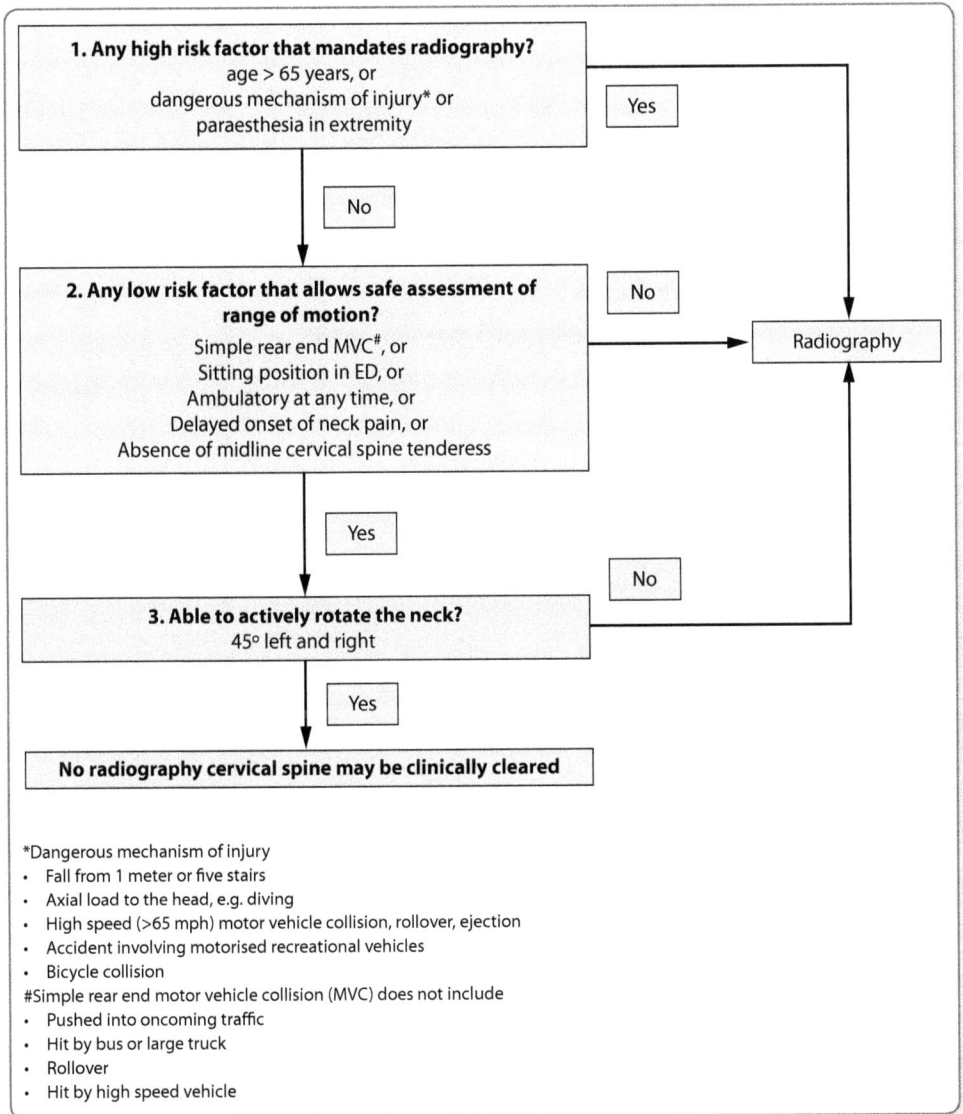

Figure 6.7.1 Summary of Canadian C-spine rules.

Scenario

A 37-year-old man has been brought in with his cervical spine fully immobilised following a car accident. He is otherwise well and did not need any pre-hospital resuscitation. Assess his cervical spine and manage him appropriately.

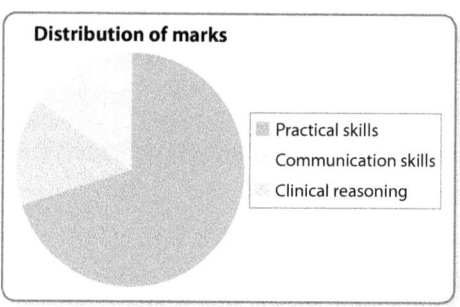

Distribution of marks
- Practical skills
- Communication skills
- Clinical reasoning

Mark sheet	Achieved	Not achieved
Introduces self to patient appropriately		
Confirms patient identity		
Explains purpose of discussion		
Asks about presence of pain and offers analgesia		
Asks about the mechanism of accident to identify high risk and low risk features		
Asks about injuries suffered		
Asks about new neurological symptoms		
Asks about intoxication and illicit drug use		
Briefly asks about medical history, medication and allergies		
Obtains consent for examination		
Cleans hands		
Performs screening neurological examination		
Examines neck for midline tenderness		
Correctly identifies patient as low risk for a cervical spine injury		
Tests range of movement in cervical spine		
Clears cervical spine		
Offers post neck-injury advice		
Invites questions		
Global mark from patient		
Global mark from examiner		

Suggested reading

Hoffman JR, Mower WR, Wolfson AB, et al. Validity of a set of clinical criteria to rule out injury to the cervical spine in patients with blunt trauma. National Emergency X-Radiography Utilization Study Group. N Engl J Med 2000; 343:94–99.

Management of co-operative, adult patients with potential cervical spine injury in the Emergency Department. College of Emergency Medicine. Clinical Effectiveness Committee, 2007.

National Institute for Health and Care Excellence (NICE) Head Injury. Clinical guideline 176. London: NICE; 2014.

Stiell IG, Wells GA, Vandemheen KL, et al. The Canadian C-spine rule for radiography in alert and stable trauma patients. JAMA 2001; 286:1841–1848.

6.8 Non-invasive ventilation

Non-invasive ventilation (NIV) is provided by bi-level positive airway pressure (BiPAP). Continuous positive airway pressure (CPAP) will not ventilate the patient although it increases mean airway pressure and overcomes intrinsic positive end-expiratory pressure (PEEP) and therefore improves oxygenation and reduces work of breathing.

Indications

- An acute exacerbation of chronic obstructive pulmonary disease (COPD) with a respiratory acidosis (pH 7.25–7.35)
- Type II respiratory failure secondary to chest wall deformity or neuromuscular disease
- Cardiogenic pulmonary oedema which is unresponsive to CPAP

Contraindications

- Facial burns/trauma/recent facial or upper airway surgery
- Vomiting
- Fixed upper airway obstruction
- The presence of an undrained pneumothorax
- Relative contraindications include:
  - Recent upper gastrointestinal surgery
  - Severe co-morbidities
  - Confusion/agitation/decreased level of consciousness
  - Bowel obstruction

Complications

- Failure of treatment
- Haemodynamic compromise
- Poor tolerance
- Pneumothorax
- Aspiration

Pre-procedure check

- Use of controlled FIO_2 using venturi mask to maintain SO_2 between 88% and 92%.
- Ensure an arterial blood gas (ABG) has been obtained to confirm the indication to start NIV as stated above
- Chest X-ray to exclude a pneumothorax has been performed and reviewed
- Equipment needed is available:
  - NIV machine
  - Circuit
  - Filter
  - Face mask appropriately sized to the patient
- The required monitoring is connected (non-invasive blood pressure, ECG, pulse oximetry)
- A plan for treatment failure must be made prior to commencing NIV. The clinician is required to decide what further interventions would be appropriate. Is NIV the maximum

appropriate treatment for the patient or would they be a candidate for intubation and ventilation? Clearly this decision should be made with the involvement of the relevant hospital specialists (respiratory physician/intensivist), and the patient if appropriate.

Technique

Consent the patient and explain to them the process. The patient should be sitting forwards or in a semi-recumbent position. The procedure of having a mask fitted should be explained to them prior to placing the mask. Many patients (who are already struggling to breathe) find the mask very claustrophobic and can panic. This leads to poor tolerance of NIV and a higher failure rate for the treatment. The best way to pre-empt this is to reassuringly explain to the patient what the procedure involves (initiating the ventilation on lower pressures can also improve comfort and tolerance of the treatment).

The next step is to correctly size the face mask that the patient will require. Masks are normally available in three sizes – small, medium and large. The size is determined with a triangular hole that is present on all NIV circuit packaging. Place this hole on patient's face in such a way that the apex of the triangle sits on the bridge of the nose and the base is just below the lower lip with both angles just outside the angle of the mouth. It must not encroach on the corner of the eyes.

Set up the NIV machine with BiPAP selection and a starting pressure of 10 mmH$_2$O of inspiratory positive airway pressure (IPAP) and 4 mmH$_2$O of expiratory positive airway pressure (EPAP). Connect the circuit to the machine outlet with a bacterial filter in between. Hold the face mask on the patient's face and let them acclimatise to it. Add additional oxygen to the circuit aiming to maintain SO$_2$ between 88% and 92%. Once the patient appears comfortable with the mask, tighten the face mask ensuring firm grip on the face and even distribution of pressure on the face. Check for any air leaks around the face mask and adjust the mask. The expiration port on the circuit should be pointed away from the patient.

This initial pressure setting should help the patient get used to the NIV, but it will not do much to ventilate the patient. Increase IPAP in increments to 20 or according to patient comfort.

Ensure the patient is comfortable. They will need frequent observation and reassurance. Plan to repeat an ABG after an hour of starting on NIV. Further planning must be made as to where the patient will be managed and what further interventions would be appropriate if the NIV was unsuccessful. For some patients it is appropriate to consider intubation and ventilation while for others NIV may be the maximum treatment that may be considered appropriate.

Scenario

A 65-year-old patient with known COPD has just arrived in ED. He is looking cyanosed and is tachypnoeic. He can't speak in full sentences and is very wheezy. His initial observations show an oxygen saturation of 70% on air, pulse of 118 beats per minute, blood pressure of 150/96 mmHg and respiratory rate of 48 breaths per minute. His arterial blood gas on air shows a pH of 7.01, pO$_2$ of 5.9 kPa, pCO$_2$ of 12.4 kPa, HCO$_3^-$ of 22.1 mmol/L and base excess of -2. Start the patient on non-invasive ventilation.

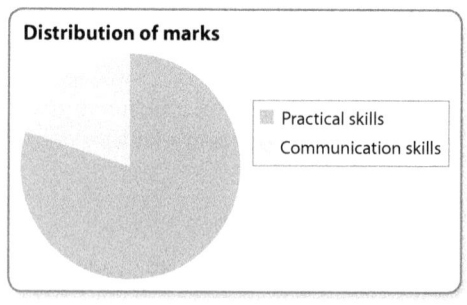

Distribution of marks

- Practical skills
- Communication skills

Mark sheet	Achieved	Not achieved
Introduces self appropriately		
Cleans hands		
Obtains consent for examination		
Examine the chest for signs of pneumothorax, heart failure		
Asks for pulse oximetry, blood pressure and ECG monitoring		
Aims for oxygen saturation between 88% and 92%		
Reviews chest X-ray		
Checks arterial blood gas results		
Explains the procedure to the patient		
Correctly sizes the face mask using gauge on mask pack		
Connects filter to the machine, then the circuit		
Checks for poor skin contact		
Starts NIV machine with sensible choice of EPAP (4 mm H_2O) and IPAP (10 mm H_2O)		
Connects supplemental oxygen to maintain SO_2 between 88% and 92%		
Holds the mask to acclimatise the patient		
Secures mask correctly		
Checks for air leak		
Ensures the expiration port is pointing away from the patient		
Changes pressure settings according to clinical response		
Plans to repeat arterial blood gas in an hour		
Discusses escalation of care in case of failure of NIV		
Plans for admission to appropriate area		
Global mark from patient		
Global mark from examiner		

Suggested reading

Benger J, Nolan J, Clancy M. Emergency Airway Management. Cambridge: Cambridge University Press, 2009.
British Thoracic Society (BTS)/Intensive Care Society (ICS) Acute Hypercapnic Respiratory Failure Guideline Development Group. BTS/ICS guidelines for the ventilatory management of acute hypercapnic respiratory failure. Thorax 2016; 71:ii1–ii35.

6.9 Direct current cardioversion

Indications

In the emergency setting direct current (DC) cardioversion is required when a patient with either a broad-complex or narrow-complex tachycardia displays adverse signs, as indicated by:
- Shock:
  - Pallor, sweating, cold and clammy extremities
  - Impaired consciousness,
  - Blood pressure <90 mmHg
- Syncope:
  - Loss of consciousness
- Heart failure:
  - Pulmonary oedema
  - Raised jugular venous pressure
  - Hepatic engorgement
- Myocardial ischaemia:
  - Angina
  - ECG changes (silent ischaemia)

DC cardioversion may also be an appropriate treatment for individuals without adverse signs who have failed to respond to pharmacological treatment.

Contraindications

- Absent central pulse (patient needs cardiopulmonary resuscitation)
- Patients who are not anticoagulated and have atrial fibrillation of an uncertain duration are at increased risk of stroke if cardioverted. This risk must be borne in mind when considering DC cardioversion, which may still be appropriate if the patients display adverse signs (as stated above)

Complications

- Pain in an awake patient
- Can induce ventricular fibrillation (shock needs to be synchronised to the R wave)

Pre-procedure check

- Full resuscitation facilities must be available
- Sedation or general anaesthetic to facilitate the procedure
- Clinician able to manage the patient's airway
- Oxygen and suction
- Intravenous access
- Monitoring (ECG, blood pressure, pulse oximetry)

Pad/paddle position

- Sternal – apical position as represented in the diagram below (**Figure 6.9.1**)

Figure 6.9.1 Defibrillator pad position.

Technique

The patient should already be in a resuscitation area and connected to a defibrillator. For the purpose of cardioversion the synchronised mode on the defibrillator should be activated (this may need to be done after each shock that is required). This is indicated by a small marker appearing near the R wave on the monitor.

Appropriate procedural sedation will be required. Midazolam (0.05–0.1 mg/kg) and fentanyl (0.5–1 µg/kg), or propofol titrated as required are commonly used alternatives for this purpose. The choice of agent is less important than safe sedation technique and use of a safe dose for the clinical situation (see Section 6.32).

Broad complex tachycardia requires higher energies. Start with 120–150 joules on a biphasic machine or 200 joules on a monophasic machine. Increase the energy stepwise if there is no response to the first shock.

Atrial fibrillation also needs higher energies similar to that for broad complex tachycardia. However, other narrow complex tachycardias such as atrial flutter and supraventricular tachycardia generally require less energy. Start with 70–120 joules biphasic or 100 joules monophasic.

In case of failure of three shocks current guidelines advise giving 300 mg amiodarone over 10–20 minutes and then repeating the shock if necessary.

Check that the cardioversion had worked. The patient will need a full ABCDE assessment. Repeat a 12-lead ECG. Continue monitoring ECG, blood pressure and oxygen saturation. If necessary discuss with a cardiologist for further management of the patient.

Scenario

A nurse calls you to see Mrs Roberts, a 75-year-old woman in the ED complaining of chest tightness. The nurse has cannulated the patient and performed an ECG. She shows you the following ECG (**Figure 6.9.2**). Manage the patient appropriately (a manikin will be used for this scenario).

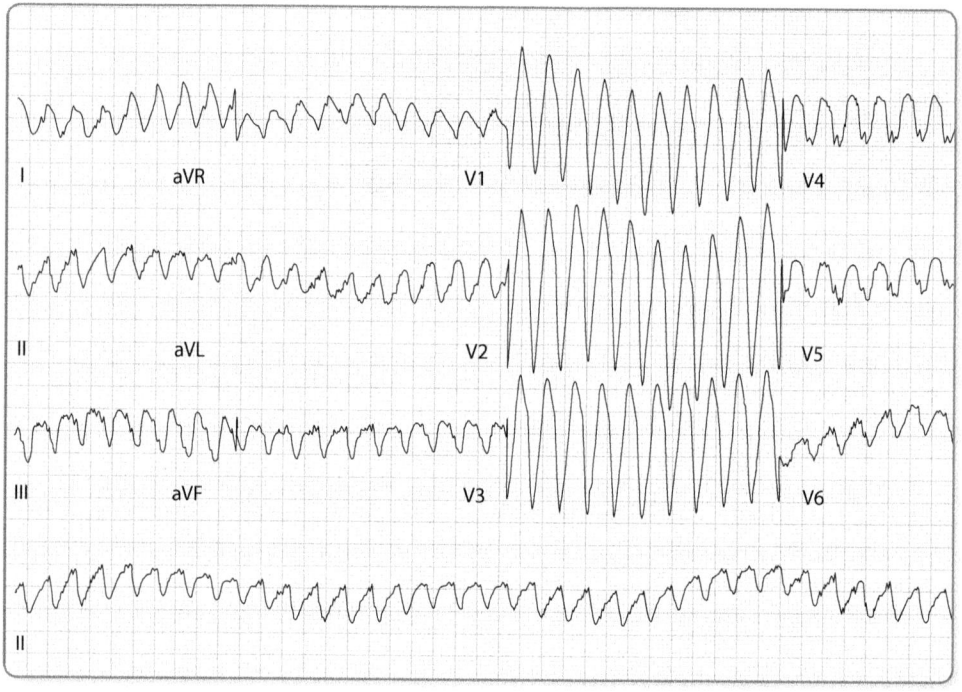

Figure 6.9.2 Mrs Roberts' ECG.

Guidance on scenario

The ECG clearly shows a broad complex tachyarrhythmia and the patient will be hypotensive and have a GCS of 13 (eyes 3, motor 6, verbal 4). There will be no help available and if assistance is requested for sedation there will be no-one available for 30 minutes. If the candidate suggests waiting for assistance the patient will develop chest pain and hypotension. It the candidate attempts to proceed without sedation the nurse will voice concerns.

Mark sheet	Achieved	Not achieved
Introduces themselves to the nurse and confirms patient identity		
Briefly enquires about the history and presentation		
Interprets the ECG rhythm correctly (VT)		
Cleans hands and wears gloves		
Performs initial ABCDE assessment		
Establishes that the patient has reduced GCS and can't give consent		
States the need for DC cardioversion		
Attaches patient to oxygen and appropriate monitoring		
Ensures intravenous access, blood samples for urgent full blood count, biochemistry and blood gas		
Selects appropriate drugs for sedation and analgesia		
Asks for anaesthetist or other doctor		
Checks airway equipment		
Checks defibrillator in sync mode		
Chooses appropriate energy for cardioversion		
Safely delivers shock		
Checks post shock rhythm		
Checks pulse, performs ABCDE assessment		
Asks for repeat 12-lead ECG		
Invites questions from nurse		
Global mark from examiner		
Global mark from nurse		

Suggested reading

Resuscitation guidelines. Resuscitation Council (UK), London, 2010.

6.10 Focused assessment with sonography in trauma, aorta and vascular access ultrasound

The core level 1 ultrasound curriculum expects trainees to be level 1 competent by the end of ST6 or higher training. Focused assessment with sonography in trauma (FAST), assessment of the abdominal aorta and IVC, vascular access and echocardiography in life support are the four main areas of competence. Up until now, there has not been an objective structured clinical examinations (OSCE) station on performing these scans, but it is possible that there will be in the future.

Focused assessment with sonography in trauma

The FAST is used as part of primary survey in a trauma patient. The assessment aims to answer a single question of whether there is free fluid present or not. It is most useful in a haemodynamically unstable patient where the demonstration of fluid in the abdominal or pleural or pericardial cavity suggests the presence of blood and mandates the need for definitive treatment, e.g. laparotomy.

Indications
- Blunt or penetrating trauma

Contraindications
- None

Advantages
- Can be performed in an unstable patient
- Portable
- Quick and easy to perform, non-invasive
- Repeatable
- High specificity

Disadvantages
- Cannot rule out pathology
- Does not identify any organ injury/site of bleeding
- Cannot distinguish blood from other fluids (e.g. ascites)
- Can be technically difficult in some individuals, e.g. obese patient

Pre-procedure check
- Equipment:
  - Portable ultrasound machine
  - Low frequency curvilinear probe
- Ultrasound gel
- Ensure that the probe is clean and personal protective equipment is worn

Standard views
Four views are obtained as part of a standard FAST scan:
- Right upper quadrant (RUQ) view to include Morrison's pouch, and right costophrenic pleural recess
- Left upper quadrant (LUQ) view to include splenorenal recess and the left costophrenic pleural recess
- Subcostal or parasternal view for the pericardial sac
- Pelvic cavity in both transverse and sagittal planes

Technique
The patient is positioned supine. The marker on the probe is always pointing to the head or the right side of the patient.
- **RUQ view (Figures 6.10.1a and 6.10.1b)**: the probe is positioned on the right side in the coronal plane in the mid-axillary line, at the level of the xiphisternum with the marker pointing towards the head. Abduct the patient's arm to allow space to position the probe. The probe is angled slightly posteriorly to visualise the renal capsule and the liver

Figure 6.10.1a and 6.10.1b RUQ view

- **LUQ view (Figures 6.10.2a and 6.10.2b)**: again abduct the patient's arm to allow space to position the probe. This view is a little more difficult to obtain as the left kidney is slightly higher that the right. Position the probe in the similar manner to the right, but slightly higher up towards the axilla and also more posteriorly

Figure 6.10.2a and 6.10.2b LUQ view

- Subcostal view (Figures 6.10.3a and 6.10.3b): the probe is placed in the subxiphoid position, pressing down but pointing upwards towards the heart. The depth may have to be increased for this view

Figure 6.10.3a and 6.10.3b Subcostal view

- Pelvic view (Figures 6.10.4a and 6.10.4b): position the probe a couple of centimetres above the pubic symphysis first in the transverse and then in the sagittal plane

Figure 6.10.4a and 6.10.4b Pelvic view

Post-procedure steps

Fluid is demonstrated as a black area on ultrasound. If fluid is not visualised, consider repeating the scan at regular intervals or (more likely) proceeding to a CT scan. It is important to understand that this is not a definitive scan. The absence of visible fluid (blood) does not meet there has not been significant injury. Save the images, appropriately annotated. The decision-making process with regard to FAST scan results can be complicated. FAST scans may not add any benefit in patients who are stable enough to undergo a CT scan; however, demonstrating the presence of blood early is valuable in case the patient deteriorates prior to CT and also allows the early mobilisation of operating theatre resources.

Assessment of abdominal aorta

Just like FAST, the assessment here is to answer the single question of whether an abdominal aortic aneurysm (AAA) is present (aorta more than 3 cm wide) or not. Clinical assessment of the aorta can be unreliable and an emergency scan can help identify an aneurysm earlier and more reliably.

Indications

Any presentation where an AAA needs to be excluded:
- Unexplained back or abdominal pain in an older patient
- Renal colic in an older patient
- Syncopal episode in an older patient
- Clinical examination indicates the presence of an aneurysm

Contraindications

- None

Advantages

- Earlier and reliable identification of an AAA
- Earlier diagnosis leading to earlier definitive treatment

Disadvantages

- Does not identify whether the aneurysm is bleeding or not
- Does not give further information as to the possible cause of symptoms

Standard views

- Transverse views at the level of celiac axis, superior mesenteric artery (SMA) and aortic bifurcation
- Longitudinal view of the entire abdominal aorta

Technique

Position the patient supine: start with the transverse view with the probe in the epigastric region, marker pointing to the right. The aorta is present anterior to the vertebral body. Characteristics of aorta are:

- On the left side
- Round shape
- Pulsatile
- Thick walled
- Non-compressible
- Bifurcates at or just below the umbilicus
- With colour-mode: If the probe is angled towards the heart so that blood flow is away or towards the probe, veins will be blue colour as the blood flows away from the probe [the acronym is Blue Away, Red Towards (BART)]

For the longitudinal view rotate the probe in the sagittal plane and visualise the aorta in its entire length. The vessel runs deep to the liver around the diaphragm and the depth may need to be increased to visualise this part.

Measuring the aortic diameter – this should be measured from outer wall to outer wall ignoring any clot present in the lumen. On transverse view measure the diameter in the anteroposterior (rather than side to side) direction as the lateral borders of the aorta are ill defined due to artefact.

Post-procedure steps
These are as described for FAST above.

Ultrasound-guided vascular access

The National Institute for Health and Care Excellence (NICE) recommends using a 2D ultrasound in most situations when inserting a central line. It is also very useful to gain peripheral access in patients who are difficult to cannulate, e.g. post-chemotherapy, intravenous drug users, very dehydrated, previous multiple attempts at cannulation, etc. The basilic vein is the most useful in this situation.

Indications
- For central venous access in any situation
- In difficult peripheral access

Contraindications
(these are relative rather than absolute)
- Time critical situations, e.g. cardiac arrest

Advantages
- Direct visualisation of the vessels
- Cannulation under direct vision
- Decreases complications
- Increases first time success
- Decreases the number of attempts required

Disadvantages
The skills are operator dependent.

Technique

For central cannulation, the steps are the same as for standard landmark technique. The ultrasound can be used to both confirm the anatomy and then proceed with the landmark technique or it can be used to cannulate under direct vision. Important points to consider:
- Choose a high frequency linear probe and set the depth depending on the site. This is usually 5 cm for internal jugular, 4 cm for femoral and 3 cm for basilic vein cannulation.
- Characteristics of a vein:
  - Oval
  - Thin walled
  - Compressible
  - Non-pulsatile
  - Internal jugular vein: Increases in diameter with Valsalva manoeuvre
  - With colour-mode: If the probe is angled towards the heart so that blood flow is away or towards the probe, veins will be blue colour as the blood flows away from the probe (the acronym is BART).
- Avoid too much zoom otherwise one cannot visualise the skin surface
- When cannulating under direct vision the longitudinal section long axis view is preferred as this allows direct visualisation of the vessel and the needle entering the lumen. Initially visualise the vein in the transverse section, then rotate the probe so that the vein is visualised in the longitudinal section
- Angle the needle relatively parallel to the skin as the needle will not be visualised if it is too steep

Scenario

A 29-year-old patient has been involved in a road traffic incident. He is a motorcyclist and was hit by a car. He landed approximately 5 feet away from the site of impact. He has been conscious with stable observations pre-hospital. He is triple immobilised. You have been asked to do a FAST scan by the team leader.

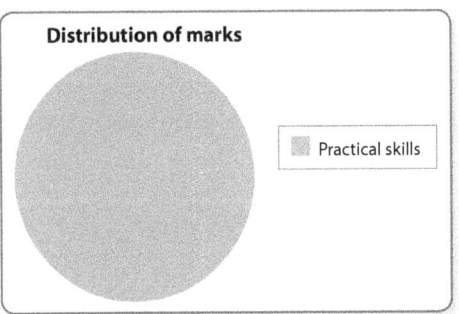

Distribution of marks

■ Practical skills

Mark sheet	Achieved	Not achieved
Introduces himself to the patient and confirms patient identity		
Enquires about any immediate discomfort or pain relief		
Established the need for FAST scan		
Positions the patient correctly		
Obtains consent for examination		
Cleans hands		
Sets up the machine correctly:		
– patient details		

Cont'd...

Cont'd...

Mark sheet	Achieved	Not achieved
– correct probe selection		
– correct probe orientation		
Correct technique for FAST scan		
Demonstrates:		
– Morrison's pouch		
– splenorenal recess		
– pleural recesses on both sides		
– pericardial sac in subcostal or parasternal view		
– pelvic views		
Acquires best possible image		
Identifies gain or artefact and suitably corrects the image		
Knows when to scan		
Appropriate speed of the procedure		
Informs the team appropriately – not a definitive scan		
Interprets the findings appropriately – communicates to the team leader		
Demonstrates appropriate attitude and professional manner		
Thanks the patient and invites any questions		
Global mark from examiner		
Global mark form patient		

6.11 Hand washing

Hand hygiene is considered to be the single most effective practice in reducing infection transmission. It is something that is easily overlooked and therefore it is an easy OSCE, yet one which candidates may not be prepared for:

Before hand washing
- Expose both forearms
- Remove all wrist and hand jewellery
- Ensure finger nails are short, clean, free from artificial nails or nail products
- Cuts and abrasions should be covered with a dry dressing

Steps of hand washing
(steps a–f should last 15 seconds each)
1. Wet hands with water
2. Take enough soap to cover both hands:
    a. Palm to palm (**Figure 6.11.1**)
    b. Palm to dorsum (**Figure 6.11.2**)
    c. Palm to palm fingers interlaced (**Figure 6.11.3**)
    d. Back of fingers to opposing palms with fingers interlaced (**Figure 6.11.4**)
    e. Rotational rubbing of thumb (**Figure 6.11.5**)
    f. Rotational rubbing of clasped fingers to palm (**Figure 6.11.6**)
3. Rinse hands with water
4. Dry thoroughly with hand towel
5. Use a hand towel to turn off the tap

Figure 6.11.1 Palm to palm.

298 Practical skills and teaching

Figure 6.11.2 Palm to dorsum.

Figure 6.11.3 Palm to palm fingers interlaced.

Figure 6.11.4 Palm to dorsum fingers interlaced.

Figure 6.11.5 Rotational rubbing – palm.

Figure 6.11.6 Rotational rubbing – fingers to palm.

Five key moments of hand hygiene

- Before patient contact
- Before a clean/aseptic procedure
- After body fluid exposure risk
- After patient contact
- After contact with patient surroundings

What should be used?

Alcohol based hand rubs should be used routinely.
Liquid soap and water hand-wash is specifically used in the following circumstances:

- Visibly soiled hands
- Caring for patients with diarrhoea and vomiting
- Working in areas where patients have diarrhoea and vomiting
- After hands have come in contact with body fluids

Alcohol does not work on spores (e.g. *C. difficile*) and some viruses (e.g. norovirus), therefore use of soap and water handwashing is recommended. In addition to thorough hand washing with soap and water it is also appropriate to wear gloves and an apron when in contact with patients who require isolation due to infectious illnesses.

Scenario

You are required to examine a patient presenting with diarrhoea and vomiting for the last 3 days. He is being cared for in a side cubicle. Demonstrate the standard infection control precautions you will take prior to examining the patient.

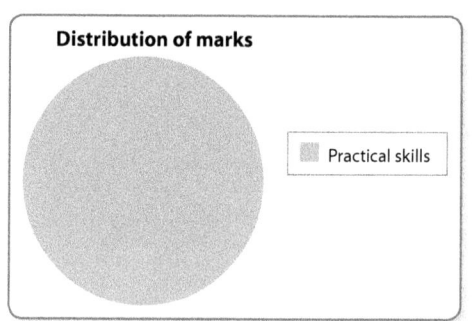

Distribution of marks

■ Practical skills

Mark sheet	Achieved	Not achieved
Removes clothing below the level of elbows		
No wrist or hand jewellery		
Short clean finger nails, with no artificial nail or nail products		
Properly dressed cuts on hands with washable dressing		
Uses of liquid soap and water		
Correctly performs steps of hand washing (including appropriate duration of each step)		
– palm to palm		
– palm to dorsum		
– palm to palm fingers interlaced		
– back of fingers to opposing palms with fingers interlaced		
– rotational rubbing of thumb		
– rotational rubbing of clasped fingers to palm		
Does not touch tap with hand after hand washing		
Wears plastic apron		
Wears non-sterile gloves		
Global mark from examiner		

6.12 Intraosseous needle insertion

Intraosseous (IO) needle insertion is a simple skill. It can be lifesaving in the resuscitation setting, allowing quick and reliable vascular access. Given its use in paediatrics it often arises in scenarios with candidates being required to perform the procedure while also explaining it to distressed parents.

Indications
In an emergency for rapid vascular access to deliver drugs, fluids, blood or blood products.

Contraindications
- A fracture proximal to the chosen site
- Ischaemic extremity
- Local trauma or infection is a relative contraindication depending on the clinical scenario

Complications
- Superficial insertion of needle resulting in extravasation of infused fluid
- Pain from needle insertion or flowing infusion
- An iatrogenic fracture or insertion of the needle through the bone
- Osteomyelitis and cellulitis
- Surrounding neurovascular injury or compartment syndrome

Common sites
- Anteromedial surface of proximal tibia
- Proximal humerus
- Distal femur
- Superior iliac crest
- Distal medial tibia

Pre-procedure check
- Local anaesthetic such as 1% lignocaine is required in a patient who is awake.
- Skin cleaning with an appropriate cleaning solution should be performed prior to needle insertion
- Equipment (**Figure 6.12.1**):
  - EZ-IO intraosseous access power driver and needle
  - EZ-connect extension set, flushed with normal saline
  - 10 mL syringe
- Sterile gloves

Figure 6.12.1 Intraosseous needle equipment (a) EZ-IO power driver ('gun') (b) needle (c) needle case (d) connector with luer lock and clamp (e) alternative manual IO needle.

Infiltration of local anaesthetic in the skin overlying the chosen site is reportedly not required as the procedure is not painful. However, an awake patient will require a 2–5 mL flush of 1% lignocaine as infusion into marrow via an IO needle is typically painful.

Insertion technique

The EZ-IO comes with 15 mm (pink), 25 mm (blue) and 45 mm (yellow) needles. Use 25 mm needles in patients more than 40 kg weight or adults. Use 45 mm needles for humeral insertion or larger patients. The needle, with its trocar, attaches to the power driver with a magnetic coupling. Position the needle perpendicular to the surface of the bone at the chosen point and gently push the needle through the skin until it rests against the bone. At this stage the 5 mm mark must always be visible above the skin for confirmation of adequate needle length to drill into bone, if this is not visible use a longer needle or different insertion point. Use gentle, steady, downward pressure and drive the needle in the bone by squeezing the trigger. Angle the needle slightly away from the physeal plate. Stop once you feel a give or have reached the desired depth. A give usually indicates that you have reached the cortex.

Remove the trocar from the needle. If the needle is stable and does not wobble, it is likely to be in the medullary cortex. Take the 10 mL syringe and aspirate. If one can aspirate blood the needle is in the right place, however, this is not always possible even when the needle is placed correctly. If samples from an IO needle are sent to the laboratory for testing, they should be clearly labelled as they are not treated the same as other blood samples.

Manual IO needles also exist. The procedure is the same for these except when inserted they require a gentle but firm rotating action until they penetrate the bone. The handle on them is connected to a central trocar and is then unscrewed leaving the needle in place. They are often preferred in neonates or very young children as some operators feel it is easier to control the amount of pressure required to ensure the needle penetrates to the correct depth.

Anteromedial tibia insertion

The landmark for this is 2 cm below (1 cm in children) and medial to the tibial tuberosity in adults. Stabilise the knee by holding the leg and keeping the knee slightly flexed. Make sure that your hand is not placed posteriorly otherwise you may get injured if the power driver slips (or in a small child if the needle goes directly through the bone).

Proximal humerus insertion

The proximal humeral insertion is preferred where injuries below the diaphragm may compromise venous return to the heart.

Position the patient's hand over the abdomen palm down (elbow adducted and humerus internally rotated). The operator should slide their thumb up the anterior shaft of the humerus until they feel the greater tubercle. This point is the surgical neck of humerus. The insertion site is on the most prominent aspect of the greater tubercle, 1–2 cm above the surgical neck. The 45 mm (yellow) needle is required for adult humeral EZ-IO insertion. The 25 mm (blue) needle may be sufficient in a child. Push the needle tip at a 45° angle to the anterior plane and posteromedial. Gently drill into the humerus 2 cm or until the hub reaches the skin in an adult. The hub of the needle should be perpendicular to the skin.

After insertion, aspiration and securing the needle, the arm must be secured in place across the abdomen. Movement back to the anatomical position may lever the needle out of position against the acromion.

Distal femur insertion

This is an alternative site to the proximal tibia for children under 6 years of age. Secure the leg out-stretched to ensure the knee does not bend. Identify the patella by palpation. The insertion site is 1 cm proximal to the patella (avoiding the growth plate) and approximately 1 cm medial to midline (avoiding the quadriceps tendon). For infants a 15-mm (pink) may be sufficient, larger children will require a 25-mm (blue) needle.

Post-procedure steps

Attach the EZ-connect and flush it with saline. This should not cause swelling in the subcutaneous tissues if the position is correct. Consider injecting a small amount of local anaesthetic through the needle to prevent pain once an infusion is flowing. The needle can be secured with a commercial stabiliser device or simply with gauze and tape. Avoid any tension on the connector set as there is an on-going risk of needle displacement. The IO needle should be used for as short a time period as possible, and should not be used for more than 24 hours or after intravenous access has been established.

Scenario

A 15-year-old patient has been brought in to the ED. He was a restrained front seat passenger in a head-on motor vehicle accident. He was trapped by compression and has suffered open fractures to both femurs. Pre-hospital intravenous access has not been established. On presentation in the ED he is maintaining his own airway with adequate breathing but has a blood pressure of 68/36 mmHg and a heart rate of 126 beats per minute. The team leader has called you to assist by inserting an IO needle.

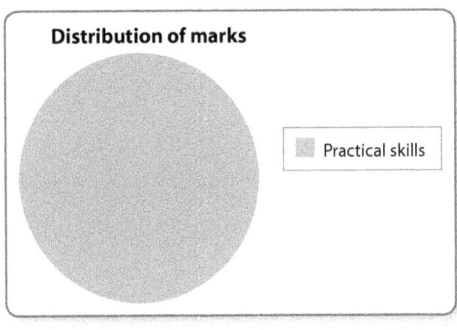

Distribution of marks

Practical skills

Mark sheet	Achieved	Not achieved
Introduces self to patient		
Explains procedure to patient		
Washes hands and wears personal protective equipment		
Chooses proximal humeral site and communicates to team leader		
Chooses 45 mm yellow sized needle		
Prepares skin with appropriate cleaning solution		
Position the patient's hand over the abdomen palm down		
Palpates surgical neck of humerus and inserts 1–2 cm proximal		
Correct technique of needle insertion		
Removes the trocar		
Attempts to aspirate needle to confirm position		
Requests samples be sent for testing		
Attaches connector and flushes with 2–5 mL Lignocaine 1%		
Secures needle		
Disposes of equipment correctly		
Global mark from examiner		

6.13 Knee aspiration

Indication
- To exclude septic arthritis

Contraindications
- Cellulitis at site of needle insertion
- Where there is an underlying knee replacement aspiration should be in theatre under sterile conditions
- Coagulopathy is a relative contraindication depending on its severity and the clinical scenario

Complications
- Introduction of infection
- Bleeding into the knee joint (haemarthrosis)
- Pain
- Damage to articular cartilage

Pre-procedure check

(See **Figure 6.13.1** below)
- Local anaesthetic such as 1% lignocaine
- Appropriate skin cleaning solution
- 20 mL syringe
- Large bore (green or white) needle
- Orange needle with 10 mL syringe for local anaesthetic
- Sterile gloves
- Dressing pack
- Universal container to collect a sample

Figure 6.13.1 Equipment for knee aspiration (a) cleaning swab (b) needle and syringe for local anaesthetic (c) needle and syringe for aspiration (d) sterile drape (e) sterile gauze (f) universal container (g) procedure tray.

Technique

Explain the procedure to the patient and obtain verbal consent. The knee can be aspirated by both medial and lateral approaches. The lateral approach avoids the bulky vastus medialis.

With the knee in extension, palpate the patella and confirm the effusion. Choose a site 2 cm lateral to the lateral (or medial, if using medial approach) border of the patella. Clean the skin with antiseptic taking standard infection control precautions and use personal protective equipment. Drape with a sterile sheet leaving the knee exposed. Inject local anaesthetic in the skin and subcutaneous tissue. Insert the larger needle at this point and direct it downwards and medially, below the surface of the patella, taking care not to hit the bone as this could damage the articular cartilage. Once in the joint there may be a palpable 'give', and also a visible flashback in the hub of the needle.

At this point aspirate as much fluid as possible. In the case of large effusions, leave the needle in place once 20 mL is aspirated and use another empty syringe to continue aspirating. Milking the fluid downwards towards the needle helps to aspirate the entire joint cavity.

Send the fluid for cytology, gram stain, crystals and culture.

Scenario

A 39-year-old man named Hitesh Patel presents to the ED with fever and rigors. He has a history of a painful knee with post-traumatic arthritis, for which he is awaiting a joint replacement. The knee has become increasingly painful despite analgesia and he can't bear weight on it. On examination, he has a swollen, painful knee and a temperature of 39°C. The orthopaedic team are busy in theatre. Perform a knee joint aspiration.

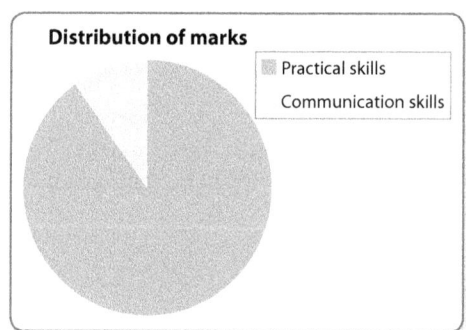

Distribution of marks
- Practical skills
- Communication skills

Mark sheet	Achieved	Not achieved
Introduces self to patient appropriately		
Confirms patient identity		
Briefly reviews the clinical history and presenting complaint		
Asks about presence of pain and offers analgesia		
Explains procedure to patient		
Obtains patient consent		
Checks equipment		
Washes hands and uses personal protective equipment		

Cont'd...

Cont'd...

Mark sheet	Achieved	Not achieved
Checks for any contraindications (surface cellulitis, joint replacement, anticoagulation)		
Chooses appropriate site for aspiration		
Adequate use of local anaesthetic		
States maximum safe dose of local anaesthetic		
Maintains sterility and uses aseptic technique		
Correct technique to aspirate joint		
Visual inspection of the fluid		
Sends the sample for microscopy, culture and sensitivity, cytology		
Dresses the puncture site		
Disposes of equipment correctly		
Explains further plan to patient		
Thanks the patient and invites any questions		
Global mark from patient		
Global mark from examiner		

6.14 Lumbar puncture

Indications

- The main indication in emergency medicine is to obtain cerebrospinal fluid (CSF) for investigation or measure the CSF opening pressure
- In anaesthesia, for spinal anaesthetic
- In oncology, for delivery of intrathecal chemotherapy

Contraindications

- Cellulitis at proposed needle insertion site
- Coagulopathy
- Reduced Glasgow Coma Score (GCS), suspected raised intracranial pressure

Complications

- Most common is a post-procedure headache, nausea or vomiting which patients should be warned about
- Less common are:
  - Infection, meningitis
  - Arachnoiditis
  - Epidural abscess or haematoma
  - Damage to spinal cord or spinal nerves

Pre-procedure check

(See **Figure 6.14.1** below)
- Local anaesthetic (1% lignocaine)
- Appropriate skin cleaning solution
- Spinal needle
- Manometer

Figure 6.14.1 Equipment for Lumbar puncture (a) sterile swab (b) needle and syringe for local anaesthetic (c) spinal needle (d) manometer components (e) sterile drape (f) sterile gauze (g) universal containers (h) glucose estimation tube (I) procedure tray.

- Four universal containers
- Fluoride oxalate tube for glucose estimation
- Brown envelope or foil to cover sample for xanthochromia testing (if required)
- Orange needle with 10 mL syringe for local anaesthetic
- Sterile gloves and gown
- Dressing pack and sterile drapes

Technique

A lumbar puncture can be performed with the patient sitting up or lying on their side. However, measurement of opening CSF pressure is only possible with the patient lying on side, and therefore this is the preferred position. Sterile gloves and gown should be worn for this procedure.

Lay the patient in the right or left lateral decubitus position with their neck and hips flexed and knees close to the chest so they are assuming the fetal position. If possible position the patient so their back is closed to the edge of the bed. An assistant is helpful to hold the patient in this position, offer reassurance and assist the procedure if necessary.

Palpate the iliac crests. A line drawn between them should correspond to the L4-L5 intervertebral space. The spinal cord ends at the lower border of L1 in adults and therefore this space contains the cauda equina and is therefore safe for the insertion of the spinal needle. Palpate this intervertebral space with the intention of inserting a needle into the space's mid-point. Some clinician's mark this point with a skin marker (though it may be wiped off when the area is cleaned).

Clean the skin with disinfectant and place a sterile drape with a window allowing access to the skin. Inject local anaesthetic at the desired space, first in the skin and then in the intended direction of the spinal needle. Direct the needle 10-15° cephalad to follow the direction of the spinous processes. Aim to judge the thickness of the subcutaneous tissue with the needle. On hitting the underlying ligament, the resistance changes and the needle is gripped firmly in the tissue.

Remove the local anaesthetic needle and insert the spinal needle with its bevel directed upwards (not towards patient's head), to split the longitudinal fibres of the dura rather than tear them.

It may be possible to feel a pop on piercing the dura and entering the subarachnoid space. The arachnoid mater is adherent to the dura and therefore the subarachnoid space is entered on piercing it.

Without moving the needle, remove the stylet from the needle and look for clear fluid entering the hub of the needle. Place the manometer with the three-way tap closed to outside to let the CSF flow into the manometer. The highest point the CSF reaches represents the opening pressure.

Take a universal container and place it underneath the manometer and close the three way tap to the CSF, letting the CSF from the manometer flow into the container. Remove the manometer once the CSF is collected from it and collect the rest of the samples directly. The following samples may be required:
1. Fluoride oxalate tube for glucose – 8-10 drops
2. Microscopy sample for cell count – 5-8 drops
3. Biochemistry sample for protein – 8-10 drops
4. Microbiology sample for gram stain – 5-8 drops
5. Biochemistry sample for xanthochromia – 8-10 drops (if required)

Post-procedure steps

Cover the sample for xanthochromia testing with foil or in a brown envelope because the pigment breaks down in sunlight and results will not be accurate.

Remove the spinal needle and put a dressing on the puncture site. Advise the patient to lay supine for at least 2 hours after the procedure.

Visually inspect the sample for colour and opacity. Normal CSF should be colourless and clear with no opacity or cells visible. Send the samples for testing. A blood sample should be sent at the same time for serum protein, bilirubin and glucose estimation.

Scenario

You review Maria Chan, a 42-year-old woman on the observation ward who was admitted last night with a sudden onset headache while lifting a heavy washing basket. She describes it as the worst headache ever in the occipital area. The pain is now controlled with analgesia and a CT of the brain was normal. The medical teams are very busy and are unable to review Miss Chan. Perform a lumbar puncture to obtain appropriate CSF samples.

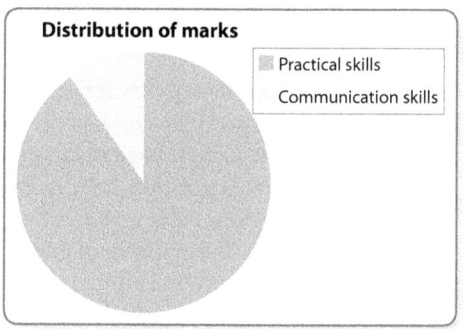

Distribution of marks
- Practical skills
- Communication skills

Mark sheet	Achieved	Not achieved
Introduces self to patient appropriately		
Confirms patient identity		
Briefly reviews the clinical scenario, patient history and treatment given until now		
Asks about presence of pain and offers analgesia		
Explains procedure to patient		
Obtains patient consent		
Checks for any contraindications (surface cellulitis on anticoagulation)		
Checks equipment		
Positions patient appropriately		
Washes hands and uses sterile gloves and gown		
Correct identification of landmarks		
Infiltrates local anaesthetic adequately		
Correct technique for lumbar puncture		
Correct use of manometer when measuring opening pressures		
Collects samples correctly		
Covers xanthochromia sample with foil or brown envelope		
Dresses the puncture site		

Cont'd...

Cont'd...

Mark sheet	Achieved	Not achieved
Appropriately disposes of equipment		
Maintains sterility and uses aseptic technique		
Informs patient of further plan (Need to stay supine for 2 hours)		
Thanks the patient and invites any questions		
Global mark from patient		
Global mark from examiner		

6.15 Anterior nasal packing

Indications
- To control epistaxis

Contraindications
- Base of skull fracture

Complications
- Pain and discomfort is the most common problem experienced with this procedure
- Uncommon complications include trauma to nasal mucosa or potentially infection if the pack is left in place for too long

Pre-procedure check
- Topical local anaesthetic:
  - 2% lignocaine with 1:200,000 adrenaline, or
  - 5% lignocaine with 0.5% phenylephrine solution available as nasal spray
- Protective face shield, apron and gloves
- Nasal speculum
- Head light or head mirror and Bull's lamp
- Tilley forceps
- Suction apparatus
- Silver nitrate cautery sticks
- Nasal pack [alternatives are commercially available nasal packs such as Merocel nasal tampons or Rapid Rhino pneumatic balloon tampon, a premade bismuth iodoform paraffin paste (BIPP) pack or simple ribbon gauze coated with petroleum jelly]
- Syringe, 10 mL saline
- Tongue depressor
- Bolster
- Gauze swabs and a kidney dish

Technique
Make the patient comfortable, sitting upright and ideally with a head support. Stand to either side of the patient with your head at the same height as the patient's and approximately 7–8 inches away.

Initially stop the bleeding by pinching the cartilaginous part of the nose for approximately 15 minutes. Use a nasal speculum to look in the nasal cavity and visualise the nasal septum from where >90% of anterior bleeds originate. Any clot in the nasal cavity should be suctioned away at this stage. Active bleeding will persist as a regular drip of fresh blood from the nose. Use suction to remove this blood and attempt to visualise the bleeding point.

Spray the nasal cavity with a topical anaesthetic and vasoconstrictor. It may help to soak a few centimetres of ribbon gauze in the local anaesthetic solution and place it in the nose with Tilley forceps. Attempt to place it against the bleeding point. Pinch the nose again and wait a few minutes. Remove the ribbon gauze and attempt to visualise the bleeding point.

The bleeding point looks like a prominent vessel or a point with adherent clot on the septum. If this can be seen then place the silver nitrate stick on the bleeding point and surrounding area to cauterise the feeding blood vessels. Avoid applying the cautery for too long as it increases the risk of septum perforation.

If the bleeding continues, or the bleeding spot cannot be seen, then proceed with nasal packing. Merocel nasal tampon is universally available and easy to use. Lubricate the tampon with water based gel and place it in the nostril. The nasal cavity runs perpendicular to the face directly backwards and a common mistake is to push the Merocel upwards leading to inadequate packing. Bear in mind the tampon starts to swell and becomes soft as soon as it comes in contact with fluids. This makes it difficult to advance it. Therefore, the tampon should be inserted promptly before it starts to swell up.

Advance the tampon all the way in the nose leaving the threads in front. The tampon can be inflated by squirting 5 mL of normal saline into the nasal cavity alongside the tampon.

A Rapid Rhino is used in a similar fashion except that it does not need to be lubricated and once in the nostril a balloon can be inflated with air to provide compression. Avoid over-inflation with 5-10 mL of air usually being sufficient.

If no nasal packing devices are available, then proceed to packing the nose with ribbon gauze. Use Tilley forceps to hold the gauze and pack the nose in layers from below upwards.

Once the pack is in place, use a tongue depressor to visualise the pharynx, any further bleeding would be seen as dripping fresh blood behind the uvula. If this is the case the, opposite nostril can be packed to provide further pressure on the septum. If the bleeding still does not stop, one may have to proceed with posterior nasal packing.

If the bleeding has stopped, place a bolster in front of the nose to avoid blood dripping down the face. Discuss the patient with the ENT specialist team for further management.

Scenario

A 72-year-old woman has been brought into the ED with epistaxis. She has no history of trauma. She has had an occasional nose bleed for the last few days stopping spontaneously, but on this occasion it has continued to bleed and she decided to call the ambulance. Paramedics have left her in the ED minors area with a nurse. The patient has adequate intravenous access. Please place an anterior nasal pack.

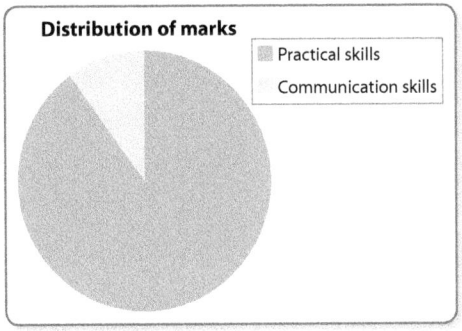

Distribution of marks
- Practical skills
- Communication skills

Mark sheet	Achieved	Not achieved
Introduces self to patient appropriately		
Confirms patient identity		
Asks about presence of pain and offers analgesia		
Briefly asks about relevant history, medication and allergies		
Explains procedure to patient		
Obtains verbal consent		
Gathers necessary equipment		
Cleans hands and uses personal protective equipment		
Examines the nasal cavity for bleeding		
Uses local anaesthetic spray		
Pinches the nose to help stop bleeding		
Prepares the tampon, lubricates with gel		
Places nasal pack correctly		
Inserts the pack fully		
Applies saline to inflate the pack		
Inspects pharyngeal wall for further bleeding		
Places a bolster on the nose		
Disposes of equipment correctly		
Reassesses patient		
Checks on patient comfort		
Comments on need to communicate with specialist team for further management		
Global mark from patient		
Global mark from examiner		

6.16 Femoral and fascia iliaca nerve blocks

A fascia iliaca compartment block is used for hip fractures in order to reduce pain, the need for systemic analgesia, and prevent delirium. Femoral nerve blocks provide quick and effective analgesia for a fractured femur, facilitating traction or splinting.

Indications
- Femoral fracture (femoral nerve block)
- Neck of femur fracture (fascia iliaca block)

Contraindications
- Allergy to local anaesthetic
- Overlying skin infection
- Anticoagulation
- Patient refusal or non-compliance

Complications
- Failure to provide adequate block
- Intravascular injection and toxicity or haematoma
- Intraneural injection
- Effective block leading to opiate analgesia 'overshoot', and subsequent respiratory depression

Procedure

In case of local anaesthetic toxicity, monitoring should be applied and a cannula placed before beginning the procedure. The first step is to position the patient appropriately, lying supine on a trolley/bed. If tolerated, the legs should be slightly apart with the affected leg slightly externally rotated. Ensuring adequate privacy for the patient, expose the appropriate area. As with all unilateral procedures stop and confirm it is the correct side.

Wearing sterile gloves, clean the patient's skin with swabs using an appropriate skin preparation. A sterile drape with a window in it should then be placed over the area.

A precalculated amount of bupivacaine (or another suitable local anaesthetic) should be drawn up into a syringe. The maximum safe dose should be checked and equates to 2 mg/kg. Remember to consider the dose carefully if bilateral nerve blocks are required. Dilute to the required volume with saline. The fascia iliac block requires 30–40 mL whereas the femoral nerve block requires 10–20 mL.

For both procedures, as the needle is advanced, aspirate to avoid an intravascular injection. Once in the correct space the local anaesthetic can be slowly injected. If there is resistance or paraesthesia, stop because this may suggest an intraneural injection. After the procedure, cover the patient up and dispose of all equipment and sharps appropriately. There is a post-procedure risk of local anaesthetic toxicity and opiate toxicity if the patient had received a lot of opiate analgesia prior to the block. The RCEM currently recommends observations at 5, 10, 15 and 30 minutes post-procedure. The site, side, dose and time of block must be documented in the patient notes.

Femoral nerve block

Initially the femoral arterial pulse should be palpated at the level of the inguinal ligament (**Figure 6.16.1**). This is represented by a line drawn between the pubic tubercle and the anterior superior iliac spine. Infiltrate insertion point with 1–2 mL of 1% lignocaine. The nerve block needle should be angled perpendicular to the skin and should puncture the skin 1 cm lateral and 1 cm distal to the pulse to a depth of approximately 3 cm. A 21G needle is appropriate for adults, while a 23G needle can be used for children.

To improve the success rate of a femoral nerve block ultrasound can be used to advance the needle to the femoral nerve sheath. A sterile ultrasound probe is used in the transverse plane at the level of the inguinal crease. The femoral nerve is identified as a hyperechoic structure lateral to the femoral artery deep to fascia lata (**Figure 6.16.2**). The needle is then inserted lateral to the probe and using an in-plane technique is advanced. Local anaesthetic is then infiltrated around the femoral nerve.

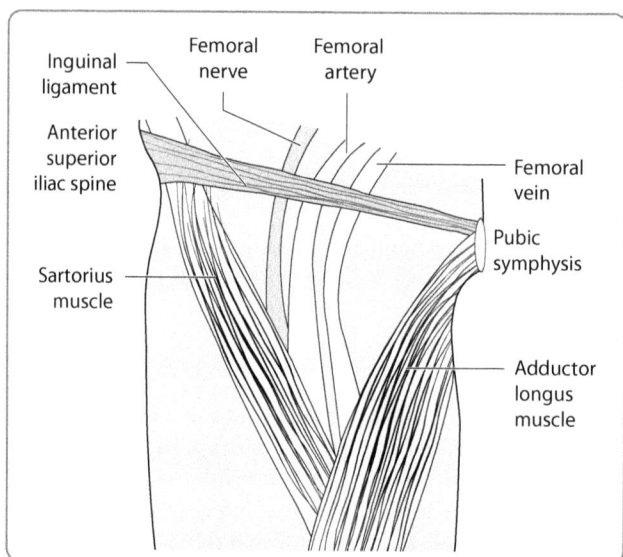

Figure 6.16.1 Femoral nerve anatomy (right side).

Figure 6.16.2 Femoral Nerve, artery and vein on ultrasound.

Fascia iliaca block

This nerve block aims to infiltrate a large volume of local anaesthetic into the fascia iliaca compartment which contains the femoral, lateral femoral cutaneous and obturator nerve. The site for puncture is found by imagining or drawing a line from the pubic tubercle to the anterior superior iliac spine, dividing it into thirds, and finding a point 2.5 cm below the junction of the middle and outer third. This point should also be at least 2.5 cm lateral to the femoral pulse, which should also be palpated for safety.

Infiltrate the insertion point with 1–2 mL of 1% lignocaine, then pierce the skin with a nerve block needle. The needle is advanced perpendicular to the skin and two 'pops' should be easily felt (the first represents the fascia lata and the second the fascia iliaca) confirming correct placement of the needle.

To improve the success rate of a fascia iliac nerve block, a sterile ultrasound probe in the transverse plane is used. The fascia lata and fascia iliaca are identified and the needle is then inserted. The operator can visualise the separation of the fascia iliaca and iliacus muscle as the local anaesthetic is administered.

Scenario

Mr Li is a 58-year-old builder who has presented with a fractured right femur. His limb is neurovascularly normal and he has no other injuries. Please administer a femoral nerve block.

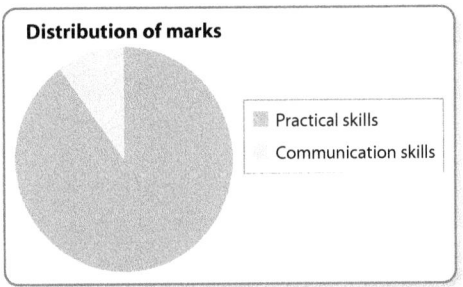

Distribution of marks
- Practical skills
- Communication skills

Mark sheet	Achieved	Not achieved
Introduces self to patient appropriately		
Confirms patient identity		
Asks about presence of pain and offers analgesia		
Briefly asks about medical history, medication and allergies		
Explains procedure to patient		
Obtains patient consent		
Cleans hands and wears gloves		
Prepares/checks equipment and doses		
States maximum safe dose of local anaesthetic		
Cleans skin		
Comments on need to use ultrasound machine or nerve stimulator		
Identifies correct landmarks for femoral nerve		
Injects local anaesthetic		
Aspirates to avoid intravascular injection		

Cont'd…

Cont'd...

Mark sheet	Achieved	Not achieved
Comments on avoiding intraneural injection		
Safe disposal of sharps		
Covers with dressing		
States need for post procedure observation		
Maintains patient dignity		
Global mark from patient		
Global mark from examiner		

Suggested reading

National Institute for Health and Care Excellence (NICE). Hip fracture management. Clinical Guideline 124. London: NICE; 2011.

6.17 Ophthalmoscopy

Ophthalmoscopy is a fundamental part of the eye examination (and cranial nerve examination) as it allows the fundus of the eye to be visualised. It is most likely to appear in the exam as a teaching station though this is not necessarily the case.
An ophthalmoscope consists of several parts (**Figure 6.17.1**):
- The handle by which it is held which also contains the power source (battery or electric cable)
- The aperture through which to look
- A dial to control the amount of light which also functions as the on/off switch
- A dial to control a series of lenses in front of the aperture to correct for any refractive error in the patient's or examiner's eyes
- A dial to change the shape and colour of the light source for different diagnostic purposes

Figure 6.17.1 Parts of the ophthalmoscope. (a) handle and battery case (b) on/off switch and brightness control (c) window showing refractive lens number (d) viewing aperture (e) refractive lens dial.

Technique

Position the patient so they are seated upright. The examination should be performed in a suitably dark room.
　Ensure the ophthalmoscope has a working light source and is functioning correctly. Before commencing select appropriate settings:
- If you wear glasses or contact lenses it may be easiest to wear them during the examination. This means you only need to select the correct refractive lens to suit the patient. Knowing what type of glasses (if any) they wear will give you an idea of which lens to select. In the absence of any refractive error the lens should be set to 0. If the

patient is short sighted (myopic) you can then rotate the dial to select a minus lens (usually red). If they are long sighted (hypermetropic) you will need to select a plus lens (normally black)
- Select the large round white beam and initially set the brightness to maximum.

Explain the procedure to the patient and warn them that you will need to get quite close to them. Ask them to remove any glasses or contact lenses.

Begin by inspecting both eyes for any deformity or abnormality.

To examine the patient's right eye stand slightly to the patient's right and hold the ophthalmoscope in you right hand and use your right eye. Ask the patient to look straight ahead or slightly to their left.

Shine the light into the patient's eye from approximately 30 cm away and look for the red reflex which is the light reflecting off the retina. Note the presence or absence of this so-called red reflex.

Having warned the patient what you are going to do place your left hand onto the patient's forehead and use your thumb to lift up their right eyelid.

Slowly move in towards the patient until you can see their retina. Then move through the refractive lenses until the retina and its vessels are in focus.

Once you identify a blood vessel you will be able to follow the vessel to the optic disc. Inspect the optic disc:
- Look at the colour of the disc. Is it pale or florid?
- Consider the size of the cup compared to the whole disc
- Are the disc's edges sharp or blurred?
- Are the vessels normal in structure and quantity?

Then look at each quadrant of the retina in turn:
- Is the retina normal in colour?
- Are the vessels normal in their structure and quantity?
- Look at the area between the vessels for haemorrhages and exudates

Next identify the macula which will be lateral to the optic disc. To do this you can ask the patient to look directly at the light source.

Once this is done move to the other side of the patient and holding the ophthalmoscope in the left hand and using your left eye examine the patient's left eye in the same manner.

During the examination the brightness of the light source may need to be reduced to maintain patient comfort and prevent excessive pupillary constriction.

One percent tropicamide can be used to dilate the pupils and provide a better view. If used always check for a history of glaucoma first and also warn the patient their vision will be blurred for some time afterwards and they will not be able to drive.

Scenario

Mr Frederick Barry is a 48-year-old man who had attended the ED with decreased visual acuity in his right eye. A medical student on placement in your ED has taken a history from Mr Barry. The student has never used an ophthalmoscope before. Teach the student how to perform an ophthalmoscope examination and discuss the clinical findings.

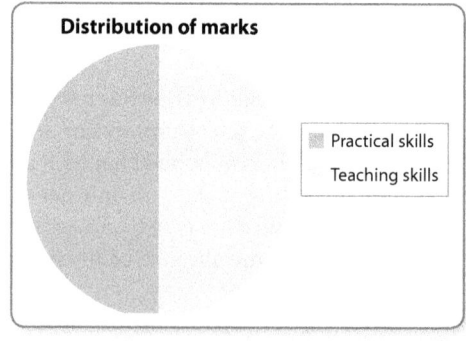

Distribution of marks
- Practical skills
- Teaching skills

Mark sheet	Achieved	Not achieved
Introduces self to medical student		
Enquires from medical student about previous experience and knowledge		
Asks him about anything specific he wants to learn		
Sets and agrees on appropriate learning objectives		
Explains rationale for performing ophthalmoscopy		
Demonstrates the ophthalmoscope and how it functions		
Demonstrates how to hold the ophthalmoscope		
Demonstrates how to position the patient correctly		
Demonstrates inspecting the external eye		
Demonstrates the red reflex		
Demonstrates examining the macula and quadrants of the retina		
Explains or demonstrates the need to examine both sides		
Correctly describes pathology in right eye		
Allows medical student to perform examination		
Comments on and corrects medical student technique where appropriate		
Checks if medical student has any questions or concerns		
Answers questions appropriately		
Agrees a plan for on-going learning		
Is non-judgemental and facilitates learning		
Global mark from examiner		
Global mark from medical student		

Instructions for actor

You are a first year clinical medical student. You have seen an ophthalmoscope used but are not really sure of when to use it or the correct technique. You are interested in how the device works and the correct technique for the examination. You are prepared to listen but also keen to use the ophthalmoscope yourself. If the candidate does not allow you to hold and use the device try and take it from them. If they do not demonstrate the correct technique before giving you the device to use you are unable to remember the steps correctly.

6.18 Otoscopy

Otoscopy is required for assessment of ear pain or discharge, hearing loss, head injury, foreign bodies and febrile illness in children. It is common for this examination to appear in exams as a teaching station.

An otoscope consists of three parts (**Figure 6.18.1**):
- The handle by which it is held which also contains the power source (battery or electric cable)
- The head which contains the magnifying lens and view finder. The lens often detaches or swings to the side to allow instruments to be passed
- The cone onto which disposable specula are placed for insertion into the external auditory canal

Figure 6.18.1 Parts of an otoscope (a) handle and battery case (b) on/off switch and brightness control (c) magnifying lens which can be moved to allow instrumentation (d) attachment for speculae (e) different sized speculae.

Technique

Position the patient so they are seated upright. Ensure the otoscope has a working light source and magnifying lens. Place a speculum onto the end.
- Stand slightly to the patient's side and begin by inspecting the outer ear for any skin changes, signs of inflammation or discharge. Holding the otoscope as you would hold a pen use your free hand to gently hold the pinna of the ear and pull it upwards and posteriorly as this manoeuvre straightens the ear canal which is normally curved. Be cautious not to hurt the patient

- Next insert the speculum of the otoscope just inside the external auditory meatus and assess the walls of the canal for any apparent changes. Any skin changes, inflammation, discharge wax or foreign body such as an insect will be seen
- As the speculum is placed deeper the tympanic membrane is seen and can be assessed
- Next examine the other ear with the same technique

Positioning children for examination

Otoscopy requires a level of compliance that young or scared children may not give. The examination is made significantly easier if the child is held in the correct way. Ask a parent or member of staff to sit normally on an upright chair. The child should then be placed on the lap so they are facing to one side. The adult places one hand on the child's head and holds it against their chest. Their other arm is wrapped around the child's body and arms so their movement is restricted. The exposed ear can then be examined. After this the child is turned to face the other side and the adult swaps their arms into the previous positions and the other ear is examined.

Scenario

A final year medical student on placement in your ED has asked you to teach him how to perform otoscopy.

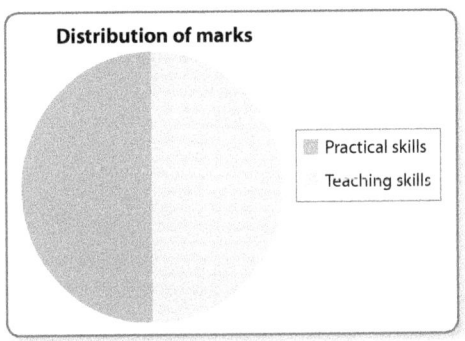

Distribution of marks
- Practical skills
- Teaching skills

Mark sheet	Achieved	Not achieved
Introduces self to medical student		
Enquires from medical student about previous experience and knowledge		
Asks him about anything specific he wants to learn		
Sets and agrees on appropriate learning objectives		
Explains rationale for performing otoscopy		
Demonstrates the otoscope and how it functions		
Demonstrates how to position the patient correctly		
Demonstrates examining the external auditory meatus		
Demonstrates examining the auditory canal		
Demonstrates examining the tympanic membrane		
Explains or demonstrates the need to examine both sides		
Allows medical student to perform examination		
Comments on and corrects medical student technique where appropriate		

Cont'd...

Cont'd...

Mark sheet	Achieved	Not achieved
Checks if medical student has any questions or concerns		
Answers questions appropriately		
Agrees a plan for on-going learning		
Is non-judgemental and facilitates learning		
Global mark from medical student		
Global mark from examiner		

Instructions for actor

You are a first year clinical medical student. You have never seen an otoscope used but have read about it. You are interested in how the device works and the correct technique for the examination. You want to know how it works and how to use it. On your first attempt you hold the device incorrectly and do not hold the ear with your free hand. If the doctor corrects you take their advice and change your technique. At the end of the session you also ask how to examine a child's ears because you've heard this can be very important but do not imagine they sit still for the examination.

6.19 Paediatric asthma – discharge planning and spacer technique

After an acute asthma exacerbation, children can be discharged once stable on 3-4 hourly inhaled bronchodilators which can be continued at home. Peak expiratory flow (PEF) and forced expiratory volume over one second (FEV1) should be >75% of best or predicted with saturations >94%.

The early use of steroids in the ED and assessment units can reduce the need for hospital admission and prevent a relapse of symptoms after initial presentation with benefits in 3-4 hours. Oral prednisolone is preferred unless the patient is unable to tolerate the dose. Use a dose of 10 mg under 2 years of age, 20 mg for children aged 2-5 years and 30-40 mg for children older than 5 years. Treatment for up to 3 days is usually sufficient and does not require tapering.

An 8-week trial of preventer (moderate inhaled corticosteroid) is indicated in children with asthma related symptoms 3 times a week, asthma uncontrolled with a short acting beta-agonist or asthma causing waking at night. Many children with recurrent episodes of wheeze triggered by viruses do not go on to develop atopic asthma and do not require preventers.

Acute asthma attacks should be considered a failure of preventive therapy and discharge plans should help families avoid further severe episodes by addressing:
- The diagnosis – documenting diagnostic criteria
- Teaching correct inhaler technique
- Consider preventative treatment or adjusting the previously prescribed preventative
- Provide a written personalised asthma action plan for subsequent asthma attacks with clear instructions regarding the use of bronchodilators and the need to seek urgent medical attention in the event of worsening symptoms
- Assess exposure to environmental tobacco smoke
- Identify the trigger of the acute attack plans and make for future exposure
- Arrange follow-up by primary care services within 2 working days and paediatric asthma clinic within 1-2 months
- Arrange referral to a paediatric respiratory specialist if there are life-threatening features

A metered dose inhaler (MDI) consists of a pressurised canister, a metering valve and stem and a mouthpiece actuator (**Figures 6.19.1a** and **6.19.1b**). In those who cannot coordinate an adequate breath with pressing the canister to discharge a dose of an inhaler, a spacer device can be fitted to the inhaler mouthpiece. This is useful for treating children and some adults.

When a dose of medication is released into the spacer it then acts as a reservoir from which the medication can be inhaled. This significantly improves drug delivery and decreases the amount of medication deposited on the back of the throat. A spacer is recommended for any child who has difficulty squeezing the canister and inhaling at the right time (particularly children <5-6 years). In those who are unable to form a seal between their mouth and the spacer mouthpiece a mask should be fitted to the spacer device which will then form a seal around the patient's mouth and nose (**Figure 6.19.2**). Various spacer devices exist but essentially function in the same way.

Figures 6.19.1a and 6.19.1b
Inhaler and its component parts
(a) canister (b) metering valve
(c) mouthpiece (d) cover.

Figure 6.19.2 Inhaler and spacer with mask.

Paediatric asthma – discharge planning and spacer technique 6.19

The basic steps in administering an inhaled medicine through a spacer device are provided below:
1. Shake canister for 5 seconds
2. Remove mouthpiece cover and check for dirt/debris in the mouthpiece
3. Insert the inhaler into the spacer. Hold the inhaler upright with the index finger on the top of the medication canister and the thumb supporting the bottom of the inhaler. You may need to use the other hand to hold the spacer
4. For young children the spacer will be used with a mask. Hold the inhaler and spacer so the mask seals around the face
5. Press down the top of the medication canister with the index finger to release the medication
6. After each spray of the inhaler allow the child to breathe 8–10 times. During this time it is important the seal around the mask/mouthpiece is maintained
7. After 8–10 breaths a subsequent dose of the inhaler can be released and the process repeated
8. When finished remember to recap mouthpiece

It is not unusual for young children to become upset when an inhaler is administered via a spacer. In these cases, it is easiest if two adults are present. One can hold the child while the other administers the inhaler. This is achieved easily if one adult sits in an upright chair with the child on their lap. The child should be placed with their back against the adult's chest. The adult can then wrap one of their arms around the child's arms and place their other hand onto the child's forehead and hold the child's head against their chest. It should be explained to the adult that they will have to hold the child firmly to stop them wriggling away from the spacer/mask.

Scenario

Nazreen is a 3-year-old girl who has attended with her father. She is coryzal and has been seen and treated for virus-induced wheeze. Nazreen has been recurrently wheezy in recent months, with a persistent cough at night that regularly wakes her. She is now well enough to go home on regular inhalers to see her own doctor in the community. Teach her father how to administer her inhaler via a spacer device and explain her discharge medications and a discharge plan.

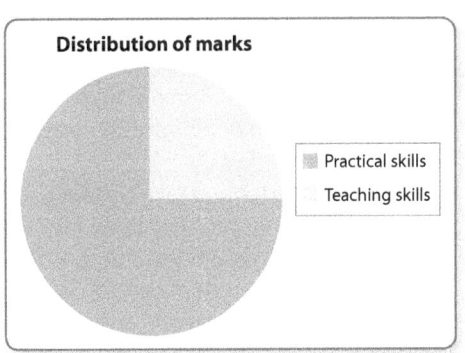

Distribution of marks

- Practical skills
- Teaching skills

Mark sheet	Achieved	Not achieved
Introduces self to the patient and father		
Confirms reason for the consultation and history of illness		
Confirm likely diagnosis (regular wheeze, cough, diurnal variation)		
Confirms treatment (tapered bronchodilator and 3 days of prednisolone)		

Cont'd...

Mark sheet	Achieved	Not achieved
Confirms patient's and father's experience of inhalers		
Explains need for good inhaler technique		
Demonstrate correct spacer technique (including face mask)		
Demonstrates shaking the inhaler and connecting to spacer		
Demonstrates achieving a good seal between mask and face		
Demonstrates administering a single puff followed by 10 breaths		
Arrange follow-up by primary care services at appropriate interval		
Explains benefits of personalised action plan orally and in writing		
Explains everyday asthma care (reliever when wheezing, coughing or having breathing difficulty)		
Explains what to do when feeling worse		
Explains what to do in an asthma attack (1 puff of reliever every minute up to 10 puffs, call ambulance if not improving)		
Allows parents and child a chance to practice and ask questions		
Global mark from father		
Global mark from examiner		

Instructions for actor

Your name is Gavi Singh. You brought your 3-year-old daughter Nazreen to the ED as she had been breathless since she woke up. She had a runny nose and cough yesterday but was fine. Today she seemed quiet, didn't eat breakfast and you noticed she had a wheeze and was breathing faster than normal. She had recurrent similar symptoms in recent months and a persistent cough worse at night which often wakes her. She was born by a normal delivery, has had all her immunisations and has never been to hospital before. No one in the household smokes.

You are comfortable to take Nazreen home but want to make sure you know what medications she requires and learn how to give her the inhaler properly.

You listen to the doctor but if they do not let you practice the technique yourself you ask them if you can have a go. When you use the spacer, after you spray the inhaler you only hold it on the face for a second and then remove it. If the doctor corrects your technique you follow them correctly. You also want to know if this episode means your daughter will get asthma. If it has not been explained to you, ask what to do if Nazreen gets worse again at home.

Suggested reading

British Thoracic Society (BTS). SIGN 153 British guideline on the management of asthma. London: BTS; 2016.

6.20 Performing an electrocardiogram

Recording a standard ECG

Position the patient so they are reclined on a trolley or bed. For placing the ECG stickers their upper body must be exposed. Attach the ten stickers as outlined below.

Limb leads

These are derived from the three limb electrodes placed on right and left arm and left leg (the black lead on the right leg is a neutral or reference electrode). They combine to form leads I, II, III, aVL, aVR and aVF. They 'look' at the heart in a coronal plane. The stickers should be placed over bony prominences to achieve the best quality trace. The exact position on a limb may vary. The quality is also improved if the stickers adhere well which may require shaving or drying the patient.

Chest leads

They are derived from chest electrodes V1 to V6. V1 and V2 are in 4th intercostals space to the right and left of the sternal border respectively. V3 is placed between V2 and V4 which is in turn placed in the 5th intercostal space in left mid-clavicular line. V5 and V6 are in the 5th intercostals space in the anterior and mid-axillary line on the left side. These leads 'look' at the heart in a horizontal plane (**Figures 6.20.1a** and **6.20.1b**).

Before recording the ECG enter the patient's details (name, date of birth, hospital number) into the machine. Ask the patient to remain still. Then press the button to initiate the ECG recording. Once complete, review the ECG. If it is adequate the leads can all be disconnected from the patient and they can redress.

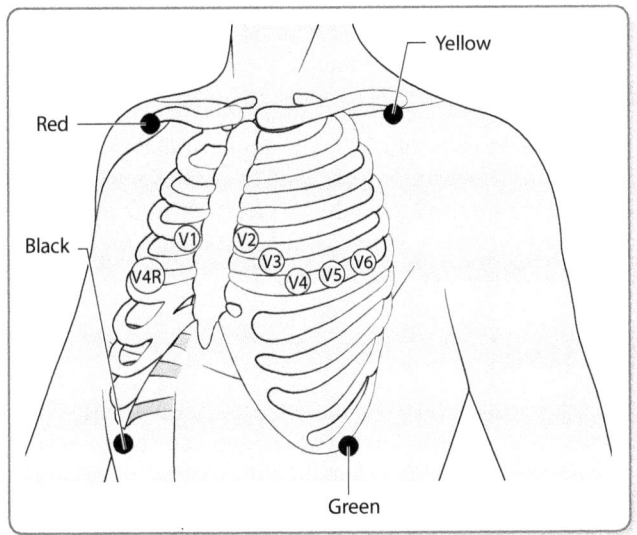

Figure 6.20.1a ECG electrode positioning.

Figure 6.20.1b Correct ECG position.

Recording right-sided ECG leads

Presence of ST elevation in V1 in association with signs of inferior myocardial infarction (MI) may indicate a right-sided MI. In this situation, a right-sided ECG can be done, most useful of which is the V4R. This is done by simply placing the V4 electrode from left to right 5th intercostal space and performing the rest of the ECG in the standard manner (**Figure 6.20.1a**). ST elevation in this lead indicates a right-sided MI.

Recording posterior ECG leads

V1, V2, V3 directly face the anterior surface of the heart (in their normal position). Any ST depression in these leads may indicate a posterior MI. In this situation posterior leads are indicated. They are done by moving the three lateral electrodes posteriorly. V4–V6 are moved to V7–V9 position. V7 is placed in posterior axillary line, V8 just under the tip of

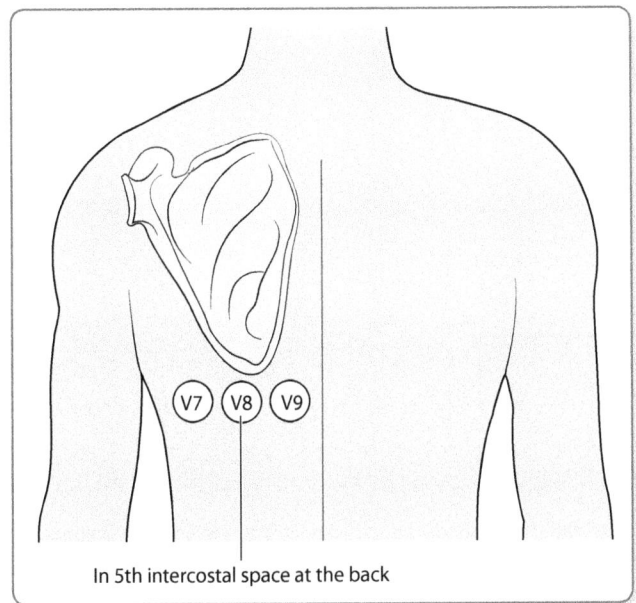

Figure 6.20.2 Posterior lead ECG electrode positioning.

In 5th intercostal space at the back

scapula and V9 between V8 and midline. The rest of the electrodes are left in the standard place. If performing a non-standard ECG, to avoid confusion ensure this is stated on the ECG (**Figure 6.20.2**).

ECG calibration

A standard ECG runs at 25 mm/s speed, recorded for 10 seconds making the standard trace 25 cm long. Each small square (1 mm on the ECG paper) on the X-axis represents 0.04 seconds. The electrical activity is measured in millivolts (mV) and the calibration is such that a 10 mm deflection on the Y-axis is equal to 1 mV. Any electrical vector towards the electrode is recorded as a positive deflection and away from the electrode is recorded as a negative deflection.

In addition, there is a rhythm strip that is usually the recording from lead II. This longer trace is used to assess any rhythm abnormalities. The rhythm strip is recorded for the whole 10 seconds whereas the other leads are recorded in groups of three for 2.5 seconds each.

ECG criteria for acute ST elevation myocardial infarction

- 1 mm ST elevation in 2 or more contiguous limb leads (i.e. I, II, III, aVL, aVF)
- 2 mm ST elevation in 2 or more contiguous chest leads (V1–V6)
- New left bundle branch block (LBBB), LBBB with a highly suggestive history or LBBB with increasing ST elevation on subsequent ECGs
- A true posterior MI may be occurring if there is ST segment depression in V1–V3
- A lateral infarct will meet the criteria if there is 1 mm ST elevation in I, and 2 mm in V6 as these are contiguous leads (although one is a limb lead and the other a chest lead) (**Figure 6.20.3**).

Figure 6.20.3 ECG territories.

Scenario

A final year medical student has seen a patient with chest pain who needs an ECG. Teach the student how to perform an ECG.

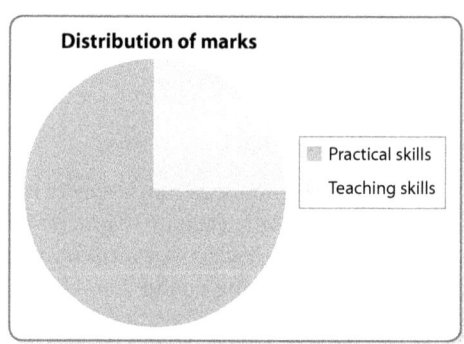

Mark sheet	Achieved	Not achieved
Introduces self to medical student		
Asks about previous knowledge and experience		
Sets learning objectives		
Explains plan to patient		
Confirms patient identity and enters data into machine		
Cleans hands		
Exposes patient adequately		
Discusses preparing patient skin (shaving or drying)		
Places ECG electrodes correctly		
Connects ECG machine to electrodes correctly		

Cont'd...

Cont'd...

Mark sheet	Achieved	Not achieved
Asks patient to remain still		
Records ECG correctly		
Reviews ECG and confirms proper trace		
Disconnects patient from machine		
Helps patient redress if necessary		
Allows medical student to repeat procedure		
Invites any questions from the medical student		
Recalls the objectives and summarises learning points		
Plan for further learning and assessment with supervisor		
Global mark from medical student		
Global mark from examiner		

Instructions for actor

You are a final year clinical medical student. You are going to become a doctor soon and have realised that you do not know how to perform an ECG. The patient you have seen attended the ED after some chest pain yesterday but is well now. They have no past medical history and take no medications.

You have asked if someone could teach you how to take an ECG. If the doctor shows you but does not offer you the chance to do the ECG yourself politely tell them you would like to do so. If offered the chance to perform an ECG, behave unsure about the sticker placement and wait for the doctor to help you. Ask them how to remember which lead is placed where. Also ask what the term "axis deviation" means and how to calculate the axis.

6.21 Blood cultures

Blood cultures permit the culture of microorganisms from blood providing essential information regarding the diagnosis of bacteraemia. They also provide information to guide appropriate antimicrobial treatment. Good technique is vital when obtaining blood cultures to prevent misleading results due to contamination.

The indication for blood cultures is suspected bacteraemia which is commonly suggested by:
- Temperature >38°C or <36°C
- Heart rate >90 beats per minute
- Respiratory rate >20 breaths per minute
- White blood cell count >12,000 mm^3 or <4,000 mm^3
- Systolic blood pressure <90 mmHg
- Clinical evidence of infection
- Chills or rigors

Technique

Begin by preparing the skin. Whenever possible take blood culture samples from a fresh site. Avoid drawing blood from peripheral lines. It is advisable to avoid the femoral vein as it is difficult to disinfect the skin in this area. When investigating potential infection related to a central line blood may be taken from the central line and from a separate peripheral site.

Clean any visibly soiled skin on the patient with soap and water and allow this to dry. Apply a disposable tourniquet and identify a suitable vein. Then clean the local area with an appropriate swab (e.g. 2% chlorhexidine in 70% isopropyl alcohol swab) and allow the area to dry. After this do not palpate the selected vein again as there is a risk of contaminating the skin.

Begin to prepare the necessary equipment. As the top of the culture bottle is not sterile remove the cap and clean the top of the bottle with a chlorhexidine and alcohol swab and allow it to dry.

There are then two accepted methods for actually taking the samples. The first method uses a butterfly needle and relies on the vacuum within the blood culture bottles. The second method uses a traditional needle and syringe.

Method 1

Clean hands appropriately and wear gloves and a gown. Attach a sterile butterfly needle to an adapter (**Figure 6.21.1**). Puncture the selected vein with the needle. Then place the adapter over the upright blood culture bottle until it pierces the lid of the bottle. The bottle will fill on its own. Fill the aerobic bottle first. Then remove the bottle and fill the anaerobic bottle in the same way. Remove the tourniquet and then withdraw the needle. Place a sterile dressing over the puncture site and apply gentle pressure to stop any oozing of blood. Discard sharps and equipment appropriately. Label the samples and complete the appropriate request for the samples to be processed.

Figure 6.21.1 (a) Blood culture bottles (b) Vacutainer adapter (c) Vacutainer needle (d) butterfly needle (e) skin cleaning swab.

Method 2

Clean hands appropriately and wear gloves and a gown. Connect a needle to an appropriately sized syringe (**Figure 6.21.2**). Puncture the selected vein with the needle and aspirate the required amount of blood. Remove the tourniquet and then withdraw the needle. Place a sterile dressing over the puncture site and apply gentle pressure to stop any oozing of blood. Discard sharps and equipment appropriately. Label the samples and complete the appropriate paperwork for the samples to be processed.

Figure 6.21.2 (a) Blood culture bottles (b) syringe (c) butterfly needle (d) skin cleaning swab.

Scenario

A student nurse in your department has observed you treating a septic patient. He has asked if you can teach him how to take blood cultures as this is something, he has never seen done. He only wishes to observe the procedure while you talk him through it.

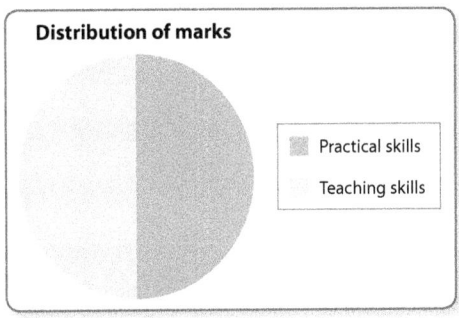

Distribution of marks

- Practical skills
- Teaching skills

Mark sheet	Achieved	Not achieved
Introduces self to student nurse		
Enquires from student nurse about previous experience and knowledge		
Asks them about anything specific they want to learn		
Sets and agrees on appropriate learning objectives		
Explains rationale for performing blood cultures		
Introduces self to patient		
Explains intended procedure		
Obtains verbal consent		
Washes hands and wears gloves and apron		
Prepares and checks appropriate equipment		
Applies tourniquet and selects suitable vein		
Cleans skin appropriately		
Cleans hands and wears gloves		
Performs venepuncture successfully		
Fills blood culture bottles correctly		
Removes tourniquet and dresses puncture site		
Disposes of sharps and equipment correctly		
Labels blood bottles and indicates the need to send samples		
Checks if student nurse has any questions or concerns		
Answers questions appropriately		
Agrees a plan for nursing student's on-going learning		
Is non-judgemental and facilitates learning		
Global mark from examiner		
Global mark from student nurse		

Instructions for actor

You are a final-year nursing student on placement in the ED. You have just had a talk about managing patients with severe sepsis and are interested to see how blood cultures are taken. You know they are used to 'grow any bacteria in the blood'. You are familiar with how to take normal blood samples but cannot do it yourself. When you observe the procedure you ask why it is different from when normal blood samples are taken. You have also heard about 'false-positive results' and ask the doctor what it means.

6.22 Backslab application

A plaster backslab is used to temporarily immobilise part of a limb following an injury. In the case of more serious injuries it stabilises the injured area thus providing analgesia and preventing further soft tissue damage. In other cases a backslab is used to provide temporary immobilisation which can accommodate further limb swelling until more definitive management when a full circumferential cast may be applied.

Though in many clinical situations the doctor may not apply the backslab themselves this is a fundamental skill all emergency clinicians should be capable of:

Basic principles

- Always provide adequate analgesia
- Remove any rings/circumferential jewellery from injured limbs as soon as possible
- Be conscious of exposed edges of the plaster cast rubbing at the edges and in the thumb web space
- Use only warm but never hot water for wetting the plaster bandage as it will heat up further when setting
- Squeezing the plaster bandage excessively removes the plaster and will weaken the cast
- Always smooth out the plaster with the palm of your hand as any irregular dents left by your fingers can cause pressure sores on the underlying skin
- Ensure no circumferential layers of the cast are applied too tightly
- Always provide verbal and written advice and consider VTE prophylaxis

Technique for below elbow backslab

The backslab extends from approximately 5 cm distal to the olecranon to a level just proximal to the metacarpophalangeal joints on the dorsal surface of the hand.

- Measure this distance using a tape measure or a strip of bandage
- Cut a piece of stockinette bandage approximately 8–10 cm longer than the distance measured. Slide this onto the forearm. The extra few centimetres should be equal at either end. These ends will ultimately be folded back over the plaster bandage to cover its rough edge. Cut a hole in it for the thumb (**Figure 6.22.1**)
- Starting at either end wrap the limb in a single layer of padding including the thumb's webspace but not the thumb itself (**Figure 6.22.2**)
- For the average adult use 6–8 layers of 15 cm wide plaster bandage cut to the above length
- Dip the plaster bandage into water, gently squeeze some of the water out of the bandage and then apply it to the area measured on the dorsal aspect of the forearm (**Figure 6.22.3**)
- Gently smooth the plaster bandage on to the limb to bond the layers together (**Figure 6.22.4**)
- Roll the extra centimetres of stockinette back over the plaster ends. This will prevent the rough plaster edges rubbing against the skin (**Figure 6.22.5**)
- Wrap a bandage around the limb and plaster backslab to secure it in place. Be cautious not to use too much tension as this can compromise blood flow in the distal limb
- Secure the bandage in place with tape (**Figure 6.22.6**)
- The fingers should be free to move fully at the metacarpophalangeal joints
- Equipment for plaster application is shown in **Figure 6.22.7**

338 Practical skills and teaching

Figure 6.22.1 The applied stockinette.

Figure 6.22.2 Stockinette and padding applied.

Figure 6.22.3 Wet plaster applied onto other layers.

Figure 6.22.4 Smoothing the plaster into place.

Figure 6.22.5 Folding back the stockinette at each end.

Figure 6.22.6 The final backslab.

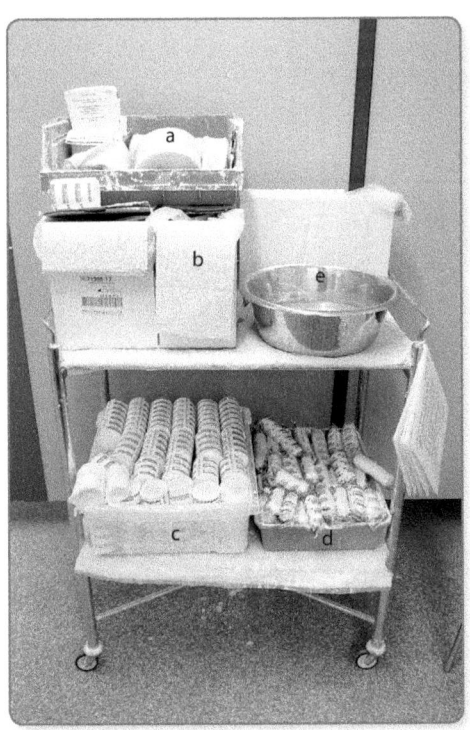

Figure 6.22.7 Equipment for plaster application (a) stockinette (b) plaster bandage (c) padding (d) bandage (e) warm water.

Technique for a Colles' backslab

In most ways the technique required is the same for applying a below elbow backslab. For a Colles' fracture the distal fragment must be stabilised in the backslab to prevent it displacing (particularly if it has been reduced). This is achieved by moulding the cast before it is set to give the wrist approximately 25° of dorsiflexion and 15° to 20° of ulna deviation.

Technique for an above-elbow backslab

This backslab extends from the mid-humerus to a level just proximal to the metacarpophalangeal joints (knuckles) on the dorsum of the hand.
- A plaster bandage (approximately 6–8 layers of 15 cm width) of the above length is prepared
- With the patient's elbow flexed to approximately 90° the stockinette and soft padding layers are applied as above
- The plaster bandage is then dipped in the water and applied to the posterior aspect of the arm at the mid-humerus and extending to the dorsum of the hand proximal to the metacarpophalangeal joints
- Make a transverse slit it the plaster bandage at the level of the elbow on both sides. Overlap the cut edges and smooth them out
- The remaining steps are as above for the below elbow backslab

Scenario

Ms Burton is a 72-year-old woman who fell in the street and was brought to the ED by ambulance. She has been assessed and has been diagnosed with a minimally displaced left Colles' fracture which does not require manipulation. She is otherwise safe for discharge home with her family. The junior doctor who has seen Miss Burton has never applied a backslab before. Teach the junior doctor how to apply a below-elbow backslab to Ms Burton's left arm.

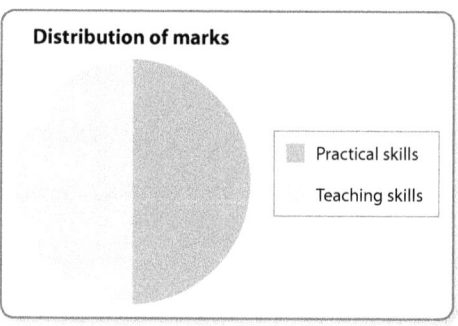

Distribution of marks
- Practical skills
- Teaching skills

Mark sheet	Achieved	Not achieved
Introduces self to junior doctor		
Enquires from junior doctor about previous experience and knowledge		
Asks them about anything specific they want to learn		
Sets and agrees on appropriate learning objectives		
Explains rationale for using a backslab		
Introduces self to patient		
Explains intended procedure		

Cont'd...

Cont'd...

Mark sheet	Achieved	Not achieved
Checks X-ray and confirms which limb is involved		
Enquires about pain and offers analgesia		
Washes hands and wears gloves and an apron		
Removes patient's rings explaining the rationale for doing so		
Measures length of stockinette and plaster bandages		
Correctly applies layers of backslab		
Provides verbal and written advice		
Agrees follow-up plan with patient		
Checks patient comfortable with plan and follow-up provided		
Checks if junior doctor has any questions or concerns		
Answers questions appropriately		
Agrees a plan for junior doctor's on-going learning		
Is non-judgemental and facilitates learning		
Global mark from examiner		
Global mark from junior doctor		

Instructions for actor

You are a newly qualified doctor working in the ED. You want to be an orthopaedic surgeon and are interested to learn as much as you can. You have asked if you can watch the backslab being put on. While the procedure is happening you ask several questions if the answers haven't already been explained:
- Why is warm water used for the procedure?
- How is a standard backslab different from a Colles' backslab?
- Why use a backslab and not a full cast?
- When should thromboembolism prophylaxis be used?

6.23 Pleural aspiration

This procedure is performed to remove air or fluid from the pleural space. In the context of emergency medicine it is normally used to aspirate pneumothoraces in accordance with the British Thoracic Society guidelines which all candidates must be familiar with. Pleural aspiration is a significantly less invasive procedure than the insertion of an intercostal chest drain and reduces morbidity while potentially allowing patients to be discharged sooner.

Technique

The first step is to confirm the side of the pneumothorax/effusion. This should be done clinically and in almost all circumstances also requires checking an up-to-date chest X-ray.

The patient should be positioned so they are sitting upright on a trolley. The appropriate site of insertion is either within the safe triangle (**Figure 6.6.1**) or in the second intercostal space in the mid-clavicular line. Any needles inserted through an intercostal space should be inserted at the lower margin of the space to avoid trauma to the neurovascular bundle below each rib.

Having positioned the patient and identified the correct landmarks an appropriate dose of local anaesthetic should be infiltrated superficially and down to the pleura. A large bore cannula (16–18G) should then be inserted with a syringe attached to aspirate as the cannula is advanced. The aspiration of air (or fluid in the case of an effusion) indicates the cannula is in the correct place. Next the cannula should be advanced and the syringe and needle removed (**Figure 6.23.1**).

Figure 6.23.1 Equipment for pleural aspiration (a) large bore cannula (b) syringe (c) three way tap (d) large syringe (e) sterile drape (f) sterile gauze (g) sterile swab.

A three way tap and 50 mL syringe can then be attached to the cannula and air aspirated. The three way tap allows the expulsion of air without having to detach the syringe each time. Aspirate up to 2,500 mL of air before removing the cannula. After removal of the cannula ensure the patient is comfortable and arrange a further chest X-ray to reassess the pneumothorax. If there has been resolution and the patient is otherwise well they can possibly be discharged with outpatient follow-up. If not an intercostal chest drain may be required.

All patients who have suffered a pneumothorax should be advised not to fly for 6 weeks after it is resolved and to never dive unless they have had it treated by a pleurectomy.

Scenario

Mr Krystian Gorski is a 28-year-old pilot. He presented today with breathlessness and has been found to have a spontaneous pneumothorax on his left side (**Figure 6.23.2**). After a review of the British Thoracic Society guidelines, you have been asked to aspirate his pneumothorax.

Figure 6.23.2 Mr Gorski's chest X-ray.

Mark sheet	Achieved	Not achieved
Introduces self to patient appropriately		
Confirms patient's identity		
Reviews the chest X-ray in the cubicle		
Explains the procedure and obtains verbal consent		
Asks about pain and offers analgesia		
Positions patient appropriately		
Identifies correct landmarks		
Prepares and checks equipment		
Cleans hands and wears gloves and apron		
Infiltrates local anaesthetic, comments on maximum dose		

Cont'd...

Cont'd...

Mark sheet	Achieved	Not achieved
Selects appropriate size cannula		
Correctly aspirates air from the pleural space		
Selects and connects large syringe and three way tap		
Stops aspirating when patient begins coughing		
Disposes of sharps and equipment appropriately		
Comments on need to arrange further chest X-ray		
Demonstrates awareness of patient comfort throughout procedure		
Informs patient regarding restriction on flying and diving		
Checks patient understands and is happy with stated plan		
Global mark from patient		
Global mark from examiner		

Suggested reading

Macduff A, Arnold A, Harvey J. Management of a spontaneous pneumothorax. Thorax 2010; 65:ii18eii31.
Havelock T, Teoh R, Laws D, et al. Pleural procedures and thoracic ultrasound: British Thoracic Society pleural disease guideline. Thorax 2010; 65:ii61eii76.
Lee J. Spontaneous pneumothorax. London: RCEM Learning; 2017.

6.24 Rapid sequence induction

A rapid sequence induction (RSI) involves the use of an induction agent followed by a neuromuscular blocking agent to allow urgent endotracheal intubation.
The main indications are:
- To protect the airway
- To pre-empt deterioration in airway patency
- To ventilate those with respiratory failure
- To facilitate safe or humane transfer

Technique

Having identified the need for an RSI the first requirement is to inform the team of the plan and allocate appropriate roles. If additional help is necessary it should be called for. Ideally there will be at least three members of the team. One to perform the intubation, one to connect monitoring and perform cricoid pressure, and a third to administer drugs and perform any other tasks that arise.

The patient's head must be positioned adequately to facilitate intubation (assuming triple immobilisation of the cervical spine is not required) in a 'sniffing the morning air position'. This is flexion at the neck and extension of the head, with the tragus at the level of sternal notch. All the required equipment should be checked (suction, bag and mask, endotracheal tubes, laryngoscopes, syringe) and oxygen and monitoring (ECG, blood pressure, pulse oximetry, end-tidal CO_2 monitoring) connected. Also ensure intravenous access is adequate (**Figure 6.24.1**).

Pre-oxygenating the patient increases the duration of time before they begin to desaturate during attempted intubation. Pre-oxygenation is performed by given the highest percentage of oxygen available for 3 minutes with assisted ventilation if the patient's breathing is inadequate.

At this point, the induction drug is given and followed by the muscle relaxant and a large flush of normal saline. Once the induction drug is given an assistant must apply cricoid

Figure 6.24.1 Equipment for intubation. (a) Yankauer suction (b) two laryngoscopes in case one fails (c) orotracheal tubes (d) syringe to inflate tube cuff (e) tube tie (f) bougie (g) filter (h) tubing for capnography.

pressure until they are asked to release it. To do this firm pressure is applied by the thumb and index finger over the cricoid cartilage. This compresses the oesophagus between the cricoid cartilage and cervical vertebrae, and prevents reflux of gastric contents and subsequent aspiration.

The laryngoscope blade is held in the operator's left hand and is inserted initially into the right side of the patient's mouth so when advanced it will displace the tongue to the left. The laryngoscope blade is then advanced until the epiglottis is seen. The blade is then lifted in-line with the handle to displace the jaw. Care must be taken not to use the blade as a lever as this risks damaging the patient's teeth. Under direct vision the endotracheal tube is then placed through the vocal cords and into the trachea. Next the patient is ventilated and the cuff on the tube is inflated until no leak can be heard.

During intubation additional equipment that may be required is suction to clear respiratory secretion, vomitus or blood and an intubating bougie. If the view is poor the bougie can be placed between the vocal chords and the endotracheal tube 'railroaded' over it. Use of the bougie must be coordinated with an assistant. The operator will insert the bougie under laryngoscopy and hold it in place. The assistant will then thread the endotracheal tube over the bougie. At this point, the operator takes hold of the endotracheal tube and the assistant holds the bougie in place so it is not advanced further. The operator then advances the endotracheal tube over the bougie, between the vocal cords, before the bougie is removed.

The correct position of the tube must be confirmed. This is done by confirming end-tidal carbon dioxide via capnography. Clinical methods of checking tube position are watching for symmetrical chest movement on ventilation and auscultating both axillae for equal air entry. Once it is agreed the tube is positioned correctly cricoid pressure can then be released.

The patient should now be reassessed. They can now be ventilated and are likely to require further medication to maintain sedation while they undergo further management.

Scenario

You are called because the paramedics have brought in a 35-year-old man. He had initially complained of a severe headache before vomiting and collapsing in a chair. Since then he has had a Glasgow Coma Score of 6. On initial assessment, he has noisy upper airway sounds on breathing spontaneously and is haemodynamically stable. The intensivist has been called but will be at least 20 minutes. You are required to manage the patient's airway. A staff nurse and junior doctor are available to help.

Mark sheet	Achieved	Not achieved
Introduces self to team		
Confirms history of events with paramedics		
Washes hands and wears gloves and apron		
Assesses airway		
Assesses breathing		
Assesses circulation		
Assesses disability		
Recognises need for RSI		
Calls for additional help (intensivist/anaesthetist)		
Explains need for RSI to team		
Allocates roles to members of team		
Prepares and checks equipment		
States plan for unsuccessful intubation		
Preoxygenates patient		
Uses correct drugs and doses		
Uses cricoid pressure		
Correct insertion of endotracheal tube		
Confirms tube position appropriately and secures it		
Comments on need to connect ventilator with appropriate settings		
Comments on need for further drugs to maintain sedation		
Arranges ongoing management (CT of the brain and intensivist review)		
Comments on need for neuroprotective measures		
Global mark from team		
Global mark from examiner		

Suggested reading

Benger J, Nolan J, Clancy M. Emergency Airway Management. Cambridge: Cambridge University Press; 2009.
Jones J. Difficult Airway Management. London: RCEM Learning; 2016.

6.25 Surgical airway

Needle or surgical cricothyroidotomy are emergency procedures to manage airway obstruction above the level of the larynx in cases where endotracheal intubation is not possible. Common reasons this may occur are maxillofacial trauma, soft tissue swelling (burns/anaphylaxis/infection) or foreign body.

Indications

Upper airway obstruction where endotracheal intubation is not possible.

Contraindications

Because needle or surgical cricothyroidotomy are to be attempted when all other measures have failed, there is no absolute contraindication. However, in those with significant deformity where the landmarks cannot be identified the success rate for the procedure may be very low.

Complications

- Subcutaneous placement of needle or tube
- Haemorrhage
- Posterior perforation of trachea or oesophagus
- Laryngeal stenosis

Initial management

A cricothyroidotomy is the last resort after all other management options have been exhausted. In an OSCE setting it is important the candidate demonstrates their knowledge of the alternatives for managing an airway to avoid a cricothyroidotomy. It is reasonable to demonstrate this knowledge by discussing the options and attempting those which seem appropriate. Never forget the basics of airway manoeuvres, suctioning, airway adjuncts and the possibility of attempting endotracheal intubation.

Having recognised that the obstructed airway cannot be dealt with by endotracheal intubation the whole team should be informed of the need for a cricothyroidotomy and the appropriate equipment requested. If the patient requires their cervical spine to be immobilised it will be necessary to remove any collar and have an assistant kneel at the head of the bed and maintain in-line immobilisation.

Depending on the circumstances either a needle or surgical cricothyroidotomy can be performed.

Needle cricothyroidotomy

This is a temporary measure that allows oxygenation (but not ventilation) through a cannula placed into the trachea. It will allow time for additional equipment or experienced

staff to be prepared. A pre-packed needle cricothyroidotomy kit may be available. If not a large bore cannula attached to a 5 mL or 10 mL syringe can be used. The steps of the procedure are:
- Wear appropriate personal protective equipment
- Identify the cricothyroid membrane between the thyroid and cricoid cartilages
- Clean the skin and if required infiltrate local anaesthetic
- Insert the needle through the skin angled at 45° caudally
- As the needle is slowly advance aspirate continually. The aspiration of air indicates the needle lies in the trachea
- Advance the needle slightly further and then slide the cannula off the needle
- Connect the cannula to a Y-connector or similar device to allow intermittent jet insufflation with high flow oxygen
- Oxygenate the patient for 1 in every 5 seconds. The chest wall should be seen to rise. During the following 4 seconds gases are able to escape through the patient's own airway
- Once the patient is being oxygenated a primary survey should be completed and preparation should begin to obtain a definitive airway

Surgical cricothyroidotomy

This procedure allows a cuffed tube to be placed in the trachea. The steps of the procedure are:
- Wear appropriate personal protective equipment
- Identify the cricothyroid membrane between the thyroid and cricoid cartilages
- Clean the skin and if required infiltrate local anaesthetic
- With your non-dominant hand stabilise the thyroid or cricoid cartilage
- Using your other hand make a horizontal incision through the cricothyroid membrane. Do not withdraw the blade from the incision until an instrument for dilating is inserted (this will avoid the formation of a false passage and subcutaneous tube placement)
- Using forceps (or a finger) dilate the incision into the trachea and insert a paediatric bougie
- Insert a tracheal or tracheostomy tube into the trachea and remove the introducer or bougie. Caution should be exercised if a tracheostomy tube is used as a small tube may not occlude an adult trachea even with the cuff inflated
- Inflate the cuff and secure the tube in place
- Confirm correct placement of the tube by ventilating the patient and auscultating their lung fields. If possible capnography and a ventilator should also be connected. The primary survey can now be completed

Seldinger method

Some manufacturers prepare kits where the above procedures are combined by the use of a Seldinger kit where a needle is passed into the trachea followed by a guidewire, a dilator and then a definitive tube (**Figure 6.25.1**).

Figure 6.25.1 (a) Guidewire (b) needle (c) syringe (d) blade (e) dilator (f) tracheal tube (g) tube tie.

Scenario

You are called to the resuscitation area to prepare to see a 23-year-old man who is being brought in by paramedics. He has gone over the handlebars of his bicycle and landed on his face sustaining severe facial injuries with heavy ongoing bleeding. He was not wearing a helmet. He is only responding to pain by localising. His respiratory rate is 6 breaths per minute with oxygen saturation on high-flow oxygen of 75%. His heart rate is 46 beats per minute with a blood pressure of 186/96 mmHg. His cervical spine is immobilised. Perform an initial assessment and manage his airway. You have 2 minutes to prepare your team (one trained and one untrained nurse) before he arrives.

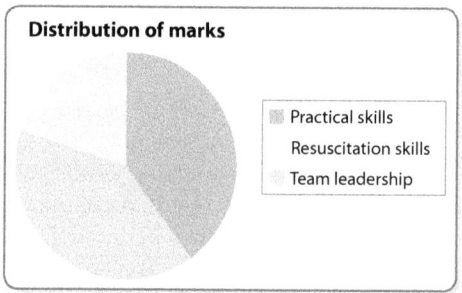

Distribution of marks

- Practical skills
- Resuscitation skills
- Team leadership

Mark sheet	Achieved	Not achieved
Introduces self to team		
Confirms history of events with paramedics		
Briefs team and allocates roles/prepares equipment		
Calls for help/trauma team		
Cleans hands and uses personal protective equipment		
Assesses airway and recognises need to protect airway		
Applies high flow oxygen and monitoring to patient		
Maintains cervical spine immobilisation throughout		
Attempts suctioning airway, recognises on-going bleeding		
Attempts airway manoeuvres/placing oropharyngeal airway – (does not attempt nasopharyngeal airway)		

Cont'd...

Cont'd...

Mark sheet	Achieved	Not achieved
Attempts ventilating patient with bag/valve/mask		
Considers (or attempts) laryngoscopy		
Recognises need for cricothyroidotomy		
Informs team of plan		
Correctly identifies landmarks for procedure		
Correctly performs procedure – needle or surgical cricothyroidotomy		
Oxygenates/ventilates patient		
Hands patient over adequately when intensivist/anaesthetist arrives		
Comments on need to complete primary survey		
Discusses on-going management – CT of the brain/face/cervical spine/maxillofacial review urgently		
Global mark from team		
Global mark from examiner		

Suggested reading

Benger J, Nolan J, Clancy M. Emergency Airway Management. Cambridge University Press, 2009.
Guidelines for management of unanticipated difficult Intubation in Adults. Difficult Airway Society. London, 2015.

6.26 Lateral cervical spine X-ray interpretation

Teaching a junior colleague how to interpret an X-ray is a common task in the exam. This can be any routine X-ray you would expect to see in the ED. This will include cervical spine, chest, pelvis, elbow, hand and foot X-rays. Others are possible but less likely. It is vital to have revised the relevant anatomy, and rehearsed your routine for interpreting these X-rays so it can be articulated clearly in the exam.

Begin the interpretation of every investigation by confirming it belongs to the correct patient and the time it was taken. It is all too easy in a busy department to make management decisions on a result that is either from another patient or a previous date.

Having done this, note the adequacy of the image. With regard to a lateral cervical spine the view must be from C1 to the superior border of T1 (**Figure 6.26.1**). If this is not the case the whole cervical spine has not been imaged and further imaging is needed. This is often a 'swimmer's view' which visualises the lower cervical spine though there are other alternatives.

To assess alignment of the cervical spine three smooth lines can be visualised (**Figure 6.26.2**):
- Line 1: this runs along the anterior surface of the vertebral bodies and the anterior surface of the odontoid peg
- Line 2: this runs along the posterior surface of the vertebral bodies and the posterior surface of the odontoid peg
- Line 3: this runs along the base of the spinous processes

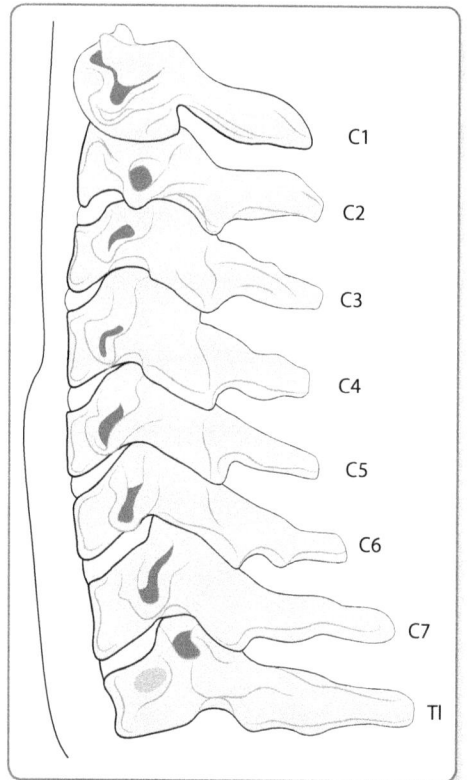

Figure 6.26.1 Lateral cervical spine.

A step or break in the continuity of one or more of these lines may indicate disruption to the normal structure and warrants further scrutiny (**Figure 6.26.3**).

Next each vertebral body should be assessed individually. From C2 they should each appear relatively rectangular with an adjoining and intact spinous process. Each intervertebral disc space should also be assessed and each should be the same height.

An increase in the soft tissue shadowing anterior to the vertebral bodies can be a valuable sign where increased soft tissue swelling may indicate an injury at that level. For this reason knowledge of the amount of soft tissue considered normal is also necessary. Between the level of C1 and C4 this should be less than 7 mm and from C5 distally may be up to 22 mm.

Having assessed the lateral cervical spine X-ray it is also required to assess an AP view and 'peg' view where the odontoid peg of C2 and the articular surface of C1 and C2 are visualised on an image through the patient's mouth.

Always remember that even with no abnormal finding on X-rays the patient still needs to be assessed clinically (see Section 6.7) because if there is ongoing clinical concern further imaging may be required before the cervical spine can be mobilised.

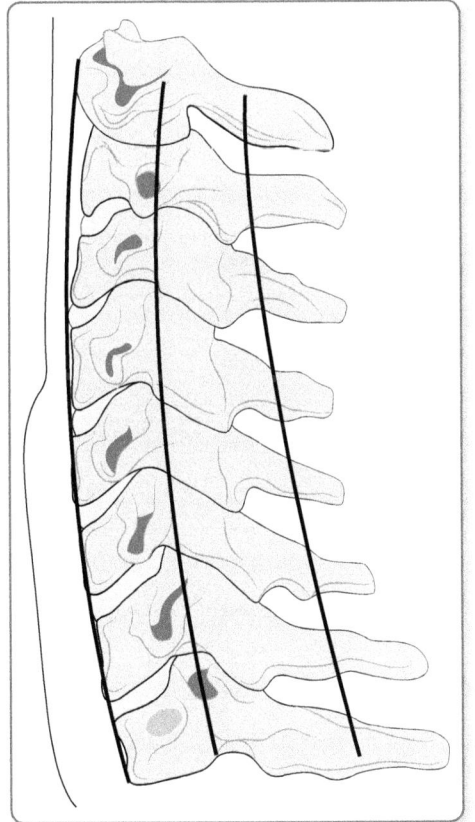

Figure 6.26.2 Cervical spine lines of alignment (a) anterior vertebral line (b) posterior vertebral line (c) spinous processes.

354 Practical skills and teaching

Figure 6.26.3 Abnormal alignment of cervical spine at C6-C7.

Scenario

A new doctor in the ED asks you to teach her how to interpret a lateral cervical spine X-ray for a patient who fell off his bicycle. Teach her how to do this and recommend a plan for the patient.

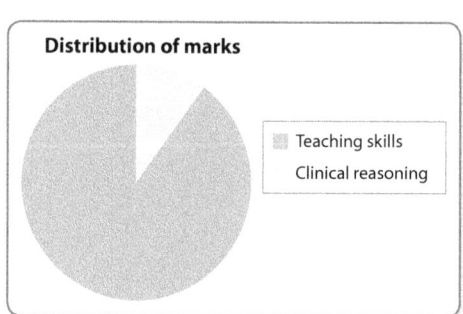

Distribution of marks
- Teaching skills
- Clinical reasoning

Mark sheet	Achieved	Not achieved
Introduces self to junior doctor		
Enquires from junior doctor about previous experience and knowledge		
Asks them about anything specific they want to learn		
Sets and agrees on appropriate learning objectives		
Asks for the history/mechanism of injury		
Checks patient requires no immediate treatment		

Cont'd...

Cont'd...

Mark sheet	Achieved	Not achieved
Explains need to check:		
– patient name and time of X-ray		
– adequacy		
– alignment		
– each vertebral body		
– joint space		
– degree of soft tissue swelling		
– need to check additional views		
Correctly interprets lateral view as adequate and normal		
Checks if junior doctor has any questions or concerns		
Agrees a plan for managing the patient		
Answers questions appropriately		
Agrees a plan for junior doctor's on-going learning		
Is non-judgemental and facilitates learning		
Global mark from examiner		
Global mark from junior doctor		

Instructions for actor

You are a junior doctor who has just started working in the ED. You are seeing a 21-year-old man who has fallen off his bicycle and arrived by ambulance triple immobilised. He was wearing a helmet, has no other injuries and all his observations are normal. He is complaining of some neck pain. You haven't felt his neck but have excluded any other injuries. He has only had a lateral view so far as the radiographers were called to an emergency.

You have not interpreted a lateral cervical spine X-ray and would like to be taught how to do so. Afterwards ask the doctor what a swimmer's view is and when it is used.

Suggested reading

Raby N, Berman L, de Lacey G. Accident and Emergency Radiology, A survival guide, 2nd edn. Elsevier Saunders, 2005.

6.27 Thomas splint application

A Thomas splint is a traction splint commonly used for fractures of the femoral shaft. The splint applies traction to the leg thereby helping reduce the fracture and the potential space for blood loss. The immobilisation also provides a degree of analgesia for the patient.

A Thomas splint consists of a full or half ring that sits around the proximal thigh and connects to two rigid rods that extend to the ankle. The lower limb is then secured by bandages to the distal portion of the two rods and traction is applied. Proximally the splint applies pressure to the buttocks and groin and distally does so through its contact with the skin of the distal limb. A femoral nerve block is often a valuable adjunct to maximise the degree of analgesia achieved and may be necessary to facilitate the splint's application.

Though various forms of this device exist the principles by which they work are very similar (**Figure 6.27.1**).

Figure 6.27.1 Equipment for Thomas splint. (a) Hip ring (with folding rods) (b) metal frame (c) frame padding (d) frame 'slings' to support leg (e) skin traction with traction cords (f) bandage for skin traction (g) device to tighten traction cords.

Technique

Explain to the patient that their leg is going to be placed in a splint to stabilise it. Ensure adequate analgesia including the consideration of a femoral nerve block. Expose the entire leg.

Prepare the splint by attaching the metal frame to the hip ring (**Figure 6.27.2**). Small slings should be positioned along the length of the splint from one rod to the other (**Figure 6.27.3**). These slings may be pre-packed or prepared from crepe bandage and will form a suspended layer of material for the leg to rest on.

Begin by applying skin traction. This requires a single piece of strapping to be run down the lateral lower leg, across the sole and then back up the medial lower leg (**Figure 6.27.4**). Commercial brands have traction cords that emanate from the middle portion of the strapping which lies over the sole of the foot. The strapping is then secured in place by crepe bandage which is wrapped around it and the lower leg (**Figure 6.27.5**).

The splint itself is an elongated rigid frame in a U-shape which attaches to a proximal ring. The size should be checked to ensure the ring is slightly wider than the upper thigh to

Figure 6.27.2 Frame and hip ring attached.

Figure 6.27.3 The splint with slings in place.

Figure 6.27.4 Applying skin traction.

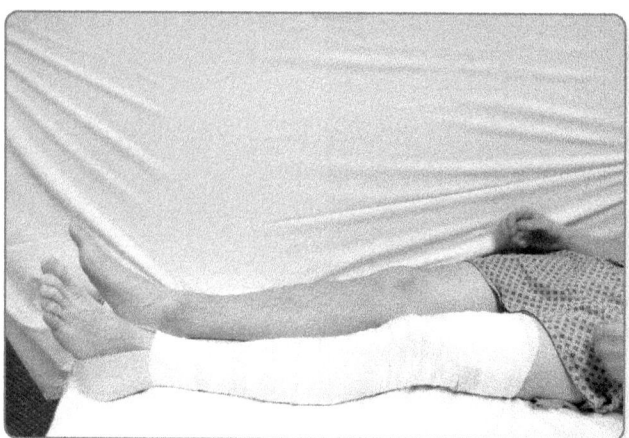

Figure 6.27.5 Skin traction secured to leg.

Figure 6.27.6 Lifting the leg to place splint.

allow for ongoing thigh swelling. This can be done by measuring the circumference of the contralateral thigh.

The leg should be gently lifted so that the splint can be slid underneath (**Figure 6.27.6**). The splint should be advanced upwards until it sits against the ischial tuberosity or perineum with care taken not to pinch the skin or genitalia.

The traction cords can then be attached to the distal end of the splint (**Figure 6.27.7**). They are then twisted so they tighten (**Figure 6.27.8**) and apply traction and then they are secured in place (**Figure 6.27.9**).

Figure 6.27.7 Attaching traction cords to splint.

Figure 6.27.8 Tightening traction cords by twisting the white stick.

Figure 6.27.9 Traction cords tightened and locked in place.

Scenario

You are called to the resuscitation area to help treat a 59-year-old man who fell off a ladder. Mr Evans has an isolated femoral fracture and no other injuries. He has already had a femoral nerve block. Apply a femoral traction splint while explaining the procedure to the nurse who has not seen it done before.

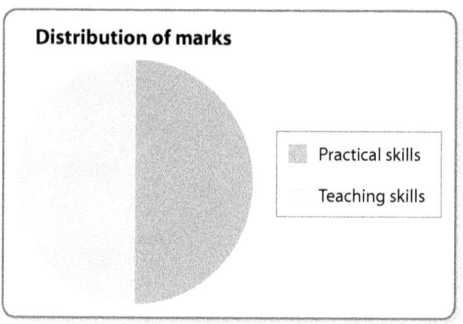

Distribution of marks

- Practical skills
- Teaching skills

Mark sheet	Achieved	Not achieved
Introduces self to nurse		
Enquires from nurse about previous experience and knowledge		
Introduces self to patient		
Cleans hands and wears gloves		
Enquires regarding presence of pain and offers analgesia		
Explains need to fit a traction splint to patient		
Obtains patient consent		
Measures circumference of thigh		
Selects appropriate size of splint		
Applies skin traction correctly		
Fits straps/slings to splint correctly		
Inserts splint under leg		
Applies traction using traction cords		
Tightens and locks traction cords in place		
Talks through each step of procedure		
Asks nurse if they have any questions		
Offers to cover patient's legs		
Global mark from examiner		

Instructions for actor

You have recently started work in the ED after working on surgical wards for several years. You are a competent nurse but have never seen a traction splint applied before. You have asked if someone could talk you through the procedure as it is done.

After the procedure, if it hasn't been discussed, you ask what the purpose of applying traction is. You also ask if there are different types of splints for the procedure and what is the most suitable type of pain relief to facilitate the splint being applied.

6.28 Male urethral catheter insertion

The catheter is inserted through the urethra so the distal end lies in the bladder and urine flows directly through the catheter into a collection bag. A size 14 or 16 standard Foley catheter is appropriate for most patients. A three way catheter is used in patient where irrigation of the bladder is required.

Indications

The main reasons for inserting a catheter are:
- Urinary obstruction whether it be acute or chronic
- Monitoring of urine output in acutely ill patients
- To facilitate bladder irrigation

Contraindications

- Suspected or actual urethral trauma
- Acute prostatitis

Complications

- Failure
- Urethral trauma
- Catheter associated infection

Technique

Having established the indication for a urethral catheter it should be ensured there are no contraindications to the procedure.

After preparing the necessary equipment (**Figure 6.28.1**) position the patient appropriately. They should be supine on a trolley in a private room with their genitalia adequately exposed.

To prevent introducing bacteria into the bladder the procedure must be done aseptically. Sterile gloves are necessary as well as full aseptic technique. To perform the procedure one hand is normally contaminated while the other remains sterile.

If right-handed the procedure is best performed standing on the right hand side of the bed with the right hand kept sterile.

Place a drape with a window over the penis so the penis protrudes through the hole in the drape. With the left hand hold the penis and retract the foreskin. Clean the penis with the normal saline and gauze ensuring the right hand is not contaminated.

Now hold the penis upright and administer the anaesthetic gel into the urethral meatus. If some of the gel leaks onto the outside of the penis it may make it difficult to hold. To prevent this it may be useful to wrap the penis in a piece of gauze and then hold it with the left hand. Allow the anaesthetic gel some time to work.

Figure 6.28.1 Male urethral catheter equipment (a) catheter (b) fluid to inject/inflate catheter balloon (c) lubricant/anaesthetic gel (d) cleaning solution (e) procedure tray (f) sterile sheet (g) sterile gauze.

Hold the catheter in the right hand. Place the distal end in the urethra and slowly advance it. If you feel any resistance it is important not to force the catheter further as this will cause trauma or make a false passage. Insert the catheter fully and check it is draining urine. Then insert the correct amount of sterile water into the port on the catheter to inflate the balloon. Next connect the catheter to a collection bag.

Before finishing the task it is vital to ensure the foreskin is replaced as this will prevent paraphimosis. Then ensure the patient is cleaned and able to redress. Help them if appropriate.

During this procedure it is important to be sensitive to patient dignity and ensure they are comfortable.

Scenario

Mr Derek Murray is a 72-year-old man who has presented with urinary obstruction. He has found it harder and harder to pass urine for some weeks and feels the flow has got much weaker. He has been unable to pass urine since yesterday. He is otherwise fit and well and does not take any medication. Catheterise Mr Murray with a urethral catheter and briefly explain a management plan to him.

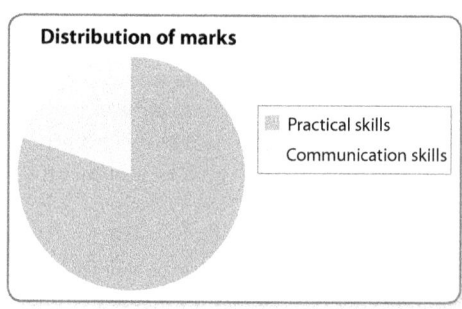

Distribution of marks
- Practical skills
- Communication skills

Mark sheet	Achieved	Not achieved
Introduces self to patient appropriately		
Confirms patient's identity		
Explains to patient the need for a catheter		
Explains what procedure involves and seeks consent		

Cont'd...

Cont'd...

Mark sheet	Achieved	Not achieved
Washes hands and wears sterile gloves		
Checks and prepares equipment correctly		
Places sterile drape		
Retracts foreskin and cleans penis		
Administers local anaesthetic gel into urethral meatus		
Correctly inserts catheter into urethra		
Checks urine is draining into catheter		
Attaches a urinary bag to the catheter		
Inflates the catheter balloon		
Replaces foreskin		
Removes sterile drape and helps patient redress		
Demonstrates aseptic technique throughout procedure		
Disposes of all equipment appropriately		
Maintains patient dignity throughout procedure		
Explains appropriate management plan to patient involving removal of the catheter and outpatient follow-up		
Global mark from patient		
Global mark from examiner		

6.29 Vaginal examination

A vaginal examination is a vital part of a gynaecological assessment. There are several clinical scenarios in which it is required including an assessment of vaginal bleeding, discharge, pain or removal of a foreign body (tampon or condom).

In the context of the exam this station tests a candidate's ability to perform an examination competently while also being sensitive to the patient and maintaining their dignity during an intimate procedure. All these elements must be dealt with to pass this station.

Initial technique

This examination has two stages, a bimanual examination and then a speculum examination.

Begin by introducing yourself, confirming the name of the patient and asking for permission to examine her. Explain what you are going to do.

Ask for a chaperone and ensure you are in a private room where the door can be locked to prevent anyone else walking in.

Ask if the patient has any pain and offer analgesia if appropriate. Put on gloves and an apron.

Ask the patient to lie supine and bend both of her knees. Then ask her to relax her legs so her knees fall apart.

Begin by inspecting the perineum for warts, ulcers, eczema, vulvitis or signs of inflammation (erythema, swelling, discharge).

Either of the following two examinations can be performed first as the initial steps and positioning remain the same for both. In the context of removing a retained foreign body if one method of examination is successful at removal the second does not need to be performed.

Bimanual vaginal examination

Using one hand separate the labia and inspect the clitoris and urethral meatus. Apply some lubricant to the middle and index finger of your other hand. Place your two fingers onto the vagina and wait for the patient to relax. Then insert both fingers into the vagina. With your other hand gently press down on the lower abdomen so the uterus or any other masses can be palpated bimanually. As with all examinations always be conscious of the level of discomfort you cause the patient and stop the examination if necessary.

Systematically assess the uterus for its position and size. Make a note of whether it feels smooth or irregular. Feel the cervix to assess if the os is open or closed. Next move your fingers into each adnexa to again palpate for masses and assess for tenderness.

The examination is complete.

Speculum examination

Consider warming the speculum in warm water to make the examination more comfortable. Then apply lubricant to it.

With one hand separate the labia and with the other rest the speculum on the vagina. As the patient relaxes slowly insert the speculum as far as it will go. Gently open the speculum and the cervix will appear in the view. If the cervix cannot be seen close and then reposition the speculum. Be careful not to pinch any tissue when closing/repositioning the speculum. Once open hold the speculum in position by tightening the screw (**Figure 6.29.1**).

The vaginal wall and cervix can now be inspected. Swabs may be performed or foreign bodies removed. After the examination gently unscrew and then close the speculum taking care not to trap any tissue or hair in it. It can now be removed.

Figure 6.29.1 Disposable speculum (a) speculum (b) handle (c) screw to lock speculum open.

Closing the examination

To end the examinations offer the patient some tissues. Allow her to dress in private and dispose of all equipment appropriately.

Communication and maintaining patient dignity

Given the intimate nature of the examination there are several additional points that must be considered to gain marks. It is always good practice for all doctors performing intimate procedures to ask for a chaperone. In the exam, though one may not be available there is likely to be a mark for the candidate mentioning a chaperone. Also given the nature of the examination it is worth commenting that you would use a private room for the examination.

To help the patient prepare for the examination explain to her what is going to happen. Take extra notice of her level of comfort during the procedure.

During the examination itself keep conversation to the minimum and afterwards allow the patient to get dressed in private.

The lost condom

This is a common OSCE as it tests practical skills, communication and professionalism when dealing with a sensitive/awkward task. Either (or both) methods of examination can be used to remove a foreign body. Direct visualisation with a speculum may be preferable to ensure a foreign body is removed intact.

It may also be necessary in these cases to give further birth control advice, which may involve the morning after pill. It is also appropriate to recommend screening for sexually transmitted infections and even post-exposure prophylaxis for HIV. Brief discussion with the patient should establish the need for these extra measures.

Scenario

Pippa Martin is a 24-year-old woman who has attended the ED, complaining of having a retained condom after sexual intercourse. Examine Miss Martin and remove the condom. You do not need to take a full history but may ask any important questions and offer appropriate advice.

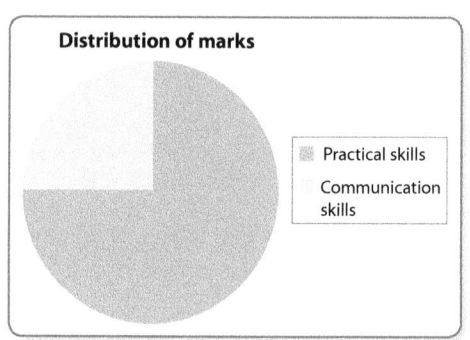

Distribution of marks
- Practical skills
- Communication skills

Mark sheet	Achieved	Not achieved
Introduces self to patient appropriately		
Confirms patient's identity		
Ensures privacy by closing curtain or door		
Takes brief history of events		
Explains what procedure involves and seeks consent		
Cleans hands and wears gloves		
Enquires regarding presence of pain and offers analgesia if needed		
Checks and prepares equipment correctly		
Requests a chaperone		
Successfully removes condom using digital or speculum examination with appropriate technique		
Minimises patient anxiety and discomfort during examination		
Keeps conversation to a minimum while performing examination		
Maintains patient dignity throughout examination		
Discusses and offers emergency contraception		
Discusses risk of sexually transmitted infections and recommends follow-up in genitourinary medicine clinic		
Global mark from patient		
Global mark from examiner		

6.30 Fitting a cervical spine collar

The purpose of the collar is to protect the cervical spine (cervical spine) in cases where there is suspected or known injury. The collar is only truly effective if the correct size is used for the patient. It is a commonly used piece of equipment in the ED. Though it is often applied pre-hospital or by nursing staff when patients arrive, doctors must be capable of sizing and fitting a collar themselves.

Technique

There is significant variation in how to assemble/prepare different collars for use. Some which are packaged flat for convenience need to be assembled (very easily) and are made in specific sizes. With others the size of the collar can be adjusted to fit various individuals. Familiarity with what is available in a particular department is necessary, though it is normally quite intuitive to prepare any collar for use.

The principle of sizing a collar remains the same for most types. The measurement required is the distance from the patient's trapezium muscle to the beginning of the jaw line. For the sake of convenience this is commonly measured by using one's hand and counting the number of fingers between these landmarks (**Figure 6.30.1**).

The collar being used is then checked to confirm its vertical height on the side corresponds to this distance (**Figure 6.30.2**). Most collars have a marker where this distance is measured. Only the rigid part of the collar should be included in this measurement as additional foam padding may be present, but is purely for patient comfort and skin protection rather than immobilisation.

Until the correct collar is available and fitted in place the patient in question should have their cervical spine manually immobilised by someone able to do so. Once the correct size collar is identified this is slid under (or if the patient is sitting up placed behind) the patient's neck until the back portion of the collar is in the midline. It is then wrapped around the patient's neck and secured so it is firmly supporting their cervical spine (**Figure 6.30.3**). With the patient supine blocks and tape may then be applied before the person manually immobilising the cervical spine releases their hands (**Figure 6.30.4**).

If X-rays are to be performed it is best to try and remove earrings, jewellery and broken glass prior to applying the collar. This prevents artefact on the X-rays and also improves patient comfort.

Figure 6.30.1 Measuring for a cervical spine collar.

Figure 6.30.2 Checking correct collar size.

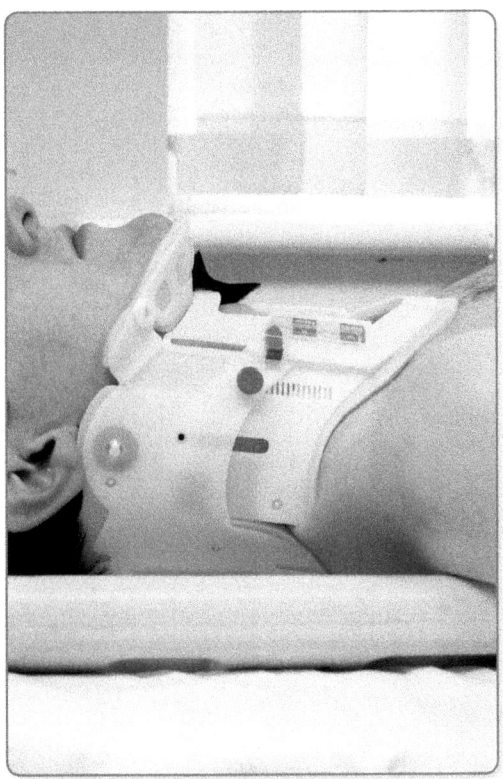

Figure 6.30.3 The collar once applied.

Figure 6.30.4 Triple immobilisation with collar, blocks and tape.

Scenario

There is a new doctor on placement in your ED. You ask him to apply a cervical spine collar to a patient and he tells you he does not know how to do it. You arrange to meet him later in the shift to teach him how to apply the collar.

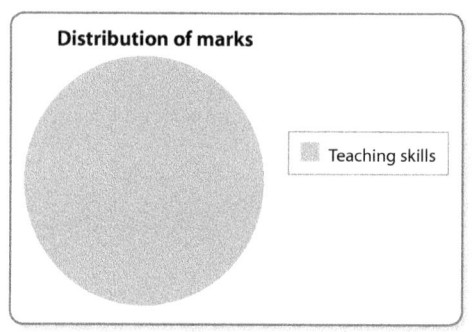

Distribution of marks

Teaching skills

Mark sheet	Achieved	Not achieved
Introduces self to doctor		
Enquires from doctor about previous experience and knowledge		
Asks him about anything specific he wants to learn		
Sets and agrees on appropriate learning objectives		
Explains rationale for use of a cervical spine collar		
Demonstrates the collar and important parts		
Demonstrates how to size the collar correctly		
Demonstrates applying and securing the collar		
Discusses the use of blocks and tape		
Discusses method of clearing a cervical spine briefly		
Allows doctor opportunity to repeat task		
Comments on and corrects doctor's technique where appropriate		
Checks if doctor has any questions or concerns		
Answers questions appropriately		
Agrees a plan for on-going learning		
Is non-judgemental and facilitates learning		
Global mark from examiner		
Global mark from doctor		

Instructions for actor

You are a junior doctor who qualified 3 years ago but have never worked in the ED or orthopaedics. You have never applied a cervical spine collar and were not sure how to measure or fit it. You watch the doctor demonstrate how to fit the collar and are keen to try for yourself. Initially you put it on too loose but amend this if the doctor corrects you. You have seen several different collars and ask what the main differences are. You also ask what to do if an immobilised patient feels sick or starts to vomit. Finally you ask whether hard collars are still needed as you've heard some places do not use them at all.

6.31 Head injury guidelines

You may be asked to demonstrate or teach information relating to a guideline or a scoring system. This may take you by surprise if you are expecting a practical teaching station rather than one based purely on teaching information. However, the teaching process is much the same and relies on basic teaching principles discussed in this chapter's introduction.

It may be stressful if you feel you cannot recall a guideline perfectly, but it will not be vital to remember every single fact in a guideline (e.g. every indication for a CT of the brain in the head injury guidelines). To gain maximum marks you should adhere to the same principles as for any other teaching station:
- Establish what the student already knows and what he/she wants to learn
- Set the objective of the teaching scenario based on the above
- Demonstrate the skill in stages (share/teach the information)
- Then ask the student to perform (repeat information), reinforcing learning
- Invite questions, clarify significant steps
- Plan for further learning and development to enhance the skill
- Point to other resources for self-learning, e.g. on-line modules or relevant papers or courses

In this OSCE, the teaching is based purely on discussion which may relate to a specific case in a scenario. There may be a whiteboard or paper provided to write some basic notes for the student which should be very brief and must not distract the student from interacting with the patient in the scenario. Remember to direct the student to sources of reference where he/she can review the material themselves.

The guidelines

The National Institute for Health and Care Excellence (NICE) clinical guideline 176 refers to patients with a head injury presenting to the ED. In addition to guidance on when to perform a CT of the brain in adults it considers several other areas:
- Pre-hospital assessment and management
- Initial management in the ED
- Indications for CT of the brain in adults and children
- Indications for cervical spine imaging in adults and children
- Ongoing care of patients with and without a significant injury

For adults the guidelines recommend a CT of the brain within 1 hour of the radiology department being informed in the case of:
- GCS <13 when first assessed in the ED
- GCS <15 when assessed in the ED 2 hours after the injury
- Suspected open or depressed skull fracture
- Signs of fracture at skull base (haemotympanum, 'panda' eyes, cerebrospinal fluid leakage from ears or nose, Battle's sign)
- Post-traumatic seizure
- Focal neurological signs
- >1 episode of vomiting
- Current warfarin treatment

In certain cases, the CT can be delayed until the following morning (or 8 hours from the time of injury) in the case of:
- Amnesia of events >30 minutes before impact (unless CT is required within 1 hour because of the presence of additional clinical findings from this list)

- Amnesia or loss of consciousness if coagulopathy (history of bleeding, clotting disorder)
- Any amnesia or loss of consciousness since the injury if age over 65 years (unless CT is required within 1 hour because of the presence of additional clinical findings from this list)
- Any amnesia or loss of consciousness since the injury if dangerous mechanism of injury (unless CT is required within 1 hour because of the presence of additional clinical findings from this list):
  - pedestrian or cyclist struck by a vehicle
  - occupant ejected from a vehicle
  - fall from >1 m or 5 stairs

For children, the guidelines recommend CT of the brain within 1 hour of the radiology department being informed in the case of:

- GCS <14 when first assessed in the ED (<15 if under 1 year of age)
- GCS <15 when assessed in the ED 2 hours after the injury
- Suspected open or depressed skull fracture or a tense fontanelle
- Signs of fracture at skull base (haemotympanum, 'panda' eyes, cerebrospinal fluid leakage from ears or nose, Battle's sign)
- Suspicion of non-accidental injury
- Post-traumatic seizure with no history of epilepsy
- Bruise, swelling or laceration >5 cm on the head
- Focal neurological signs

Additionally, for children the guidelines recommend a CT of the brain if more than one of the following risk factors are present:

- Loss of consciousness lasting more than 5 minutes (witnessed)
- Abnormal drowsiness
- Three or more discrete episodes of vomiting
- Dangerous mechanism of injury (high-speed road traffic accident either as pedestrian, cyclist or vehicle occupant, fall from a height of greater than 3 metres, high-speed injury from a projectile or other object)
- Amnesia (antegrade or retrograde) lasting more than 5 minutes

Children with only one of the risk factors should be observed for a minimum of 4 hours after the head injury, and a CT scan performed if any other risk factors develop.

Scenario

A new doctor in the ED has seen a 6-year-old boy with no medical history or medication who fell off a climbing frame and hit his head. He was unconscious for 'a few minutes' but is now recovered. He has a small graze to his forehead, but thorough examination has been normal. He does not have amnesia, has not vomited, there is no evidence of a seizure. The boy presents with his mother who witnessed the event. There are no concerns of non-accidental injury. The new doctor is unsure if a CT of the brain should be performed. Teach the indications for a CT of the brain and discuss a plan for this patient.

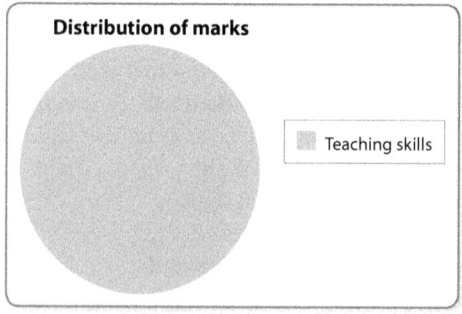
Distribution of marks — Teaching skills

Mark sheet	Achieved	Not achieved
Introduces self to junior doctor		
Enquires from junior doctor previous experience and knowledge		
Clarifies what they want wants to learn		
Sets and agrees on appropriate learning objectives		
Explains rationale and use of CT of the brain guidelines		
Explains guideline indications for a CT of the brain		
Explains other elements of the guidelines including criteria to image cervical spines		
Allows junior doctor opportunity to state their understanding		
Comments on and corrects junior doctor where appropriate		
Correctly states the patient does not need a CT scan		
Discusses plan for patient (explains safe discharge versus observation – either acceptable if justified)		
Checks if junior doctor has any questions or concerns		
Answers questions appropriately		
Agrees a plan for ongoing learning		
Is non-judgemental and facilitates learning		
Global mark from examiner		
Global mark from junior doctor		

Instructions for actor

You are a junior doctor who has been working in the ED for a few weeks but have only dealt with one or two patients with a head injury. With one of them you called the radiologist to arrange a CT of the brain, but the radiologist said they did not need one. Today after seeing a patient you have asked for some advice. You are not aware of the head injury guidelines but are grateful once they are explained to you.

If not explained to you already, ask where you can find the guidelines. Also ask what the signs of a base of skull fracture are.

If it has not been made clear, ask what you should do with your patient.

Suggested reading

National Institute for Health and Care Excellence (NICE). Head injury: assessment and early management. CG176. London: NICE; 2014.

6.32 Procedural sedation

Procedural sedation is the administration of sedatives and/or analgesics to allow the patient to tolerate painful procedures while independently maintaining cardiorespiratory function. The aim is to facilitate a short but unpleasant or painful procedure by achieving a reduced level of consciousness, while the patient maintains their airway and ventilatory control.

Indications
- Short-duration painful procedures in the emergency setting

Contraindications
- Procedures that need to be carried out in theatre
- Contraindicatory patient factors – high anaesthetic risk, predicted difficult airway
- Children less than 1 year of age
- Resource issues – inadequate staff, non-availability of adequate monitoring, unfamiliar drugs

Complications
- Deeper level of sedation than anticipated, possibly resulting in respiratory arrest
- Hypoxia and/or hypercarbia
- Hypotension can occur and is more likely in elderly patients or patients with existing haemodynamic compromise
- Airway obstruction due to secretions, loss of airway tone or laryngospasm
- Vomiting and aspiration
- Post-sedation emergence phenomenon which may occur with drugs such as ketamine
- Failure of the procedure
- Inadequate sedation

Common procedures needing sedation
Procedural sedation can be used to facilitate various procedures. Some of the most common are:
- Reduction of fractures (e.g. Colles' or mid-forearm) or dislocations (e.g. shoulder or ankle)
- Suturing of simple wounds in children
- Wound exploration and debridement
- Incision and drainage of superficial abscesses
- DC cardioversion

Pre-procedure checks
Clearly patient safety is vital during any sedation. The following checks are fundamental in ensuring any risks to the patient are minimised:
- Pre-anaesthetic assessment of the patient must include:

- Adequate medical and drug history, including allergies, anaesthetic history, any use of recreational drugs and alcohol consumption
  - Fasting status – though it may be worth enquiring regarding fasting status recent evidence shows the risk of aspiration is minimal
  - Airway assessment – does the patient have predictors of difficult airway or ventilation?
- Check that the necessary resources are available – 'staff, stuff, space'
  - 'Staff':
    - A second person to perform the procedure
    - A dedicated nurse to help with sedation
  - 'Stuff':
    - Appropriate choice of drugs
    - Working suction equipment and rescue airway devices
    - Monitoring equipment – non-invasive blood pressure cycling at 5-minute intervals, saturation probe, ECG monitor and end-tidal CO_2 monitoring
    - Choice of oxygen delivery – face mask or nasal prongs
    - Oro- or nasopharyngeal airway adjuncts appropriately sized
    - Self-inflating resuscitator bag (e.g. Ambu bag) with an appropriate-sized face mask, connected to oxygen
    - Adequately stocked adult or paediatric airway trolley
    - Reversal agents, in particular naloxone if opioid sedation is being used
  - 'Space':
    - Available resuscitation bay
- The patient should be prepared appropriately by ensuring:
  - The patient's body weight has been checked and recorded
  - Consent has been obtained and documented
  - Intravenous access has been set up with intravenous fluids connected if required
  - The patient is connected to the required monitoring and at least one set of observations have already been recorded

Commonly used sedative drugs

A degree of familiarity is required with the use of all these sedative agents. Choice of drug varies depending on various factors, including the medical practitioner's experience/skill set, the patient's comorbidities and departmental staffing. Individual departments often have their own guidance for drug selection and use based on their own local governance frameworks. Often the starting dose is lowered for elderly patients and then, if there is an inadequate response, smaller additional increments are given until the desired effect is achieved.

Propofol

One percent propofol is very commonly used. It provides adequate sedation, has predictable onset time and a short duration of action. However, it suppresses respiration and can cause significant hypotension, especially in elderly patients. It has no analgesic properties and is often used in conjunction with a short-acting opiate such as fentanyl. In a healthy adult patient, a starting dose is 1 mg/kg. In elderly patients this is often reduced to 0.25 mg/kg.

Fentanyl

This is a synthetic opioid that has a rapid onset and a short duration of action. It should be given 2–3 minutes before the sedative agent. It usually has some sedative properties in addition to being a potent analgesic. The usual dose is 10 μg/kg. This should be given slowly as it may otherwise cause chest wall rigidity. It is used in conjunction with a sedative such as propofol or midazolam.

Ketamine

This acts as an antagonist at N-methyl-D-aspartate (NDMA) receptors and produces a dissociative state. It is a potent sedative and analgesic, maintains airway reflexes and is very haemodynamically stable. It does increase airway secretion; however, there is no evidence that it increases the incidence of laryngospasm. It is associated with emergence phenomenon whereby patients may experience visual hallucinations. This is more common in adults and is never seen in children. It may be administered by the intramuscular or intravenous route. The benefit of intravenous use is that it is more predictable in onset, can be repeated and has a shorter duration of action. The usual intravenous starting dose is 0.75–1 mg/kg of 1% ketamine.

Midazolam

This is a short-acting benzodiazepine that has a rapid onset of action. It has strong anxiolytic, sedative and amnesic properties. However, it has an unreliable onset of action, and at doses needed to produce adequate sedation it may cause significant respiratory depression. It can also produce paradoxical excitation in children and elderly. The usual dose is 0.05–0.1 mg/kg of a 1 mg/mL dilution. A low dose is often given during ketamine sedation as this may assist in preventing/treating emergence phenomenon.

Ketofol

This is a combination of ketamine and propofol in a 1:1 ratio. It is usually prepared by mixing 10 mL each of 1% propofol and 1% ketamine in a 20 mL syringe. The dose is 1 mL/kg which delivers half of each of propofol and ketamine. Theoretically this minimises the side-effect profile of both drugs and provides good sedation and analgesia.

Depth of sedation

The American Society of Anesthesiologists (ASA) classification of the depth of sedation is described below. In most patients, the aim of procedural sedation is to achieve moderate sedation, or conscious sedation as described here:
- Minimal sedation (anxiolysis) – normal response to verbal stimulus, impaired cognitive function
- Moderate sedation/analgesia (conscious sedation) depression of consciousness, purposeful response to verbal stimulus, maintains airway and ventilatory control
- Deep sedation/analgesia – depression of consciousness, purposeful response to repeated or painful stimulus, may lose airway and ventilatory control
- General anaesthesia – depression of consciousness with no arousal to repeated painful stimulus, loss of airway control and ventilatory function, may need circulatory support

Post-sedation

After sedation the patient should be monitored in the procedure area until their vital signs have normalised, they have recovered a normal level of consciousness, have a normal response to verbal stimulus and normal reflexes with no significant adverse symptoms.

Patients should be discharged with an appropriate advice leaflet and, depending on the circumstances, in the care of another adult.

Scenario

John Ibrahim is a 14-year-old boy. He fell while kicking a football. He has a deformed ankle which needs reduction and plaster (**Figure 6.32.1**). You have been asked to teach a junior doctor how to perform conscious sedation to facilitate this procedure. Talk through how to prepare for and administer conscious sedation.

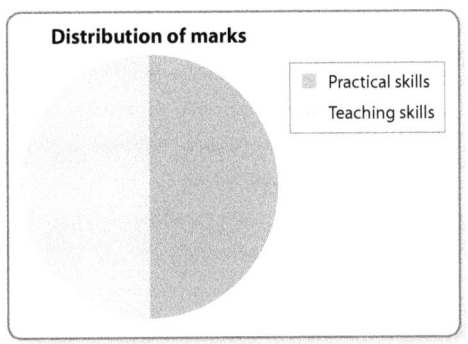

Mark sheet	Achieved	Not achieved
Introduces self to the junior doctor		
Enquires from junior doctor about previous experience		
Asks them about anything specific they want to learn		
Sets and agrees on appropriate learning objectives		
Discusses the following:		
– administration of appropriate analgesia		
– checks limb – confirms dislocation		
– checks limb – confirms neurovascular status		
– checks limb – X-ray confirming dislocation		
– procedural sedation – discusses need for		
– procedural sedation – discusses benefit of		
– procedural sedation – discusses risk of		
– procedural sedation – need to gain consent		
– patient assessment – last meal time		
– patient assessment – medical history		
– patient assessment – medications		
– patient assessment – allergies		
– patient assessment – weight		
– patient assessment – airway assessment		
– resources – adequate number of staff		
– resources – drug choice		

Cont'd...

Cont'd...

Mark sheet	Achieved	Not achieved
– resources – airway trolley		
– resources – suction		
– resources – monitoring (BP, ECG monitoring, pulse oximetry, end-tidal CO_2)		
– resources – oxygen delivery – mask and Ambu bag		
– resources – resus room		
– pre-procedure check – one set of observations		
– pre-procedure check – running IV line and fluids		
– sedation – appropriate dose of sedative agent chosen		
– sedation – discusses end point of conscious sedation		
– sedation – performance of ankle reduction		
– sedation – post sedation advice		
Checks if junior doctor has any questions or concerns		
Answers questions appropriately		
Is non-judgemental and facilitates learning		
Agrees a plan for on-going learning		
Global marks from junior doctor		
Global marks from examiner		

Figure 6.32.1 Mr Ibrahim's ankle.

Suggested reading

Safe Sedation of Adults in the Emergency Department. London: Royal College of Anaesthetists and Royal College of Emergency Medicine, 2012.

Royal College of Emergency Medicine (RCEM). Best practice guideline: pharmacological agents for procedural sedation and analgesia in the emergency department. London: RCEM; 2016.

Royal College of Emergency Medicine (RCEM). Guideline for ketamine sedation of children in the emergency department. London: RCEM; 2009.

National Institute of Health and Care Excellence (NICE). Sedation in Children and Young People. CG112. London: NICE; 2010.

6.33 Slit lamp examination

In addition to a systematic eye examination and fundoscopy, the ability to do a basic slit lamp examination is also a requirement of the College's curriculum. A slit lamp combines a low-power microscope with a high-intensity light that is shaped as a narrow slit, illuminating only a narrow 'slice' of the eye at any one time.

A slit lamp examination is essential for any eye examination, especially for assessing the anterior structures of the eye. Most patients with corneal foreign bodies, suspected eye injuries, corneal abrasions or loss of vision will need to be assessed using a slit lamp.

Candidates should familiarise themselves with the equipment at their places of work to ensure familiarity with the equipment controls and thus ensure smooth examination technique.

Technique

In addition to a working slit lamp, you will also need:
- A cotton bud
- Fluorescein drops or strips
- Local anaesthetic eye drops

The steps in using a slit lamp are:
1. Position yourself on the seat and adjust it to a comfortable height and sitting posture
2. Set the binoculars at the correct inter-pupillary distance for you
3. Set the eyepieces at the correct diopter – start with 0 on both eyes
4. Turn the light on at the lowest voltage
5. Set the light filter to neutral; this reduces glare
6. Start with the light and the binoculars in the same axis. Change to an angled beam (by moving the light across) when examining transparent media such as the cornea, anterior chamber and lens
7. Seat the patient on their side of the slit lamp
8. Place the patient's chin on the chinrest and adjust the chinrest height so that the black mark is aligned with the lateral canthus. The patient's forehead should be forward against the bar (**Figure 6.33.1**).
9. The patient can stabilise themselves by holding on to the side handles
10. Adjust the width, height and angle of light beam, to obtain a slit on the eye
11. Move the microscope forward with the joystick and bring the cornea into focus
12. Systematically examine the following areas of the eye:
    a. External eye – look around the eye (cheek, nose, brow)
    b. Lid margin, eye lashes
    c. Inside the lower eye lid – evert it using a cotton bud
    d. Conjunctiva and sclera
    e. Cornea – look for surface irregularities and foreign bodies (use a long narrow beam of light) (**Figure 6.33.2a**)
    f. Anterior chamber – use an angled beam and make the slit short and wide (**Figure 6.33.2b**)
    g. Iris and pupil
    h. Lens – use an angled beam and make the slit short and wide
    i. Examine the cornea with blue filtered light using fluorescein
    j. Continue to the Seidel test for corneal perforation: fluid escaping from a corneal perforation washes away the fluorescein stain on the cornea
        1. Repeat all these steps for the other eye
        2. Finish the examination and summarise your findings

Practical skills and teaching

Figure 6.33.1 Patient positioning (A) for the slit lamp examination; the basic controls are for changing the width of the beam (B), the magnification (C), the filter (D) and the length of the beam (E).

Figure 6.33.2 Slit lamp examination. (a) Narrow beam and (b) Wide beam illumination.

Scenario

Simon is a final-year medical student who is observing in the minors area of the ED. Teach him how to use the slit lamp on the model provided.

Distribution of marks
- Teaching skills
- Examination skills

Slit lamp examination 6.33

Mark sheet	Achieved	Not achieved
Introduces self to the medical student		
Enquires from medical student about previous experience and knowledge		
Asks about anything specific they want to learn		
Sets and agrees on appropriate learning objectives		
Explains rationale for using slit lamp		
Demonstrates controls on slit lamp – power, voltage, binoculars, slit and light controls		
Demonstrates how to position self		
Demonstrates how to position patient correctly		
Instils local anaesthetic eye drops		
Demonstrates examination systematically:		
– external eye (peri-ocular structures)		
– lids, lashes – everts lower eye lid		
– conjunctiva and sclera		
– cornea		
– anterior chamber		
– pupil and iris		
– lens		
Uses fluorescein staining to examine cornea		
Allows medical student to perform examination		
Comments on and corrects technique where appropriate		
Checks if medical student has any questions or concerns		
Answers questions appropriately		
Agrees a plan for ongoing learning		
Is non-judgemental and facilitates learning		
Discusses appropriate management for corneal abrasion		
Global mark from examiner		
Global mark from medical student		

Instructions for actor

You are a keen final year medical student. You have spent a few days in the ED and want to learn about slit lamp examination. You have seen a junior doctor use it for removal of a foreign body. You don't know how to operate it. You are not sure how to control the light and magnification and would like to do it yourself once shown.

6.34 Wound assessment and suturing

Management of traumatic wounds is an essential emergency skill. It frequently presents as an OSCE. Candidates are expected to safely assess the wound, determine the tetanus risk, discuss follow-up plans and demonstrate good suturing technique. Clearly there is a lot to cover in the short period of time and it is easy to run out of time. All elements of this station must be well practised and familiar so that it is possible to complete all the necessary discussion while simultaneously performing the suturing. Practising beforehand will ensure that a few sutures can be demonstrated with a no-touch technique in a competent fashion.

Factors to consider

Time since injury and mechanism

This information may be provided in any given scenario. Usually wounds sustained within 8–10 hours can be closed primarily. If they are on the lower limbs, extensively contaminated or contain a lot of crushed or necrotic tissue the time-window for wound closure should be shortened according to the circumstances. Conversely, for wounds on the face the time window may be extended.

Wound characteristics

Information regarding the nature of a wound may be provided.

A clean wound with no crushed or degloved tissue and no underlying (neurovascular, tendon, bone or joint) damage is suitable for primary closure. If this information is not provided, you need to demonstrate that you have assessed for these complications.

Depth of wound – which layers are involved? Can you see the base of the wound clearly?

Suspected foreign bodies – a common scenario is the patient who has cut their hand on glass. Consider an X-ray for retained glass before suturing.

Site – while a laceration over a joint is likely to need suturing (due to continuous movement) a pretibial laceration is managed by Steri-Strips or tissue glue (there is high incidence of skin necrosis if this friable tissue is sutured).

Tetanus risk (also see section 2.11) – for tetanus risk, wounds are classified as described in **Table 6.34.1**.

Patient characteristics

From the patient it is important to identify both their:
1. **Past medical history:** systemic disease (e.g. diabetes mellitus or chronic renal failure), immunosuppressive medications, steroids, intravenous drug abuse and old age may result in increased risk of infection and wound breakdown
2. **Tetanus immunisation status:** universal tetanus immunisation was started in 1961 in the UK. Before this it was only available to armed forces personnel. Therefore, some patients born before this date have not received any tetanus immunisation. Patients are classified into one of three groups as shown in **Table 6.34.2**.

Table 6.34.1 Classification of wounds: tetanus risk

Clean wound	Tetanus-prone wound	High-risk wound
No tetanus-prone or high-risk features	Puncture-type injuries acquired in a contaminated environment and likely therefore to contain tetanus spores, e.g. gardening injuries Wounds containing foreign bodies such as wound splinters Open fractures Wounds/burns with systemic sepsis Certain animal bites and scratches	Heavy contamination with material likely to contain tetanus spores, e.g. soil, manure Wounds/burns that show extensive devitalised tissue Wounds/burns that require surgical intervention that is delayed for >6 hours

Decision on immunisation and immunoglobulin

The decision as to whether to administer a tetanus vaccine or tetanus immunoglobulin is based on consideration of both the tetanus risk of the wound and the tetanus immunisation status of the patient, as shown in **Table 6.34.2**.

Table 6.34.2 Indications for tetanus immunisation and prophylaxis after injury

	Clean wound	Tetanus prone wound	High-risk wound
Aged 11 years and over, who have received an adequate priming course of tetanus vaccine (3 doses) with the last dose within 10 years OR Aged 5–10 years who have received priming course and pre-school booster OR Aged under 5 years who have received an adequate priming course	No treatment	No treatment	No treatment
Received adequate priming course of tetanus vaccine but last dose <10 years ago OR Children aged 5–10 years who have received an adequate priming course but no pre-school booster (Including UK born after 1961 with history of accepting vaccinations)	No treatment (unless next dose of vaccine due and convenient to administer)	Immediate reinforcing dose of vaccine	Immediate reinforcing dose of vaccine And One dose of human tetanus immunoglobulin at a different site
Not received adequate priming course of tetanus vaccine (including uncertain immunisation status and/or born before 1961)	Immediate reinforcing dose of vaccine	Immediate reinforcing dose of vaccine And One dose of human tetanus immunoglobulin at a different site	Immediate reinforcing dose of vaccine And One dose of human tetanus immunoglobulin at a different site

The recommended dose of intramuscular TIG is: 250 (IU) for most uses or 500 IU if >24 hours have elapsed or there is risk of heavy contamination or following burns. The dose is the same for both adults and children.

Pre-procedure check

Ensure the following equipment is available:
- Clean trolley to place equipment on
- Sterile suturing kit with toothed and plain forceps, needle holder and scissors
- Appropriate suture
- Local anaesthetic, syringe and needle for infiltration
- Saline, 20 mL syringe and blunt needle for irrigation
- Sterile gloves
- Dressing set – with drape and gauze
- Cleaning solution – povidone–iodine (Betadine) or chlorhexidine for cleaning the skin
- Dressing to cover the wound

Technique

- Local anaesthetic – lignocaine 1% in a maximum dose of 3 mg/kg or lignocaine with adrenaline (maximum 7 mg/kg) are most commonly used. Don't use adrenaline on digits or peripheries
- Wound irrigation, debridement and exploration – normal saline is the most commonly used fluid for wound irrigation. It is recommended that iodine or other agents are not used, because they interfere with wound healing. Ensure removal of all foreign material from the wound. Confirm the depth of the wound
- Haemostasis – oozing of blood from lacerated wound margins should stop once the wound is sutured. Veins may need to be ligated. Significant arterial bleeding may need operative intervention
- Standard aseptic non-touch technique must be used – ensure that the wound does not come in contact with any item that is not sterile. The principle is that the key site (the wound) should come into contact only with the key part (the needle tip, sterile gloves, tip of forceps, etc.). Maintain an aseptic field around the wound and keep sterile equipment and dressings within this area
- Suturing – interrupted suture placement using non-absorbable sutures is the most commonly used technique. Vary the suture size and removal time according to the site of injury (**Table 6.34.3**). A full description of suturing technique is outside the scope of this book, and candidates should ensure they are well acquainted with the technique before the exam. Examples are shown in **Figures 6.34.1** and **6.34.2**. Often the wound provided in the exam is a V shape and candidates are expected to demonstrate a technique that distributes the tension evenly.
- Dressing – apply a suitably sized sterile dressing

Post-procedure steps

It is best practice to provide post-procedure advice for the patient in writing. Include the following topics: when and where to get sutures removed, avoiding getting the wound wet for the first 48 hours and the need to seek further attention if developing any signs of infection. Provide some spare dressings. Prescribe antibiotics if the wound is contaminated or the patient is in a high-risk group. Give advice regarding analgesia and signs suggestive of infection.

Table 6.34.4 Suture site, size and time of removal

Site	Suture size	Remove by
Face	6/0	5 days
Scalp	3/0 – 4/0	7–10 days
Upper limb, proximal lower limbs	4/0 – 5/0 (hands)	8–10 days
Foot	3/0 (sole) to 5/0 (dorsum)	10–14 days
Back, abdomen, chest	3/0 – 4/0	8–12 days

  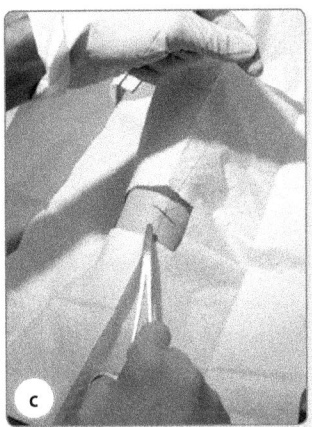

Figure 6.34.1 Suturing. (a) Orient yourself parallel to the wound. (b) Placement of needle holder for tying a knot. (c) Final knot position.

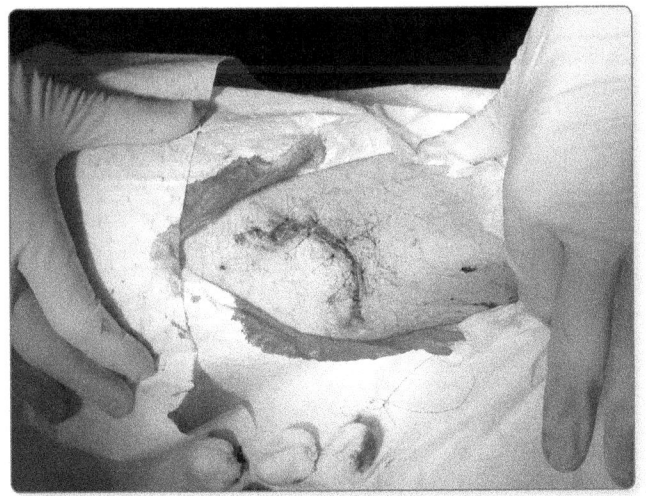

Figure 6.34.2 Sutured wound.

Scenario

A 24-year-old patient, Mr Richard Sangahan, sustained a forearm laceration when he fell and pushed his arm through a window at home. He did not sustain any other injury, is usually healthy and is well. He does not have any distal neurovascular injury and all tendons are normal on examination. The wound has been assessed and needs to be sutured because it is gaping. Suture the wound appropriately and provide any further management and advice as required.

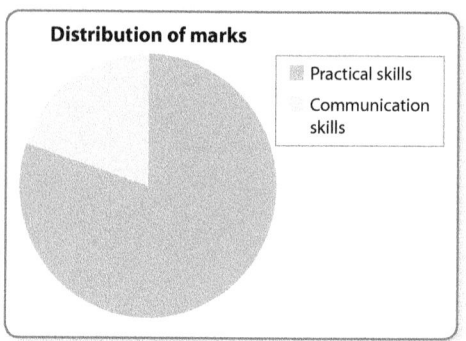

Distribution of marks
- Practical skills
- Communication skills

Mark sheet	Achieved	Not achieved
Introduces self to the patient		
Confirms patient identity		
Enquires regarding presence of pain and offers analgesia		
Explains need to suture the wound		
Obtains patient consent		
Prepares and checks equipment		
Cleans hands and applies sterile gloves		
Cleans skin with cleaning solution		
Establishes a sterile field using sterile drape		
Injects local anaesthetic appropriately		
States correct dose of anaesthetic		
Explores the wound and confirms depth		
Irrigates the wound with saline – appropriate volume		
Checks for any foreign bodies		
Appropriate technique – interrupted sutures		
Places appropriate number of sutures		
Avoids tension on skin, overlapping of skin edges		
Ensures skin edges evert		
Leaves adequate length of suture for easy removal		
Maintains non-touch technique		
Applies dressing		
Disposes of equipment/sharps appropriately		
Advises against tetanus immunisation		
Post procedure advice – no antibiotics		
Global mark from examiner		
Global mark from patient		

Instructions for actor

Your name is Richard Sangahan. You were walking through your home, when you slipped and fell. Your arm went through a window causing a wound to your forearm. You applied a towel as a bandage and came to the hospital. You are able to move the fingers well and have normal sensation in your hand. The window margin was clean and painted. You are healthy and well, don't take any medications, are right handed and have had all your immunisations as far as you know. You are worried that the wound may get infected and would like to get the wound stitched and ask for some antibiotics. If the doctor explains their plan clearly you are satisfied with whatever they suggest.

Suggested reading

Cole E. Wound management in the A&E department. Nursing Standard 2003; 17:45–52.
DeBoard RH, Rondeau DF, Kang CS, Sabbaj A, McManus JG. Principles of basic wound evaluation and management in the emergency department. Emerg Med Clin North Am 2007; 25:23–39.
Salisbury D, Ramsay M. Chapter 30: Tetanus. Immunisation against infectious disease ['The Green Book']. London: Public Health England, 2018.

Chapter 7

Adult acute presentations

- 7.1 Introduction
- 7.2 Basic life support
- 7.3 Advanced life support: non-shockable rhythms
- 7.4 Advanced life support: shockable rhythms
- 7.5 Advanced life support: special circumstances
- 7.6 Bradyarrhythmias
- 7.7 Tachyarrhythmias
- 7.8 Adult anaphylaxis
- 7.9 Stopping resuscitation efforts
- 7.10 Preeclampsia
- 7.11 Delivering a baby
- 7.12 Upper gastrointestinal bleed with massive haemorrhage

7.1 Introduction

The examination normally contains two resuscitation style objectively structured clinical examinations (OSCEs). These are usually double stations, which are allocated twice the time of other stations. As a result, being unsuccessful in these OSCEs would mean failing two stations at once. Unless stated in the text all remaining scenarios in this book are the length of two OSCE scenarios. These OSCEs are similar, though more challenging, to the test scenarios at the end of standard life support provider courses that all candidates will be familiar with. Therefore, with thorough preparation it should be possible to pass these OSCEs easily. As well as reading this introduction candidates are encouraged to read and reflect on the discussion of non-technical skills in the introduction to this book.

Applying an ABCDE style approach to assessing these cases is recommended. In basic terms the approach is the same as in other stations, i.e. preparation, running the scenario using an ABCDE assessment style and then closure.

Preparation

Often the OSCE will begin with a pre-alert that a patient who is unwell is due to arrive in the ED by ambulance, allowing the candidate time to prepare. On occasion, however, the scenario may involve assessing and managing a patient who is already in the ED. In any of these circumstances, a degree of logical preparation or at least a mental tick box exercise is useful. To run a successful resuscitation scenario the candidate should consider the following:

1. **People**
   In the scenario anticipate what tasks will need to be performed. What are the skills of the staff present and what other skills and staff will (or may) be needed?
   Introduce yourself, know your team's names, ask them what their level of competence is and assign specific tasks that they are able to perform. For example, if you have a student nurse with you, it is appropriate to ask her to start chest compressions while you take charge of the airway. On the other hand, if there is another doctor with airway skills, they can take care of the airway and you can perform other tasks. Or indeed if there are multiple staff present can you be team leader and take a hands-off approach? State your thoughts and your plan out loud. It provides clarity for your team as to what is expected. Think ahead to anticipate further help from other people in the department, i.e. senior ED staff, or critical care, paediatrics, paediatric intensive care or obstetrics and neonatology for a pregnant woman in cardiac arrest. Always call for help early.

2. **Monitoring**
   Check your equipment (monitor, oxygen saturation probe, non-invasive blood pressure, capnography and defibrillator). It is also appropriate to ask if there is someone competent to use the defibrillator. If this task is going to fall to you it may be helpful to have a quick look at the machine to ensure familiarity with its controls.

3. **Equipment**
   Personal protective equipment:
   - Do not forget to clean hands and wear gloves and aprons as appropriate
   - Ask additional staff to do the same

   Airway:
   - Oxygen – (so basic it is easy to forget)

- Working suction
- Airway trolley with airway adjuncts and equipment for intubation

Breathing:
- Self-inflating Ambu bag with reservoir bag, connected to oxygen

Circulation:
- Defibrillator, pads and connections
- Intravenous access, intraosseous access
- Portable ultrasound – who will do the echo?

Disability:
- Temperature probe
- Warm fluid in the case of hypothermic patients (or cooled after a ventricular fibrillation arrest)

4. **Drugs**
   - Resuscitation drugs
   - Scenario specific drugs, e.g. antidotes, antiarrhythmics
   - Rapid sequence induction drugs

   Specific drugs and equipment for the situation, e.g. chest drain kit or blood to transfuse in the case of haemorrhage.

Running the scenario

This is the main part of the station. The tasks that the candidate is required to perform can be broken down into various domains and careful attention to each of these domains will help to run a successful scenario.

1. **Medical tasks**
   - Assessment of the patient and initiation of management in a logical manner (ABCDE assessment)
   - It allows for a simple, stepwise and methodical approach which should prevent clinical findings and interventions getting missed or overlooked. In reality many tasks can be, and often are, performed simultaneously and candidates should use their experience and judgement to balance a linear ABCDE approach with a team-based simultaneous activity approach. Largely the higher the number of team members present and the higher their skill level the more activity can be delegated to happen at the same time
   - Demonstration of the knowledge of the resuscitation protocols. You should know relevant algorithms and the drugs to be used at prescribed time intervals
   - Knowledge of key diagnostic tests and when they are required (blood gas, blood sugar, X-ray, ECG and echocardiogram)

2. **Communication**
   - Think ahead and communicate with the team at crucial stages. This starts in the preparation stage and continues in the scenario. Inform them about important decisions
   - Gather information about the patient from paramedics, other medical and nursing staff, family members, patient letters or general practitioner letters
   - Family – if the family member is present in the station, then assigning one team member to the family is good practice. Empathise and explain to the family what is going on

3. **Control of the situation/leadership**
   - If staffing allows and your role is team leader stand back and take an overview of the situation
   - Provide clear and confident instructions
   - If unsure of a management step do not hesitate to discuss with the team and take decisions together. This happens in real life
   - Think ahead and inform the team of the next steps
   - Ensuring overall care – appropriate chest compressions, ratio of ventilation and compression, safe defibrillation, sharps and infection control precautions
4. **Decision making**
   - Critical decisions at each step will require experience and knowledge, e.g. airway management and which algorithm to follow, drug decisions and interpretation of investigations
   - The four Hs and Ts relating to reversible causes and the relevant interventions for each are basic and vital knowledge (see section 7.3). Remember to consider these during scenarios
   - If there is any uncertainty do not be afraid to ask your team members for help and advice, e.g. If you cannot remember the fourth reversible T or feel something has been missed

Closure

On-going care:
- Clearly state what needs to happen to the patient next. In cardiac arrest if there is successful return of spontaneous circulation (ROSC), then initiating post cardiac arrest care and a handover to critical care colleagues is important. If an ECG shows a ST elevation myocardial infarction the patient will probably need the catheter lab
- Communicate with the family about ongoing care and further management
- Thank the team

Keep an open mind

For the purpose of clarity many of the acute presentations that may arise are discussed individually in the following scenarios. You must be familiar with all the relevant algorithms, be able to change from one algorithm to another unexpectedly and be able to perform the necessary interventions. As in real life, one can never know what to expect and must not be put off if faced with something that indeed wasn't expected.

A 'resuscitation' OSCE may not involve a cardiac arrest but may instead require management of an arrhythmia. A patient in one of these scenarios may be pregnant, or hypothermic. A patient with an arrhythmia may have taken an overdose which also needs managing. Rather than achieving return of spontaneous circulation the correct management may be to agree CPR is futile and decide to stop. There may be challenging personalities or unexpected distractions.

There is no substitute for knowledge of the treatment guidelines but in addition to this a calm and logical approach is vital. Always begin with the basics of an ABCDE assessment and return to this when interventions are made or circumstances change. When there is time always consider reversible causes that need to be addressed. The approach of thinking things through one step at a time will allow for logical thought, clarity, clear communication, good leadership and successful outcomes.

Alternative scenarios

At the end of each of the following extended resuscitation stations, we have included one or more alternative scenarios. These contain a brief summary of an alternative presentation and may contain guidance on what interventions will be required. This is to encourage candidates to consider the variety of scenarios they may be faced with and prepare for them.

Candidates should expand on this further and think of challenging scenarios that could appear in the examination. Having done so it is important to rehearse how each of those scenarios should be dealt with. The more alternatives that are practiced, the less chance there is of being confronted with a case the candidate feels unprepared for.

Suggested reading

Advanced Life Support, 7th edn. Resuscitation Council (UK), 2015.

7.2 Basic life support

This station is normally structured so the candidate must manage a collapsed patient. This is likely to proceed on the lines of in-hospital resuscitation and what to do as a first responder when assessing a patient. It is important to know the algorithms, be able to demonstrate each stage and be able to explain the purpose of each intervention.

A basic life support OSCE could also be teaching based, requiring a candidate to teach a medical student or a nurse how to perform basic life support (BLS). In a teaching OSCE, pay particular attention to observing and where necessary correcting the student's technique for airway manoeuvres, ventilation and chest compressions.

Sequence for managing a collapsed patient in hospital

1. Ensure it is safe to approach. Wear personal protective equipment and check infection control precautions have been taken. If teaching on a manikin, ensure it has been cleaned between trainees
2. Call for help and assess the patient. It is important as an early responder, to ensure that help is on its way. Assess the patient by a gentle but firm shake of the shoulders and loudly asking 'Are you all right?'
3. From here further management will depend on whether there is a response from the patient or not:
   - If there is a response continue with an ABCDE assessment with appropriate interventions. Attach oxygen, blood pressure monitoring, pulse oximetry, 12-lead ECG and gain intravenous access
   - If there is no response then call for help if not already done. Turn the patient onto their back, open the airway using head-tilt, chin-lift or jaw thrust manoeuvres and look for signs of life for a maximum of 10 seconds. You are looking for chest movement, or movement of air to confirm breathing and the presence of a central pulse which is most conveniently palpated at the carotids. This can be done by keeping the airway open, placing the responder's cheek next to patient's mouth, looking tangentially down the chest and feeling for a pulse with the other hand. Agonal or occasional breathing should not be considered a sign of life
4. If there is no sign of life, start cardiopulmonary resuscitation, with chest compressions at a rate of 100–120 per minute and ventilations in a ratio of 30:2 (for every 30 chest compressions, give two ventilation breaths)
   - The correct hand position for chest compressions is in the middle of the lower half of the sternum. Compress to at least 5–6 cm and allow the chest to recoil in between compressions
   - Use airway manoeuvres and adjuncts to keep the airway patent and deliver ventilation with a self-inflating bag valve device connected to an oxygen supply. Ensure a proper seal of the facemask. Ventilate with an inspiratory time over 1 second and ensure the chest is rising
5. In cardiac arrest the priority is to identify whether there is a shockable or non-shockable rhythm. Therefore, connect the patient to a defibrillator as soon as possible. This should be followed by advanced life support as soon as possible.

Scenario (single station length)

Teach a student nurse how to manage a patient who collapses in hospital. Answer any questions they may have.

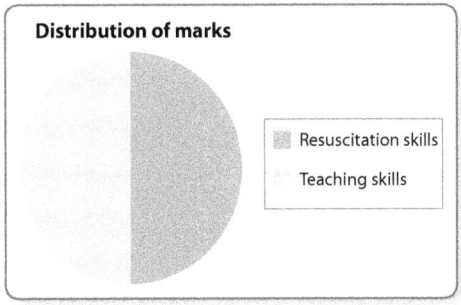

Guidance on scenario

When the student performs the task there will be some technical errors in their BLS technique. The candidate is expected not only to teach the process adequately but also to correct the student's technique.

Mark sheet	Achieved	Not achieved
Introduces self to the student and confirms identity		
Checks student's knowledge about life support, attendance at clinical scenarios		
Enquires about anything specific they want to learn		
Sets objective to learn the drill of BLS, in hospital collapsed patient		
Demonstrates the scenario in logical stages:		
– safe to approach		
– personal protective equipment and infection control precautions as appropriate		
– shouts for help		
– checks for response		
– opens airway using appropriate manoeuvre – head tilt-chin lift or jaw thrust		
– correctly checks for signs of life for maximum 10 seconds – confirms cardiac arrest		
– calls cardiac arrest team if not already done so		
– starts basic life support appropriately		
– correct technique for compressions (hand placement, frequency and depth of chest)		
– demonstrates ventilation with mask or self-inflating bag		
– correct chest compressions to ventilation ratio		
– explains need for further early defibrillation and advanced life support (ALS) management as appropriate		
Asks student to repeat the drill		
Corrects technique to manage airway and chest compressions		
Reinforces important steps		
Invites questions		

Cont'd...

Cont'd...

Mark sheet	Achieved	Not achieved
Directs the student to consolidate learning (on-line modules, resuscitation training, and visits to ED etc.)		
Plans future assessment and review		
Is non-judgmental and facilitates learning		
Global score from student		
Global score from examiner		

Alternative scenario

Teaching advanced life support: the candidate may be asked to teach the advanced life support algorithm and safe defibrillation technique.

7.3 Advanced life support: non-shockable rhythms

Pulseless electrical activity (PEA) and asystole are the two non-shockable rhythms. While both PEA and asystole have extremely poor outcomes unless a reversible cause can be found, PEA can be a very low output state where a pulse is not palpable and therefore it is more important to identify any reversible cause.

After confirming cardiac arrest, the priority is to start cardiopulmonary resuscitation. The next priority is to connect a defibrillator correctly to analyse the underlying rhythm. Further interventions are guided by whether there is a shockable rhythm or not. PEA is represented by organised electrical activity without any palpable cardiac output whereas asystole is no discernible cardiac electrical activity at all.

In an OSCE you will be expected to know the ALS algorithms and have a thorough understanding of their advanced management. As team leader it is useful to think out loud so the team are aware of your analysis of the rhythm, assessment of the patient and plan of management. This ensures clear communication and enhances team work. You are expected to follow the relevant algorithm, ensure each intervention (including chest compressions) is performed effectively, gather information from required investigations and make decisions.

Address reversible causes while resuscitation is ongoing, again it is good practice to talk these through out loud. Do not just list them but also explain why they are not relevant or if they are relevant how they are being addressed. The main consideration is which of these could be a causative factor and how can it be excluded or treated? Continue with cardiopulmonary resuscitation while all reversible causes are either dealt with or excluded.

Reversible causes

Four Hs:
- Hypoxia
- Hypovolemia
- Hypothermia
- Hypo-/hyperkalaemia, hypoglycaemia, hypercalcaemia and metabolic causes

Four Ts:
- Tension pneumothorax
- Tamponade
- Thrombosis – coronary (myocardial infarction), pulmonary (pulmonary embolism)
- Toxins

Where appropriate perform echocardiography for up to 10 seconds while a pulse check is being done. This is particularly useful in the case of PEA and will also exclude cardiac tamponade as a reversible cause.

Continue with cardiopulmonary resuscitation while all reversible causes are either dealt with or excluded.

Scenario

You are called to the resuscitation room. You are told that a 38-year-old man was just discharged by an ED locum doctor who had diagnosed a chest infection. He had originally come to the ED with dizziness but collapsed in the car park while leaving. Paramedics are bringing him back now. The doctor left to handover to a colleague and there are no notes written. You have a staff nurse and a student nurse present.

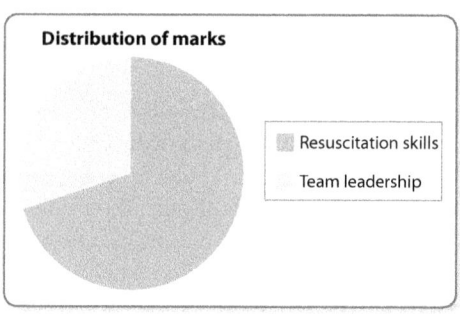

Distribution of marks
- Resuscitation skills
- Team leadership

Initial patient observations

(As the patient is assessed during the scenario these observations will be provided by the nurse)

Airway	Own airway
Breathing	Respiratory rate 50 breaths per minute. Shallow poor respiratory effort Bilateral breath sounds. Oxygen saturations 68% on air
Circulation	Weak 'thready' palpable pulse. Heart rate 160 beats per minute
Disability	GCS E2, V2, M5
Exposure	Grey, clammy, temperature 37°C

Blood gas results will be provided to the candidate by a member of staff if the candidate asks for the test to be performed.

pH	7.03
pCO_2	5.2 kPa
pO_2	6.3 kPa
Na^+	138 mmol/L
K^+	4.8 mmol/L
Cl^-	102 mmol/L
HCO_3^-	13 mmol/L
Base excess	−19 mEq/L
Lactate	9.4 mmol/L
Blood sugar	14.7 mmol/L

Guidance on scenario

The members of the team will perform tasks competently but only when directed by the candidate. The patient will undergo initial assessment. The rhythm is sinus tachycardia. Part way through the initial assessment the patient will deteriorate and suffer a cardiac arrest. There will be cardiac activity on the monitor but no central pulse. If help is called a senior trainee will attend to manage the airway.

The patient's original doctor will arrive and be extremely distressed. If the candidate calms them down they will be able to say the patient had attended with pleuritic chest pain and dizziness. They had a normal examination and ECG and were given antibiotics for a presumed chest infection. They will suggest the patient has developed septic shock.

If performed, an echocardiograph video clip will be shown to the candidate. It will demonstrate a contracting heart and an obviously dilated right ventricle. If assessed the patient has a unilateral swollen calf.

If appropriate thrombolytic therapy is given the patient will develop a pulse and their observations will slowly normalise. If not already performed they will require airway management.

Mark sheet	Achieved	Not achieved
Introduces self to the team		
Checks team member's competencies		
Briefs team on expected patient		
Prepares the resuscitation bay, specifies tasks to team members		
Ensures personal protective equipment for the team		
Tries to contact original doctor/gather information about patient		
On arrival performs appropriate initial assessment		
Ensures high-flow oxygen, monitoring, intravenous cannulation		
Recognises deterioration and declares cardiac arrest		
Calls for help (if not done earlier)		
Ensures appropriate airway management		
If not already done gains intravenous access and requests blood for urgent blood gas measurement and appropriate blood tests		
Continues uninterrupted chest compressions and ventilation at correct rate and ratio		
Speaks to original doctor in professional and sensitive manner		
Ensures adrenaline delivery every alternate cycle		
Ensures good quality compressions		
Rechecks rhythm and pulse every 2 minutes		
Goes through reversible causes – Hs and Ts		
Performs echocardiograph (or asks colleague to do so)		
Commences thrombolytic therapy in correct dose		
Continues basic resuscitation management appropriately		
Identifies presence of cardiac output		
Re-evaluates ABCDE		
Starts return of spontaneous circulation (ROSC) care		
Contacts intensivist if not already done so		
Hands over to intensivist adequately		
Global score from team		
Global score from examiner		

Alternative scenarios

Candidates should review all of the causes of a non-shockable cardiac arrest and ensure they are familiar with the advanced management for each of these. Any of these (or indeed a combination of these) may be relevant in a scenario and candidates will be expected to manage the case confidently while directing others and being confronted with distraction and conflicting information.

Hypoxic cardiac arrest: a 34-year-old woman who is known to have epilepsy had a seizure in a public place. She suffered no injuries but vomited soon after. With the paramedic crew she had a GCS of 3 and was making minimal respiratory effort. They were unable to secure a definitive airway. Her oxygen saturations fell to unrecordable and her rhythm was pulseless electrical activity. She arrives GCS 3, in PEA and with a temperature of 33°C.

7.4 Advanced life support: shockable rhythms

Managing a shockable rhythm, i.e. ventricular fibrillation (VF) or pulseless ventricular tachycardia (VT), should be straight-forward as there is clear guidance in the ALS protocol. The need for thorough practice and rehearsal of the algorithms cannot be overemphasised.

With regard to shockable rhythms, once cardiac arrest is confirmed the best chance of recovery is with early defibrillation and good quality chest compressions. Commence chest compressions and ensure the defibrillator is connected as soon as possible. Once connected analyse the rhythm and if appropriate state that a shock is required. Ask for chest compressions to continue while the defibrillator is charging. Next, deliver a shock safely. Once the shock is delivered it is recommended that chest compressions are commenced as soon as possible. Do not stop after delivering the shock to check the rhythm unless there are obvious signs of life.

Persisting VF/VT

- Confirm airway control, by endotracheal tube (ETT) or laryngeal mask airway (LMA) (if skills unavailable effective bag valve mask ventilations are acceptable initially), and good quality uninterrupted CPR
- 1 mg of adrenaline should be given every second cycle after the third shock
- Amiodarone 300 mg should be given after the third shock, and a further 150 mg can be used for refractory VF/VT. If amiodarone is not available, use Lidocaine 1 mg/kg, but not if amiodarone has been given already
- Consider changing the defibrillator pads to an anteroposterior position if shocks are unsuccessful at converting the rhythm
- Review the four Hs and Ts (see section 7.3) and aggressively manage any identifiable reversible cause
- Use sodium bicarbonate (50 mL of 8.4% or 50 mmol) if poisoning by tricyclic antidepressants, sodium channel blocking drugs or hyperkalaemia is suspected
- Consider use of mechanical device for chest compressions as these may be prolonged resuscitation attempts and are generally continued while VF/VT persist
- In suitable patients it may be appropriate to transfer a patient in VF to the catheter lab for coronary intervention. The standard ALS algorithm can be followed during transfer

Scenario

A 52-year-old man is on his way to the ED with paramedics. He was at a meeting, where he developed chest pain and then felt clammy and short of breath. He is alert but the paramedics have called ahead as he is grey and looks very unwell. The phone call cut out before any further information was provided. They are due to arrive in 1 minute. There are two experienced nurses available to help when the patient arrives.

Distribution of marks
- Resuscitation skills
- Clinical reasoning
- Team leadership

Initial patient observations

The patient and his wife are brought into the resuscitation bay. He has repeatedly asked for her to stay with him.

(As the patient is assessed during the scenario these observations will be provided by the nurse or by the monitoring)

Airway	Self-maintained
Breathing	Respiratory rate 28 breaths per minute. Bibasal crackles
	Oxygen saturation 100% on high flow oxygen
Circulation	Heart rate 170 beats per minute. Blood pressure 74/48 mmHg. Capillary refill time 5 seconds
Disability	Glasgow coma score 15
Exposure	Temperature 35°C. Clammy and grey
Blood sugar	11.6 mmol/L

A blood gas is unavailable as the machine is broken.

Guidance on scenario

As the initial assessment is proceeding the patient will deteriorate. They will not have a palpable pulse and if monitoring was attached early it will demonstrate a broad complex regular tachycardia. It is expected that standard ALS protocols will be followed. Immediately prior to defibrillation the defibrillator screen will go blank and the machine will stop working. The staff nurse will get another defibrillator from the next bay and attach it quickly. During this time there will be no choice but to continue with basic life support. When the new defibrillator is attached the rhythm is Ventricular Fibrillation (**Figure 7.4.1**). This will revert to a pulseless Ventricular Tachycardia after two shocks and cycles of resuscitation. When the pulse is checked there will no palpable central pulse. By this point a team of helpers will have arrived and should be used appropriately. Clinical findings and results will not suggest any reversible causes that can be addressed further. After two further cycles and shocks being delivered the patient will cardiovert to sinus rhythm and have a weak palpable pulse.

Figure 7.4.1 Initial rhythm strip.

The candidate will also be expected to communicate with the patient's wife who is understandably distressed and asking what is going on. She is not disruptive once a member of staff is allocated to support her.

After the difficulty with the defibrillator the additional team members will appear very stressed but will perform tasks competently when directed by the candidate. The patient's ECG suggests an ST elevation myocardial infarction (**Figure 7.4.2**). The candidate is expected to coordinate immediate transfer to the cardiology 'Cath lab' prior to the end of the scenario.

Figure 7.4.2 ECG post ROSC.

Mark sheet	Achieved	Not achieved
Introduces self to the team, confirms their competencies		
Takes adequate infection control precautions		
Asks to prepare resuscitation bay		
Makes plan and delegates roles to nurses		
On arrival performs appropriate ABCDE assessment		
Recognises deterioration and reassesses appropriately		
Calls for help (if not already done so)		
Correctly identifies rhythm and need for defibrillation		
Allows measures to be taken to permit early defibrillation with alternative machine		
Ensures airway is managed appropriately		
Manages resuscitation algorithm correctly		
Correct use of adrenaline and amiodarone		
Delegates roles to team and supervises them adequately		
Considers reversible causes of cardiac arrest		
Communicates with wife appropriately and allocates team member to support her		
Identifies change in rhythm		
Recognises return of spontaneous circulation (ROSC)		
Initiates post ROSC care		
Asks for 12-lead ECG		
Recognises ST elevation myocardial infarction		
States need for patient to go to catheter lab		
Calls cardiologist and intensivist		
Hands over patient to specialist efficiently		
Global score from team		
Global score from examiner		

Alternative scenarios

As for the previous section the candidate must be familiar with the advanced management of all reversible causes for a cardiac arrest with a shockable rhythm. They must demonstrate the ability to initiate and oversee high quality advanced life support and at the same time be able to manage the underlying cause to a high standard. Candidates are encouraged to reflect on every reversible cause and consider how these should be managed if they present individually or in combination in a scenario.

Refractory VF: a 42-year-old man has collapsed and his rhythm is VF. He is normally fit and well but has a strong family history of ischaemic heart disease. He has received three shocks with paramedics but remains in VF. Regardless of intervention in the ED he remains in VF. The cardiology team eventually suggest he can be taken to the 'cath lab' while in VF using an automated chest compression device.

7.5 Advanced life support: special circumstances

Electrolyte disorders, poisoning, drowning, hypo-/hyperthermia, pregnancy are important non-traumatic special circumstances that can arise as part of an advanced life support (ALS) scenario. Initially these situations may seem daunting. In all cases, however, a logical and stepwise approach coupled with certain specific knowledge is all a candidate requires to be successful.

Starting with the basics, early intubation, good quality cardiopulmonary resuscitation and chest compressions form the basis for these scenarios. Initial principles are the same as those outlined for the ALS shockable and non-shockable rhythms discussed above. In addition to these, knowledge of required specific treatments for the condition at hand is needed. Often the required specific interventions can be considered at the same time that a candidate would normally consider the four Hs and Ts. Outlined below are the main specific considerations that are required under certain special circumstances.

Pregnancy

- Call for expert help early for the mother and unborn child (neonatology, obstetrics, intensive care and anaesthetics)
- Start good quality cardiopulmonary resuscitation, minimising interruptions to chest compression
- For women over 20 weeks gestation, manually displace the uterus to the left or if feasible add left lateral tilt (aim for between 15° and 30° of tilt). This decompresses the vena cava and increases venous return
- Control the airway earlier as there is a higher risk of aspiration
- During the ongoing ALS algorithm consider the standard reversible causes as well as those specific to pregnancy which are now discussed in turn
- Manage haemorrhage with good fluid resuscitation and O negative blood. If possible use a rapid infusion system and consider the following: oxytocin and prostaglandin analogues, correcting any coagulopathy, tranexamic acid and uterine interventions or hysterectomy
- Pulmonary embolism requires the consideration of thrombolysis if the diagnosis is strongly suspected
- Urgent caesarean section should be considered as soon as possible for women over 20 weeks gestation. Between 20–23 weeks this is with the intention of saving the mother, whereas over 24 weeks there may be a good outcome for both the mother and child
- Once a pregnant woman suffers a cardiac arrest a caesarean section should be completed within 5 minutes to achieve the best possible outcome for both mother and fetus. Clearly to facilitate this help must be called for as early as possible

Poisoning

- Consider the personal safety of the team (especially when multiple casualties are involved simultaneously or dealing with poisons like cyanide, corrosives or organophosphates)

- Manage cardiac arrest on standard algorithms and ensure good quality cardiopulmonary resuscitation
- Try to identify the poison and get help from a national poisons advice centre
- Make specific interventions and use antidotes when poisons are known, otherwise focus on supportive therapy
- Be prepared for a prolonged cardiopulmonary resuscitation. It is well recognised that a good outcome may be possible after cardiac arrest from poisoning after prolonged resuscitation
- Once the airway is controlled, consider giving a single dose of activated charcoal, depending on the type of poison and the time of ingestion, or whole bowel irrigation for poisoning with prolonged release or enteric-coated drugs
- Haemodialysis, haemoperfusion or extracorporeal membrane oxygenation should be considered in discussion with poisons centre and the critical care team

Hypothermia

Hypothermia has been shown to be neuroprotective as it reduces the oxygen consumption of the brain. Also hypothermia itself may produce a very slow and low volume pulse with an un-recordable blood pressure. Therefore, beware of diagnosing death in cardiac arrest during hypothermia even if there are no signs of life, as they are unreliable.

- Look for signs of life for up to 1 minute before concluding that there is no cardiac output. If possible use echocardiography or Doppler to establish whether there is any cardiac activity or peripheral blood flow
- Warming must begin early and be as effective as possible. Remove all wet clothes and if necessary dry the body. Actively warm the patient, using warm intravenous fluids at 40°C, warm humidified gases to ventilate and a warming blanket. Bladder, gastric, pleural and peritoneal lavage with warm fluids are effective interventions. If facilities are available extracorporeal warming (cardiopulmonary bypass) is also a possibility
- Large amounts of intravenous fluids are required when rewarming as the intravascular space expands
- Ventilation may be difficult as the chest can become very stiff, therefore, attempt early intubation
- Use a low reading thermometer and preferably a rectal or oesophageal probe to measure core body temperature
- In the case of shockable rhythms if ventricular fibrillation or ventricular tachycardia is detected, attempt defibrillation with up to three shocks at maximum energy level. If the rhythm persists do not give another shock until core body temperature is above 30°C
- Drugs should be withheld until the core body temperature is higher than 30°C, and then double the intervals between drug doses. Only after the temperature has risen to above 35°C should standard timings be used for drugs

Drowning

- The primary cause of cardiac arrest in drowning is hypoxia and correction of hypoxaemia is critical for any chance of ROSC
- Rescue breaths, good quality basic life support (BLS) at the scene with attempted

ventilation, (as compression only cardiopulmonary resuscitation is unlikely to improve hypoxia)
- Cervical spine immobilisation is indicated when signs of injury are apparent or there is a history of diving, signs of trauma or alcohol intoxication
- Attempt early airway control, with a cuffed endotracheal tube, use suction to remove pulmonary oedema fluid
- Once the airway is secured, a high positive end expiratory pressure (PEEP) may be needed
- Victims may be hypovolaemic due to hypothermia and the hydrostatic pressure of the water on the body. This should be corrected with intravenous fluids

Scenario

A pregnant woman of 33 weeks gestation is on her way to the ED after collapsing at home following an episode of heavy vaginal bleeding. On arrival of the paramedics her rhythm was pulseless electrical activity (PEA). She received one cycle of CPR and a litre of crystalloid fluid prior to a palpable pulse being felt. She has been cannulated and is having her breathing assisted via a supraglottic airway device. You have an ALS trained nurse, an untrained nurse and an experienced ED doctor to help.

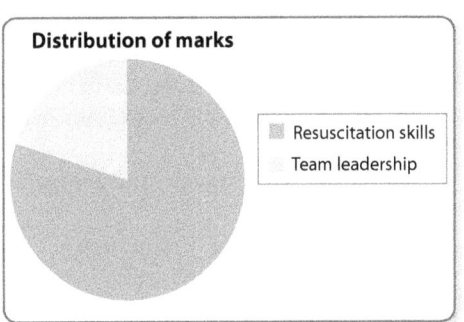

Distribution of marks

- Resuscitation skills
- Team leadership

Initial patient observations

(As the patient is assessed during the scenario these observations will be provided by the nurse)

Airway	Supraglottic airway device achieving poor ventilation due to large leak
Breathing	Respiratory rate 20 breaths per minute via Bag-valve-mask. Clear lung fields. Oxygen saturation – no trace achieved
Circulation	No palpable peripheral or central pulse, Sinus tachycardia on monitor Uterus not displaced
Disability	Glasgow coma score E1, V2, M4
Exposure	Temp 35.5°C
Blood sugar	9.3 mmol/L

Guidance on scenario

With the history provided the candidate is expected to make adequate preparation for an antepartum haemorrhage including recruiting other teams immediately. This should include critical care staff, an obstetrician and if delivery is anticipated (as it should be) a paediatric/neonatal team. An adequate number of staff will arrive individually as required for the scenario to proceed. The history and clinical findings will indicate the cause of cardiac arrest to be haemorrhage.

It will be noted early that the airway device is not allowing ventilation and this must be changed to an endotracheal tube. A single cannula will have been pulled out when the patient was removed from the ambulance.

There will be ongoing heavy bleeding and the patient will not have a pulse when they are assessed.

After a major transfusion is commenced and the uterus has been displaced to the left by an appropriate method there will still be no output. An ultrasound/echo machine will not be available and the full team will not arrive until after the patient has arrested.

The candidate will be expected to brief the team and coordinate a perimortem caesarean section. The obstetric registrar will be reluctant and say they have never had to do this before. If the reason for the procedure is explained they will agree to perform the procedure and complete it quickly. A second team must be formed from staff available to address the needs of the child after delivery. The child will be removed from the scenario. After delivery if the transfusion is continued the patient will develop an output.

The patient must be reviewed from an ABCDE perspective prior to being transferred to theatre.

All staff will be competent and perform tasks asked of them efficiently.

Mark sheet	Achieved	Not achieved
Introduces self to the team, confirms their competencies		
Calls for appropriate additional help		
Takes adequate infection control precautions		
Asks to set up resuscitation bay and prepare for major transfusion		
Coordinates team to perform initial ABCDE assessment		
Recognises and declares cardiac arrest, initiates CPR		
Confirms need for endotracheal intubation		
Supervises placement of intraosseous needles, (does not pursue intravenous access)		
Reasseses post intubation		
Coordinates CPR while blood is being transfused		
Leads CPR management correctly		
Ensures uterus is displaced appropriately		
Reassesses and declares need for Peri-mortem caesarean section		
Explains plan to team adequately		
Directs and supports obstetric registrar to perform task		
Ensures appropriate plan for care of delivered child		
Continues resuscitation and transfusion of patient/mother		
Recognises cardiac output		
Reassesses patient		
Initiates appropriate post resuscitation care		
Plans for transfer to theatre		
Keeps calm and manages team appropriately		
Takes timely and clear decisions		
Global score from team		
Global score from examiner		

Alternative scenario

Candidates must be prepared to demonstrate their knowledge of the advanced management of each of the respective special circumstances. Any of these causes for cardiac arrest may present independently or in combination.

Hypothermic overdose: a patient arrives having been found in a cold bath tub and with an empty bottle of amitryptiline. Core temperature is 29°C and the patient has a broad complex tachycardia.

Suggested reading

Antepartum Haemorrhage. Green top guideline 63. The Royal College of Obstetricians and Gynaecologists, 2011.

The acute management of thrombosis and embolism during pregnancy and the puerperium. Green top guideline 37b. The Royal College of Obstetricians and Gynaecologists, 2015.

7.6 Bradyarrhythmias

The candidate may be asked to establish non-invasive pacing as part of a peri-arrest scenario or after successful ROSC. It is useful to remember the algorithm for bradycardia management and be familiar with and confident when initiating external pacing.

Also consider and treat whatever has caused the bradycardia. Look for any clues in the history provided. Could the patient be having a myocardial infarction? Could they have taken an overdose of a beta-blocker or digoxin? Knowledge of the advanced management of these overdoses will also be expected.

Recognition

Extreme bradycardia is defined as heart rate <40 beats per minute. Ensure the patient is in the resuscitation area. If there is no cardiac output, start cardiopulmonary resuscitation as per ALS.

Commence an ABCDE assessment and look for adverse features. Request a 12-lead ECG as soon as it is appropriate to do so. Adverse features are:
- Shock (systolic blood pressure <90 mmHg, clammy, sweaty, reduced level of consciousness)
- Syncope
- Myocardial ischaemia
- Heart failure

Check a 12-lead ECG for complete heart block, Mobitz type II heart block or ventricular pauses of over 3 seconds. These (or a recent history of asystole) are indications that the patient is at a higher risk of asystole.

If there are adverse signs or a risk of asystole intervention is required.

Interventions

Give oxygen, establish intravenous access, and connect the patient to appropriate monitoring (blood pressure, pulse oximetry, cardiac monitor/defibrillator).
- The first-line treatment is intravenous atropine 500 mcg. This can be repeated to a maximum dose of 3 mg. Absence of a satisfactory response is an indication for pacing
- Transcutaneous pacing can easily be established in the ED using a defibrillator with a pacing function. There is no requirement for a central line and the procedure can be life-saving, allowing time for definitive measures to be planned. Patients will often feel the shock from external pacing and therefore some degree of sedation will be required
- Consider starting patients on an isoprenaline infusion via a central line. It is usually a 10 mg/mL preparation started at 3 mL/h

Technique

- Most defibrillators can pace. Ensure the one the patient is attached to has this capability
- Use appropriate drugs for sedation. Midazolam and fentanyl are most commonly used During the scenario continue to remain aware of the patient's clinical condition and level of comfort. Depending on the skills available find out if an anaesthetist is available to manage the airway and sedation

- Connect the patient to the defibrillator using the self-adhesive pads in an AP position. The sternal-apical position is preferable in cardiac arrest as there is no need to turn the patient
- Also attach the defibrillator's ECG electrodes. These are needed so that the defibrillator can interpret the rhythm during pacing. Ensure clean and dry skin when applying the pads
- Switch the defibrillator to pacing mode. It will select a default pacing current and frequency. Each pacing potential is seen as a spike on ECG. Once pacing is effective this spike should be followed by a QRS complex and a T wave which indicate electrical capture. If there is no QRS complex, increase the current slowly to achieve electrical capture. This usually occurs in the range of 50–100 mA
- Once electrical capture is established you must reassess the patient. Check for mechanical capture by palpating for a central pulse
- If maximum current settings are reached and there is no electrical capture, change the position of the pads. If still there is no electrical capture, it may indicate a non-viable myocardium. Involve the cardiology team as soon as possible

Scenario

A 48-year-old man is about to arrive having been found collapsed at home after a presumed overdose as he was found with a suicide note. He had vomited once prior to the paramedics arrival. With the paramedics he lost his output and was in PEA. He required two cycles of CPR and received a single dose of adrenaline before regaining a weak pulse. He has a history of atrial fibrillation and his medication packaging has been brought with him. You have 1 minute to prepare before the patient arrives in the ED. There is an experienced staff nurse, a student nurse and a competent junior anaesthetist available to assist you. Assess and manage the patient appropriately.

Distribution of marks
- Resuscitation skills
- Team leadership

Initial patient observations

(As the patient is assessed during the scenario these observations will be provided by the nurse)

Airway	Supraglottic airway device with vomit around face
Breathing	Respiratory rate 22 breaths per minute, clear lung fields
	Oxygen saturation 92% on high flow oxygen
Circulation	Pulse 15 beats per minute, blood pressure 60/34 mmHg
	Capillary refill time 4 seconds, ECG provided when asked for (**Figure 7.6.1**)
Disability	Glasgow coma score 7 (eyes 1, verbal 2, motor 4)
	Pupils equal and reactive
Exposure	Temperature 36°C
Blood sugar	9.3 mmol/L

Figure 7.6.1 Patient's initial ECG

Blood gas results will be provided to the candidate by a member of staff after the candidate has asked for the test to be performed.

pH	6.93
pCO_2	11.2 kPa
pO_2	24.3 kPa
Na^+	138 mmol/L
K^+	7.7 mmol/L
Cl^-	97 mmol/L
HCO_3	−13 mmol/L
BE	−19 mEq/L
Lactate	9.4 mmol/L
Blood sugar	12.7 mmol/L

Guidance on scenario

The paramedics do not know what the patient has taken. A few minutes into the scenario the daughter arrives and states the patient suffers from depression and alcohol dependence. She has found empty drug packaging in the patient's home which is for Digoxin 250 mcg and a new box was issued yesterday.

If the patient is not managed promptly and correctly they will suffer a further PEA arrest.

The patient must have their airway protected early in the scenario. Digoxin levels may be checked by the candidate but the candidate will be informed results will take several hours.

Atropine and intravenous fluids make have no effect on the patient. The patient must be treated for digoxin toxicity and for hyperkalaemia. Digoxin specific antibody will be available if requested. An emergency dosing chart will also be available and the nurse will be able to calculate the dose. Once commenced there will be a slow gradual improvement in heart rate and blood pressure. Calcium chloride and an insulin/dextrose infusion in correct doses will also have a beneficial effect. Sodium bicarbonate may also be given.

Vasopressors (in an appropriate dose) or transcutaneous pacing will not be effective as initial treatments. If initiated after the medical treatments in the paragraph above both will improve the patient's parameters further (but are unlikely to be achieved in the time provided). If no sedation is given the patient will become distressed by the repetitive shocks.

This settles with appropriate sedation and analgesia.

Haemodialysis is unlikely to improve digoxin elimination as the drug has a large volume of distribution and is highly protein bound. It may be considered in the case of associated renal failure or acidosis, however.

Time permitting the candidate will be prompted to speak to the patient's daughter or an intensivist to summarise the management so far and ongoing plan.

Mark sheet	Achieved	Not achieved
Introduces self to the team, checks experience and provides a team brief		
Ensures adequate personal protective equipment for all staff		
Takes appropriate hand over from paramedics		
Ensures pulse check on patient arrival		
Appropriate initial ABCDE assessment		
Requests definitive airway and supervises/coordinates procedure		
Obtains intravenous access and requests appropriate blood tests		
Recognises digoxin toxicity as primary problem		
Initiates treatment to address hyperkalaemia		
Initiates treatment with digoxin specific antibody		
Performs correct measures in reasonable timeframe		
Uses safe technique and doses for all interventions attempted		
Gives appropriate sedation and analgesia		
Reassesses patient appropriately		
Obtains appropriate history from daughter		
Summarises plan accurately		
Global mark from examiner		
Global mark from team		

Alternative scenarios

Beta-blocker overdose: the patient will present after an intentional overdose of propranolol. They will have an altered level of consciousness and severe hypotension. They will go on to have a seizure and subsequent cardiac arrest. They will require airway management and appropriate medical therapies and will finaly stabilize on an inotrope infusion.

Inferior myocardial infarction: the patient will present following a collapse. They will display slow pulseless electrical activity, and after resuscitation will have an output with a heart rate of 18 beats per minute and inferior ST elevation on the monitor and on an ECG if performed. They will require airway management, transcutaneous pacing and transfer to the catheter laboratory.

7.7 Tachyarrhythmias

Readers should refer to section 6.9 regarding direct current (DC) cardioversion when reading this section.

Like all conditions in this chapter, this scenario may arise in an OSCE to test peri-arrest arrhythmia management or may form a small section of a broader OSCE and candidates should be prepared for either eventuality.

The patient should be in a resuscitation bay with appropriate monitoring (blood pressure, pulse oximetry) and a defibrillator attached. When managing a patient with a tachyarrhythmia, commence as always with an ABCDE assessment.

Look for adverse signs during the initial assessment:
- Shock (systolic blood pressure <90 mmHg, clammy, sweaty, reduced level of consciousness)
- Syncope
- Myocardial ischaemia
- Heart failure

Interventions

Administer high flow oxygen, establish intravenous access, and connect the patient to appropriate monitoring (blood pressure, pulse oximetry, cardiac monitor/defibrillator).

Obtain a 12-lead ECG and check electrolytes with point of care tests. During the initial assessment consider and treat the cause of the tachycardia. Look for any clues in the history provided. Could the patient have deranged renal function? Hyperkalaemia can cause a broad complex tachycardia. Could they have taken an overdose of tricyclic antidepressants? Knowledge of the how to manage these conditions will also be required.

If the patient displays any adverse signs the treatment of choice is synchronised DC cardioversion. This is regardless of whether the cause is a narrow or a broad complex tachycardia. Patients will need some form of sedation and/or analgesia to facilitate this, e.g. midazolam and fentanyl. Depending on the skills available and urgency find out if an anaesthetist is available to manage the airway and sedation.

If adverse signs are present attempt DC cardioversion with up to three individual synchronised shocks. If this fails to restore sinus rhythm the recommendations are intravenous amiodarone 300 mg and a further shock.

If there are no adverse signs then intervention depends on the rhythm. It must be decided as to whether it is a broad or narrow complex tachycardia and then for each whether it is regular or irregular.

A broad complex irregular tachycardia is likely to be atrial fibrillation (with bundle branch block or pre-excitation) or polymorphic ventricular tachycardia. While a broad complex regular tachycardia is probably ventricular tachycardia or a supraventricular tachycardia with bundle branch block.

A narrow complex, irregular tachycardia is likely to be atrial fibrillation, whereas a narrow complex regular tachycardia is probably a supraventricular tachycardia.

Each of these arrhythmias will need specific management and may require the involvement of a cardiologist.

Scenario

You are asked to urgently review a 24-year-old woman brought to the resuscitation area. Paramedics report significant blood loss and progressively decreased level of consciousness. She has been found at home having cut both her wrists. There is a nurse, an experienced senior ED trainee and another junior trainee available to assist you.

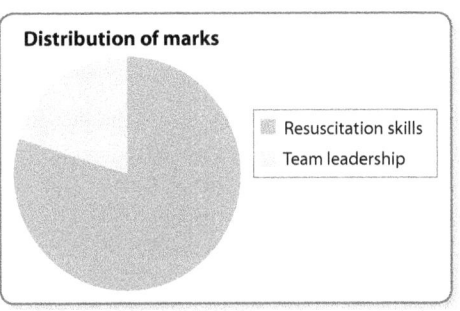

Initial patient observations

(As the patient is assessed during the scenario these observations will be provided by the nurse)

Airway	Patent
Breathing	Respiratory rate 26 breaths per minute, clear lung fields bilaterally
	Oxygen saturation 92% on air. 100% on high flow oxygen
Circulation	Pulse 164 beats per minute, blood pressure 64/40 mmHg
	Capillary refill time 5 seconds,
	ECG handed to candidate (**Figure 7.7.1**)
Disability	Glasgow coma score 9 (eyes 2, verbal 2, motor 5)
Exposure	Temperature 35°C, bleeding wounds to both wrists
Blood sugar	6.7 mmol/L

Figure 7.7.1 Patient's initial ECG.

Blood gas results will be provided to the candidate by a member of staff after the candidate has asked for the test to be performed.

pH	7.03
pCO_2	7.2 kPa
pO_2	24.3 kPa
Na^+	138 mmol/L
K^+	4.8 mmol/L
Cl^-	97 mmol/L
HCO_3	−13 mmol/L
BE	−15 mEq/L
Lactate	7.4 mmol/L
Hb	74
Blood sugar	7.7 mmol/L

Guidance on scenario

The candidate must ensure that pressure is applied to both wrists early to prevent further bleeding. They must commence a blood transfusion while competing an initial ABCDE assessment. There will be no palpable pulses in the left hand. If this is not recognized a team member will comment on the left hand later in the scenario.

The patient will have a sinus tachycardia with broad QRS complexes (if this is not noted and an ECG is not requested a team member will comment on the QRS morphology on the ECG monitor). The patient will deteriorate and will be pulseless with a broad complex tachycardia requiring defibrillation after which they will have a GCS of 3. They will need their airway secured. The candidate is expected to treat the patient for blood loss and a suspected tricyclic antidepressant overdose. The rhythm and physiological markers will improve once the patient is given sodium bicarbonate. Once intubated and ventilated if the patient is hyperventilated to achieve a respiratory alkalosis they QRS morphology will normalize further.

The candidate must make a plan for the patient to be stabilised and be transferred to theatre for vascular surgery.

Mark sheet	Achieved	Not achieved
Introduces self to the team, checks experience and provides a team brief		
Ensures adequate personal protective equipment for all staff		
Takes appropriate hand over from paramedics		
Ensures pulse check on patient arrival		
Prevents further blood loss from wounds		
Appropriate initial ABCDE assessment		
Requests definitive airway and supervises/coordinates procedure		
Obtains intravenous access and requests appropriate blood tests		
Administers blood in appropriate volume		
Correctly delivers DC shock		
Recognises significance of ECG and blood gas		

Cont'd...

Cont'd...

Mark sheet	Achieved	Not achieved
Initiates treatment with Sodium bicarbonate		
Performs correct measures in reasonable timeframe		
Uses safe technique and doses for all interventions attempted		
Reassesses patient appropriately		
Arranges for urgent vascular surgical review		
Hands patient over to anaesthetist and surgeon appropriately		
Global mark from examiner		
Global mark from team		

Alternative scenarios

Torsades and hypokalaemia: the patient has a complicated and unclear history of bowel pathology with multiple operations. She presented after three days of vomiting. Her rhythm is Torsades de pointes and she is unconscious. She cardioverts to sinus rhythm after each shock but her rhythm soon deteriorates again. Her potassium is 1.5 mmol/L.

Supraventricular tachycardia: the patient is haemodynamically normal. They do not respond to vagal manoeuvres, or an initial dose of adenosine and then start to decompensate with chest pain and hypotension. After attempted DC cardioversion their rhythm is pulseless VT.

7.8 Adult anaphylaxis

Anaphylaxis is a severe, life-threatening, generalised or systemic hypersensitivity reaction. In the examination, the scenario may not always make it clear that the problem is anaphylaxis (see also the scenario in section 8.2). It is always important to consider what has caused the reaction and ensure the cause is removed.

Recognition
Anaphylaxis is likely when the following three criteria are met:
- Sudden onset of symptoms that are rapidly progressing
- Life-threatening A-airway, B-breathing or C-circulation problem
- Skin and/or mucosal changes (urticaria, angioedema, flushing)

In addition the presence of a trigger (allergen) supports the diagnosis. This could be intravenous fluid, antibiotics, a new drug, food or an insect sting.

Life-threatening problems to identify
- Airway – Intraoral swelling, hoarse voice, stridor, palatal oedema, swollen tongue.
- Breathing – Rapid breathing, wheeze, fatigue, cyanosis, hypoxia with $SO_2 < 92\%$.
- Circulation – Cold clammy peripheries, hypotension, faint, drowsy, coma.
- Skin changes may or may not always present at the same time or may not be obvious. Expose the patient to look for a rash.

Interventions
Once the diagnosis is made, then follow the resuscitation council algorithm and College of Emergency Medicine guidelines for anaphylaxis. Important points to consider are:
- Call for help early and remove the trigger if readily identifiable, e.g. stop the intravenous infusion of penicillin being given
- Adrenaline is the drug of choice in this situation. Current guidance advises using 500 μg (0.5 mL of 1:1000) intramuscularly as soon as life-threatening complications are recognised. Do not wait for intravenous access to be established
- Further interventions will depend on the situation. Therefore, early intubation will be warranted where there is life-threatening airway swelling, whereas, intravenous fluids with or without inotropic support will be required for a profoundly shocked patient
- In cardiac arrest, follow the advanced life support algorithm and prolonged resuscitation is often needed
- Intravenous (or intramuscular) chlorphenamine and hydrocortisone should be used once life-threatening problems have been identified and dealt with. The standard dose for adults is intravenous chlorphenamine 10 mg and intravenous hydrocortisone 200 mg
- Mast cell tryptase helps to confirm the diagnosis. It rises soon after onset of anaphylaxis reaching peak at 1–2 hours and then falls back to baseline within 6–8 hours. Therefore, any sample collection should be carefully timed. This should not interfere with initial resuscitation. The first sample should be collected as soon as practicable, the second at 1–2 hours and another after 24 hours to check baseline levels

Scenario

An ED nurse urgently calls you to review her patient. The patient looks panicked and has suddenly become clammy and breathless while receiving treatment.

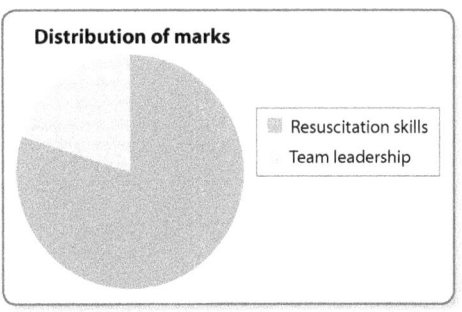

Initial patient observations

(As the patient is assessed during the scenario these observations will be provided by the nurse)

Appearance	Sweating
Airway	Speaking single words as feels unwell, airway – swollen tongue/lips
Breathing	Respiratory rate 30 breaths per minute, wheeze bilaterally
	Oxygen saturation 84% on air, 92% on high flow oxygen
Circulation	Pulse 130 beats per minute, blood pressure 60/40 mmHg
	Capillary refill time 1 second
Disability	Glasgow coma score 14 (eyes 4, verbal 4, motor 6)
Exposure	Temperature 37°C. Flushed, urticarial rash on abdomen
Blood sugar	7.3 mmol/L

Guidance on scenario

The patient is receiving intravenous antibiotics for a complicated dog bite. Anaphylaxis must be diagnosed and the antibiotics must be stopped. She does not respond to initial treatment of anaphylaxis and subsequently suffers a PEA cardiac arrest. An additional doctor with airway skills and a junior nurse will attend if help is called. Ventilation via a bag-valve-mask or supraglottic device (if attempted) will be very difficult due to bronchospasm. An assisting airway doctor will be able to achieve a definitive airway but the patient will remain hard to ventilate. During CPR each dose of adrenaline will result in a pulse which is only briefly palpable. The candidate must commence an adrenaline infusion to achieve adequate bronchodilation and sustained return of spontaneous circulation.

Mark sheet	Achieved	Not achieved
Introduces self to nurse		
Obtains brief history of events		
Calls for additional help		
Performs appropriate ABCDE initial assessment		
Diagnoses anaphylaxis		

Cont'd...

Cont'd...

Mark sheet	Achieved	Not achieved
Stops antibiotic infusion		
Applies high flow oxygen		
Initiates appropriate treatment		
Recognises cardiac arrest		
Ensures appropriate airway management		
Correct management of advanced life support algorithm		
Recognises need for and commences adrenaline infusion		
Plans for mast cell tryptase measurement		
Global score from examiner		
Global score from team		

Alternative scenario

Nut allergy: a patient with asthma and a known nut allergy has been to a party at an ice cream parlour and arrives having collapsed. The patient has arrested prior to arrival and has too much facial oedema for a definitive oral airway. They require a surgical airway and ongoing management of the advanced life support algorithm as well as an adrenaline infusion to achieve return of spontaneous circulation.

Suggested reading

Acute allergic reaction. Guidelines in Emergency Medicine Network, 2009.
Anaphylaxis. Clinical guideline 134. National Institute for Health and Care Excellence, London, 2011.

7.9 Stopping resuscitation efforts

There are a variety of factors to consider when deciding whether or not to cease attempts at resuscitation. Primarily the decision is based on whether or not there is likely to be a successful outcome. This judgement is often formed as part of a dynamic thought process that evolves as a resuscitation effort is underway.

In an examination setting a candidate normally anticipates that to perform well there will be a positive outcome. This is the very reason that a scenario where resuscitation is futile can identify candidates who are confident in their clinical decision making.

Regarding when to stop resuscitation the main considerations are the patient's comorbidities, the duration of the cardiac arrest, potential duration of cerebral hypoxia, the cardiac arrest rhythm, the response to treatment thus far, the presence of reversible causes that are yet to be addressed and the patient's wishes (if known). It is generally accepted that if all reversible causes have been dealt with, asystole persisting for 20 minutes is not likely to lead to a successful outcome. However, there are many factors that influence the chance of a successful outcome and these must all be considered.

It is also accepted that family members, who wish to, may benefit from being present during resuscitation efforts. Though this may make it more challenging for staff present it is important to support the wishes of family members. Always ensure a member of staff is allocated to support any family that may be present.

It is important to recognise that different clinicians, hospital staff, patients and family members may have different views as to what the correct decision is. With this in mind it is important to consider others during the decision making. The final decision rests with the team leader but it is helpful for the team leader to explain their clinical rationale in a sensitive and respectful manner to all of those present. In cases where the team leader is considering ending resuscitation efforts, it is likely to be helpful to state that this is the case, explain why and seek the opinions of others present. If a family member is present the team leader should communicate with them clearly and it must be explained that the family member is not being asked to give their permission for resuscitation to end. Once these steps have occurred and any concerns or questions have been dealt with the team should be given clear instructions as to when to stop. Always thank the team present for their efforts and allow a further opportunity for any questions to be answered. In cases that are likely to be particularly emotive or distressing for those present consider a 'debrief' to allow everyone the opportunity to discuss the case and any concerns or questions they may have.

Scenario

An ambulance crew is bringing a 48-year-old male patient (and his wife) to ED following a cardiac arrest. On the crew's arrival the patient's rhythm was VF. He received two shocks along standard advanced life support (ALS) protocols and had a rhythm change to PEA. After two further cycles of CPR and a dose of adrenaline the patient had a palpable pulse.

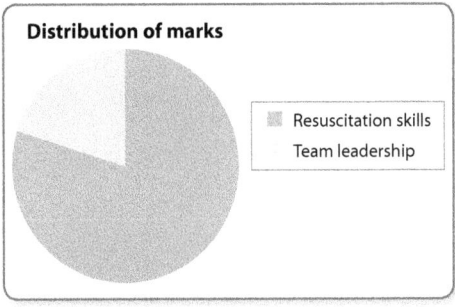

Distribution of marks
- Resuscitation skills
- Team leadership

He is cannulated. Expected time of arrival is in 2 minutes. You have one ALS trained nurse and an experienced doctor with you. Manage the patient appropriately once he arrives.

Initial patient observations

(As the patient is assessed during the scenario these observations will be provided by the nurse)

Airway	Supraglottic airway device
Breathing	No spontaneous respiratory effort
	Being ventilated via a bag-valve-mask, bilateral air entry
	Oxygen saturation maximal oxygen
Circulation	Pulse 36 beats per minute on monitor, no palpable pulse
	Capillary refill time 4 seconds
Disability	Glasgow coma score 3 (eyes 1, verbal 1, motor 1)
	Pupils fixed, unreactive
Exposure	Temperature 35.5°C
Blood sugar	7.3 mmol/L

Blood gas results will be provided to the candidate by a member of staff at an appropriate point in the scenario.

pH	6.8
pCO_2	9 kPa
pO_2	24 kPa
HCO_3	6 mmol/L
BE	−20 mEq/L
Lactate	13 mmol/L
K^+	8 mmol/L

Guidance on scenario

The patient arrives with his wife who wants to be present. He is normally fit and active but has recently been taking regular anti-inflammatories for knee pain. For the past 3 days he's had diarrhoea and vomiting. His GP had visited yesterday and diagnosed 'stomach flu'. This morning she had gone to work but returned home early to check on him.

On arrival in the ED, the patient has no cardiac output and is not receiving chest compressions. The paramedics last felt a pulse 'several' minutes ago but were distracted by a problem with the ambulance equipment before arriving at the ED. After a further cycle of CPR his rhythm progresses to asystole and will remain asystole. Clinical findings will not reveal any reversible causes other than the high potassium level. The patient's wife is understandably very distressed and the candidate will be required to explain what is happening during the scenario.

Mark sheet	Achieved	Not achieved
Introduces self to the team and checks their competencies		
Takes appropriate infection control precautions		
Briefs team on expected patient, delegates roles, prepares equipment		
On patient arrival performs pulse check		
Recognises PEA arrest and commences CPR		
Takes a handover from paramedics		
Acknowledges wife and communicates appropriately with her		
Does not try to remove wife, allocates team member to support her		
Performs logical ABC assessment		
Correctly uses ALS algorithm		
Excludes reversible causes adequately including reviewing blood gas		
Recognises ongoing CPR is futile		
Informs team and wife		
Addresses concerns voiced by wife appropriately		
Supports/directs team to stop CPR (may perform several cycles of CPR first)		
Thanks team		
Communicates with wife providing adequate explanation of events		
Global score from team		
Global score from examiner		

Alternative scenario

Distressed family: an 82-year-old independent man is brought to the ED after a collapse. His wife arrives with him and says he has been getting chest pain on walking upstairs for a couple of weeks. He remains in asystole with an unsurvivable blood gas. He was due to go on a once in a lifetime holiday next week to see his son in Australia. His wife asks that everything be done for him as she isn't ready to say goodbye.

7.10 Preeclampsia

Preeclampsia is defined as new hypertension with blood pressure above 140/90 mmHg and significant proteinuria in a woman >20 weeks pregnant. Severe preeclampsia is preeclampsia with severe hypertension (blood pressure >160/110 mmHg), additional symptoms and biochemical or haematological impairments. Eclampsia refers to convulsions associated with preeclampsia.

Fortunately, with modern obstetrics this is a relatively rare presentation, but one should be capable of recognising it and prepared to deal with it when it occurs. It has high fetal and maternal mortality and needs to be managed in association with the obstetric, anaesthetic and intensive care teams.

Features of severe preeclampsia are:
- Severe headache
- Problems with vision such as blurring or flashing lights before eyes
- Severe pain just below the ribs or vomiting
- Papilloedema
- Clonus
- Liver tenderness
- Haemolysis, elevated liver enzymes and low platelets (HELLP) syndrome
- Platelet count below 100×10^9/L
- ALT or AST rising to above 70 IU/L

In addition be aware of additional criteria requiring level two care:
- Evidence of cardiac failure
- Abnormal neurology
- Oliguria
- Hyperkalaemia
- Haemorrhage
- Seizures
- HELLP syndrome
- Intravenous therapy to control hypertension

Interventions

Controlling hypertension

Labetalol is the first-line drug for controlling hypertension. In severe preeclampsia an intravenous infusion with invasive blood pressure monitoring should be used. The initial starting dose is 50 mg over at least 1 minute, which can be repeated after 5 minutes if necessary. An infusion can be started at 20 mg/h and doubled every 30 minutes, usual maximum rate 160 mg/h. Aim to keep blood pressure <150/80–100 mmHg. Hydralazine and nifedipine can also be used.

Preventing or controlling seizures

Magnesium sulphate is the drug of choice to prevent and treat seizures. Loading dose of 4 g over 5 minutes, followed by an infusion of 1 g/h for 24 hours. If there are further seizures, 2–4 g intravenously over 5 minutes can be repeated. Diazepam or phenytoin should not be used.

Steroids to aid fetal pulmonary maturity

Betamethasone 12 mg intramuscularly repeated after 24 hours is used for fetal lung maturity if birth is likely within 7 days. It is recommended before 34 weeks' gestation and can be considered after 34 weeks.

Supportive care

Supportive interventions should be based on the ABCDE assessment. The patient may need to be intubated and ventilated. Intravenous fluids should be used judiciously. Coagulopathy may need correction, particularly if a caesarean section is to be considered.

Definitive treatment

This requires a caesarean section. The urgency of this depends on the gestation and clinical circumstances.

Scenario

A woman who is 35 weeks pregnant has arrived in the ED with a headache and abdominal pain. She has vomited once. She is a recent migrant and has not had much contact with health services. There is nurse to assist you.

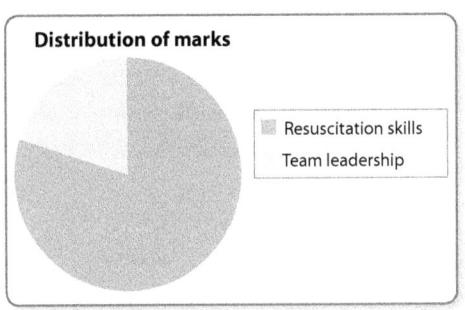

Initial patient observations

(As the patient is assessed during the scenario these observations will be provided by the nurse)

Airway	Clear
Breathing	Respiratory rate 20 breaths per minute, clear lung fields
	Oxygen saturation 100% on high flow oxygen
Circulation	Pulse 72 beats per minute, blood pressure 180/100 mmHg, capillary refill time 1s
Disability	Glasgow coma score 10 (eyes 3, verbal 2, motor 5)
Exposure	Temperature 35.5°C, appears agitated
Blood sugar	5.3 mmol/L

Guidance on scenario

During this scenario the patient will be unable to provide a history and will then have a tonic-clonic seizure which will stop spontaneously. After the seizure her GCS will be 3. This will require the patient to be reassessed with their drop in Glasgow coma score managed appropriately and the treatment for preeclampsia to be expedited.

Mark sheet	Achieved	Not achieved
Introduces self to the nurse and patient		
Takes adequate infection control precautions		
Asks nurse to connect monitor – ECG, blood pressure, pulse oximetry		
Performs logical ABCDE assessment with basic interventions		
Identifies high blood pressure, diagnoses preeclampsia		
Asks for intravenous access and sends appropriate blood samples		
Checks blood sugar		
Asks for urine sample to check proteinuria		
Manages seizure safely		
Calls for additional help (if not done earlier)		
Re-evaluates patient ABCDEs		
Glasgow coma score-E1 M1 V1		
Ensures airway is protected		
Commences intravenous magnesium in appropriate dose		
Commences intravenous labetalol to control hypertension (or suitable alternative)		
Asks for arterial line and urethral catheter		
Uses intravenous fluids appropriately		
Checks response to treatment		
Asks for ECG and chest X-ray		
Calls obstetrics and intensive care urgently		
Hands over to intensive care registrar		
Global score from team		
Global score from examiner		

Alternative scenario

Seizure: an obese female patient is prealerted as she has had a prolonged seizure and has a decreased level of consciousness. On arrival she is unconscious, hypertensive and on further assessment is pregnant. Peripheral vascular access is not possible.

Suggested reading

Hypertension in pregnancy. Clinical guideline 107. National Institute for Health and Care Excellence, London, 2010.

7.11 Delivering a baby

Faced with a delivering mother do not forget to prepare for the care of the baby: the necessary arrangements should be made for both mother and baby.

Preparation
- In the ED it is best to manage the patient in a resuscitation bay
- Call for help if there is time. The obstetrician, midwife and paediatrician should be called. In the meantime additional ED staff will be able to help
- Turn on the Resuscitaire and confirm there is working suction and towels. Open a delivery pack and check that it has umbilical clamps. Check the monitoring equipment
- Entonox is a helpful analgesic in this situation
- Check ergometrine or oxytocin is available
- Organise the team and allocate tasks

Delivery

Unless imminently delivering, it is always preferable to transfer the patient to labour ward.

Regular uterine contraction every couple of minutes with a dilated cervix indicates established labour. Once the cervix is fully dilated, the patient is in the second stage of labour.

Occipitoanterior (OA) vertex presentation is likely to proceed without complication (other presentations may lead to obstructed labour). In this situation, the flexed head emerges and then extends. This is followed by the rotation of the baby so that the shoulders lie in the anteroposterior plane and the baby faces the mother's thigh, usually the right thigh as a left OA presentation is more common than a right OA presentation. The anterior shoulder delivers first, followed by the baby's delivery.

Post-delivery care
- Mother's care: the mother is now in the third stage of labour. Give intramuscular Syntometrine (5 units oxytocin and 500 mg ergometrine). Transfer her to the labour ward for further post-delivery care
- Baby's care: ensure that the baby is crying, is pink, has a normal tone, grimaces on stimulation and has a heart rate of >100 beats per minute (**Table 7.11.1**). Clean and dry the baby with towels and keep the baby with the mother. Ensure appropriate management to prevent hypothermia. If there are any concerns remember the neonatal resuscitation algorithm. The score is normally performed at 1 and 5 minutes after birth. Scores of 7 or above are considered normal (section 8.11)
- Cord care: once the cord ceases to pulsate, keep the baby level with the mother and clamp the cord twice. Cut between the clamps a couple of centimeters from the umbilicus

Table 7.11.1 The APGAR score

	0	1	2
Appearance (Color)	Blue	Blue at extremities, body pink	No cyanosis
Pulse (Heart rate)	Absent	<100/min	≥100/min
Grimace (Reflexes)	No response to stimulation	Feeble cry when stimulated	Cry or pull away when stimulated
Activity (Tone)	None	Some flexion	Flexed arms and legs that resist extension
Respiration (Breathing)	Absent	Weak, irregular, gasping	Strong cry

Scenario

A nurse informs you that a 30-year-old woman who is 39 weeks pregnant and has abdominal pain has just arrived in the ED reception. This is her third pregnancy and she is in a lot of pain. She is being brought through to the resuscitation area. Manage her appropriately.

Distribution of marks
- Practical skills
- Communication
- Team leadership

Initial patient observations

(As the patient is assessed during the scenario these observations will be provided by the nurse)

Airway	Clear
Breathing	Respiratory rate 28 breaths per minute, clear lung fields
	Oxygen saturation 100% on high flow oxygen
Circulation	Pulse 72 beats per minute, blood pressure 128/80 mmHg
	Capillary refill time 1 second
Disability	Glasgow coma score 15
Exposure	Temperature 36°C, in pain
Blood sugar	5.3 mmol/L

Guidance on scenario

The steps to be taken in this scenario are clear. The additional specialists must be called early but will be busy and arrive as soon as they can (once the child has been delivered).

Mark sheet	Achieved	Not achieved
Introduces self to the nursing staff		
Confirms the information from ambulance phone		
Enquires regarding experience in team		
Prepares for the patient's arrival		
Asks for resuscitation bay		
Asks for obstetric and paediatric teams to be called		
Checks availability of delivery pack – cord clamps, towels, local anaesthetic for possible episiotomy		
Asks to start Resuscitaire		
Gets entonox cylinder and asks for Syntometrine		
Ensures everyone wears personal protective equipment		
Assigns reasonable roles to team members		
On patient's arrival		
Confirms established labour – regular contractions lasting a minute		
Explains imminent delivery to mother		
Offers Entonox to mother		
Establishes intravenous access, send full blood count, urea and electrolytes		
Examines perineum, confirms crowning		
Supports perineum with left hand to avoid tear		
Delivers baby's head, checks for cord around the neck		
Allows head to extend and anterior shoulder to deliver		
Delivers the baby		
Asks for syntometrine intramuscularly		
Post-delivery care		
Performs baby checks – Apgar score		
Clamps the cord appropriately		
Dries the baby and gives to mother		
Covers mother and baby to avoid hypothermia		
Hands over to obstetric registrar and midwife when they arrive		
Global score from team		
Global score from examiner		

Alternative scenario

Shoulder dystocia: there is failure to progress normally and on examination the cause is shoulder dystocia. Appropriate manoeuvre's must be attempted with the candidate explaining what actions must be taken. The obstetric registrar is competent but junior and must be directed to take action to facilitate urgent delivery of the child.

7.12 Upper gastrointestinal bleed with massive haemorrhage

Patients who experience an upper gastrointestinal bleed with massive haemorrhage are very unwell, shocked and may be peri-arrest. In addition, they are vomiting blood and at risk of aspiration. There are well-established guidelines by the National Institute for Health and Care Excellence (NICE) and the Scottish Intercollegiate Guidelines Network (SIGN), which should be used when confronted with a patient in this condition. Airway interventions may be required before you can safely manage this patient.

Priorities in this presentation are:
- completing a systematic assessment
- ensuring adequate vascular access
- resuscitation with blood and appropriate blood products
- activating a major haemorrhage policy
- correcting clotting abnormalities
- stabilising the patient and initiating medical therapies (**Table 7.12.1**)
- co-ordinating an emergency endoscopy in an appropriate setting (endoscopy or theatre)

Remember also that in an unstable patient with suspected variceal bleeding who cannot get to endoscopy because it is not available at your centre or in the scenario provided, temporising measures with balloon tamponade may be the only solution. The patient would need to be intubated prior to this procedure.

Table 7.12.1 Drug therapy for non-variceal and variceal upper gastrointestinal bleeding

Management	Suspected non-variceal bleeding	Suspected variceal bleeding
Proton pump inhibitor	Not recommended before endoscopy	Recommended before endoscopy
Antibiotics	Not recommended	Recommended
Vasoactive therapy	Not recommended	Recommended: Terlipressin 2 mg IV every 4 hours OR Octreotide 50 µg bolus followed by 50 µg/h infusion OR Somatostatin 250 µg IV bolus followed by 250 µg/h infusion
Tranexamic acid	Only as part of massive transfusion protocol	Only as part of massive transfusion protocol

Scenario

You are called to the resuscitation area to see a 45-year-old man brought in by ambulance with haematemesis. He is known to be an alcoholic. His wife called an ambulance because he started vomiting fresh blood. He is breathing by himself and paramedics have given him supplemental oxygen. They could not achieve intravenous access. There is a junior nurse available to help you.

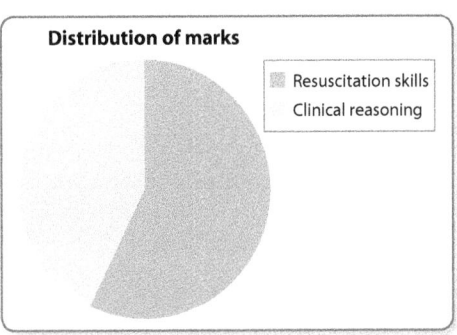

Distribution of marks
- Resuscitation skills
- Clinical reasoning

Initial patient observations

As the patient is assessed during the scenario these observations will be provided by the nurse.

Airway	Patent, fresh blood in mouth
Breathing	Respiratory rate 26 breaths per minute, clear lung fields
	Oxygen saturations 95% on air
Circulation	Pulse 148 beats per minute, blood pressure 80/40 mmHg
Disability	Glasgow coma score 13 (eyes 3, verbal 4, motor 6)
Exposure	Temperature 34.8°C, Pale
Blood sugar	4.9 mmol/L

Guidance on scenario

As the patient is assessed he vomits blood mixed with coffee ground material. His observations do not change significantly. Once vascular access is gained and blood is transfused his observations slowly improve. If an endoscopist is contacted the endoscopist asks if the patient can wait until the following morning for an endoscopy. If the patient is not kept warm and no varices-specific medication is given the nurse will suggest that these things need to be addressed.

Venous blood gas results will be given by the nurse (if they are requested):

pH	7.1
HCO_3	−16 mmol/L
BE	−10 mEq/L
Lactate	5.2 mmol/L
Haemoglobin	6.2 g/dL

Mark sheet	Achieved	Not achieved
Introduces self to nurse		
Wears personal protective equipment		
Performs appropriate ABCDE assessment with basic interventions		
Suctions vomitus/blood		

Cont'd...

Cont'd...

Mark sheet	Achieved	Not achieved
Administers high flow oxygen		
Secures two large bore IV cannulae		
Takes appropriate blood samples (including blood gas)		
Initiates volume replacement – initially crystalloid or blood		
Reassesses circulation		
Administers blood		
Activates massive transfusion protocol		
Continues volume resuscitation		
Corrects coagulopathy – vitamin K, fresh frozen plasma, platelets		
Suspects variceal bleeding		
Asks for antibiotics, terlipressin, tranexamic acid		
Inserts nasogastric tube		
Comments on need to keep patient warm		
Comments on need to insert urethral catheter		
Arranges endoscopy as an emergency procedure		
Global score from nurse		
Global score from examiner		

Alternative scenario

Unstable patient: the patient has no known varices and recently has a normal colonoscopy. They are anticoagulated. They continue to suffer haematemesis and also begin to have melaena. Even after all appropriate steps they remain haemodynamically unstable. Immediate endoscopy must be coordinated in the safest location available.

Suggested reading

Acute upper gastrointestinal bleeding: management, CG 141. London: National Institute for Health and Care Excellence, 2012.

Chapter 8

Paediatric acute presentations

- 8.1 Introduction
- 8.2 Paediatric anaphylaxis
- 8.3 Paediatric asthma
- 8.4 Paediatric advanced life support
- 8.5 Management of a child choking on a foreign body
- 8.6 Paediatric seizures
- 8.7 Paediatric septic shock
- 8.8 Paediatric supraventricular tachycardia
- 8.9 Paediatric trauma
- 8.10 Neonatal duct dependent circulation
- 8.11 Newborn baby resuscitation
- 8.12 Paediatric stridor

8.1 Introduction

The principles of how to approach a resuscitation style objectively structured clinical examination (OSCE) have been discussed already in the introduction to the adult acute presentations chapter (see section 7.1). Broadly speaking the approach can be divided into preparation for the scenario, knowledge of the drugs and specific interventions required and systematic running of the scenario followed by closure. As well as reading this introduction candidates are encouraged to read and reflect on the discussion of non-technical skills in the introduction to this book.

At the beginning of a paediatric scenario a few minutes will normally be allocated to prepare for a child's arrival in the ED. It is expected that at the start of a paediatric scenario a candidate's preparation will include making certain fundamental calculations to be able to manage interventions smoothly.

Preparation time is short and it will make the best impression if the abilities of the assistants who are present are put to good use. This is a vital part of demonstrating team leadership skills and it is, therefore, advisable for the candidate to allocate roles to each individual present (while checking their skillset) and ask them to perform certain preparatory tasks while the candidate then performs the 'WETFLAG' calculations. A whiteboard is commonly provided for the candidate to demonstrate the calculations.

The **WETFLAG** calculations are based on using the patient's age to calculate an estimated weight. Using the age and estimated weight, interventions can be prepared which are specific to the child:

Weight (estimated in kg)	<12 months	(age in months /2) + 4
	1–5 years	(age in years × 2) + 8
	>6 years	(age in years × 3) + 7
Energy		4 J/kg body weight
Endotracheal Tube width		(age in years/4) + 4
Fluids		20 mL /kg
		10 mL/kg (in trauma)
Lorazepam		0.1 mg/kg
Adrenaline		0.1 mL/kg of 1:10,000 adrenaline (10 µg/kg)
Glucose		2 mL/kg of 10% dextrose

Certain other drugs may be required and if this can be anticipated from the scenario provided (e.g. a fitting child) the relevant calculations can also be made. Any additional treatments are dealt with in the relevant sections of this chapter.

Dealing with parents/guardians

Another element specific to paediatric scenarios is dealing with the arrival of a child's parent/guardian. During the scenario a parent or guardian may accompany the child or appear part of the way through the scenario. They may be very upset or anxious and have many questions.

As in real life the candidate will need to communicate with them sensitively while maintaining their primary focus on the unwell child. It is normally expected that a candidate will thoughtfully gain any relevant history and explain the unfolding events. In addition it is best practice to allocate a member of staff who can remain with the parent/guardian and provide them with information and support.

In paediatric stations where no family members arrive it is always worth asking the paramedics or patient if anyone is expected. This demonstrates to everyone that a candidate is aware of the need to involve parents/guardians as soon as it is possible and appropriate to do so.

Alternative scenarios

At the end of each of the following extended resuscitation stations we have included one or more alternative scenarios. These contain a brief summary of an alternative presentation and may contain guidance on what interventions will be required. This is to encourage candidates to consider the variety of scenarios they may be faced with and prepare for them.

Candidates should expand on this further and think of challenging scenarios that could appear in the exam. Having done so it is important to rehearse how each of those scenarios should be dealt with. The more alternatives that are practiced, the less chance there is of being confronted with a case the candidate feels unprepared for.

Suggested reading

Advanced Paediatric Life Support, 6th edn. Advanced Life Support Group, Manchester, UK 2016.

8.2 Paediatric anaphylaxis

Always consider this in the differential for patients with respiratory distress, shock or cardiac arrest. Signs may vary but should include:
- Skin – rash, itching, oedema
- Gastrointestinal – abdominal pain, diarrhoea, vomiting
- Respiratory – wheeze, stridor
- Circulatory – shock, cardiac arrest

As soon as anaphylaxis is suspected it is vital to not only assess/resuscitate the patient but to simultaneously consider what has caused it and if possible remove the precipitant (e.g. by stopping an infusion of antibiotics or removing a bee sting).

The management of anaphylaxis can be divided into interventions at each step of an ABCDE assessment. Current guidelines recommend the following treatments and doses for treating children with anaphylaxis. In severe cases, as well as medical therapy, airway management techniques and ventilatory support must be implemented as required.

Adrenaline

Adrenaline is the main drug required in anaphylaxis. It reverses peripheral vasodilation and bronchospasm. The indication for adrenaline is respiratory distress or shock. The dose of intramuscular adrenaline is 10 µg/kg. It is accepted that either 1:1,000 or 1:10,000 may be an appropriate concentration depending on the age of the child (the volume of 1:1,000 adrenaline may be so small in young children that it is difficult to prepare/measure). The required dose therefore equates to 0.1 mL/kg of 1:10,000 or 0.01 mL/kg of 1:1,000.

In cases where shock is resistant to adrenaline, crystalloid fluid boluses should also be given and the dose of adrenaline can be repeated.

For those patients with life-threatening features and no response to intramuscular (IM) adrenaline it should then be administered intravenously. The recommended dose is 1 µg/kg administered over one minute and titrated to response. An ongoing infusion may also be required.

Hydrocortisone and chlorphenamine

Both these drugs can be administered by slow intravenous injection or if necessary intramuscularly in doses based on the child's weight. The appropriate doses based on age are stated in **Table 8.2.1**.

Table 8.2.1 Anaphylaxis drug doses

Age	Hydrocortisone	Chlorphenamine
<6 months	25 mg	250 µg/kg
6 months–6 years	50 mg	2.5 mg
6 years–12 years	100 mg	5 mg
>12 years	200 mg	10 mg

Additional therapies

- **Airway:** Nebulised adrenaline may be used and repeated as necessary. If there is complete airway obstruction endotracheal intubation or a surgical airway should be performed
- **Breathing:** Both nebulised salbutamol and intravenous magnesium are appropriate adjuncts in cases where bronchospasm is a major feature. Bag ventilation may be required in apnoeic patients
- **Circulation:** In addition to intravenous adrenaline, coordination of good quality advanced life support will be required in cardiac arrest. Effective communication and team leadership must be practiced in advance

Scenario

You have been called to the resuscitation room by a student nurse. She has just taken a phone call from a panicked radiographer to say a colleague is rushing over a 5-year-old boy who became unwell in the X-ray waiting room. He was waiting for an X-ray of his ankle and was eating a cereal bar. He was then seen to vomit and become distressed. His parent could not be found. You have a short time to prepare before the child arrives. Manage the child appropriately.

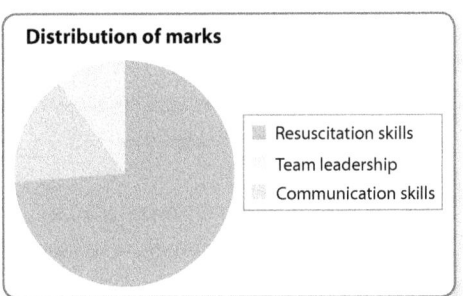

Distribution of marks
- Resuscitation skills
- Team leadership
- Communication skills

Initial patient observations

(As the patient is assessed during the scenario these observations will be provided by the nurse)

Appearance	Swollen face
Airway	Unable to speak, audible stridor, swollen tongue
Breathing	Respiratory rate 50 breaths per minute.
	Mild wheeze bilaterally, minimal air entry
	Oxygen saturations 78% on air. 92% on high flow oxygen
Circulation	Heart rate 150 beats per minute.
	Blood pressure 48/30 mmHg
	Capillary refill time 1 second
Disability	Glasgow coma score (GCS) 15. Looks exhausted, decreased tone
	Blood sugar 6.4 mmol/L
Exposure	Temperature 37°C. Red blotchy rash on body

Guidance on scenario

Initial intramuscular adrenaline, hydrocortisone and chlorphenamine (though the latter two drugs are less important in the acute setting) results in no improvement. If used nebulised adrenaline will reduce the stridor and improve the oxygen saturations but the benefit will wear off after a short period of time. If/when attempted intravenous access will not be possible and the candidate will need to insert an intraosseous (IO) needle. Repeat observations will not improve and a further dose of IM adrenaline will be required. Following two doses of IM adrenaline and crystalloid boluses the patient will not have responded. They will still be oxygenating well but have circulatory compromise. They will require an initial bolus of intravenous adrenaline.

Mark sheet	Achieved	Not achieved
Introduces self to student nurse		
Takes relevant history of events from student nurse		
Calls for additional help		
Confirms skills and experience of nurse		
Performs correct calculations		
Performs appropriate ABCDE assessment with basic interventions		
Identifies likely anaphylaxis		
Administers intramuscular adrenaline (if not already done so)		
Reassess and gives further IM adrenaline		
Gains intraosseous access		
Administers appropriate bolus of fluid at 20 mL/kg		
Additional appropriately dosed medical treatments		
Administers IV adrenaline in safe dose		
Delegates tasks to other staff appropriately		
When mother arrives is sensitive to her		
Elicits history of nut allergy in family members from mother		
Explains events and treatment to mother		
Delegates a staff member to support mother		
Contacts paediatrician/intensivist		
Global mark from examiner		
Global mark from parent		

An important part of managing the other individuals in the scenario is being prepared for different behaviour, being able to anticipate these and staying calm. Below are the types of instructions that may be provided to the other individuals. By considering them it is hoped the candidate may be better prepared for how staff or parents may behave in this and the following scenarios.

Instructions for student nurse

You are a competent final-year nurse on placement in the ED. You have just taken a phone call from a radiographer stating they are rushing a 5-year-old boy down the corridor to you. He was waiting for an ankle X-ray and was eating a cereal bar. He then became breathless and vomited once. His mother was looking for a toilet and now cannot be found.

You can perform routine observations but cannot administer medications. Perform any basic tasks as you are asked to. If asked to gain intravenous access or give medications explain that you cannot do so as you are not experienced enough.

When prompted state the observations/results as given in the initial patient observations.

Instructions for staff nurse

You are an experienced ED nurse and comfortable looking after children in the resuscitation area. Administer medications and perform any tasks as you are asked to. Explain that you are not comfortable to gain intravenous access in this child and ask the doctor to do this. If asked to contact a paediatrician or senior ED doctor, explain that you have done so and they are on their way.

When prompted state the observations/results as given in the initial patient observations.

Instructions for child's mother

You had taken your 5-year-old son Billy for an ankle X-ray as he twisted it badly. While in the X-ray waiting room you went to the toilet and when you returned you were told Billy had become very breathless and was in the ED.

When you arrive there the doctor is giving him adrenaline. You are upset and scared by all the fuss around Billy. You want to know what happened and if he is going to die. Answer any questions you are asked about Billy. He is fit and well with no medication or allergies. If not asked directly, state that both your husband and 7-year-old daughter have a nut allergy.

If you feel ignored, become more upset and anxious about Billy dying. If your questions and concerns are dealt with by the doctor or one of the nurses, become relaxed and focus on standing with Billy and supporting him.

Alternative scenario

Drug error: a 5-year-old boy was admitted for a dog bite on the forearm complicated by an open fracture. He is receiving intravenous antibiotics when he suffers an anaphylactic reaction to a penicillin-based antibiotic. His father had already stated he is allergic to penicillin and this was written on his medication chart. The nurse had accidentally prepared the wrong antibiotic and administered it. The nurse is extremely upset and unable to perform any ongoing care. The father is extremely angry. These matters must be dealt with appropriately while managing the child's cardiac arrest.

Suggested reading

Acute allergic reaction. Guidelines in Emergency Medicine Network, (on behalf of) Royal College of Emergency Medicine, London, 2009.
Anaphlyaxis. Clinical guideline 134. National Institute for Health and Care Excellence, London, 2011.
Angio-oedema and Anaphylaxis. Clinical knowledge summaries. National Institute of Health and Care Excellence. London, 2017.

8.3 Paediatric asthma

As always we recommend the initial assessment of an asthmatic patient should follow an ABCDE stepwise approach. During this assessment associated conditions (such as a pneumothorax) should be sought and excluded.

Oxygen

For patients with oxygen saturations below 94% supplementary oxygen should be administered via a face mask or nasal cannula. The flow rate can be titrated to maintain saturation between 94% and 98%.

Assessing severity

The severity of any asthma attack should be considered and classified. This guides what initial interventions are required and how quickly to escalate them. There are several similar lists of criteria dividing cases into mild, moderate, severe and life-threatening (Table 8.3.1). Note that though peak flow rate is useful it is unreliable in the acute setting as it is difficult to perform effectively.

In severe and life-threatening cases call for additional help early.

Always consider anaphylaxis and tension pneumothorax as differential or additional diagnoses which can easily be missed.

Table 8.3.1 Grading asthma severity

Acute severe asthma	Life-threatening asthma
SaO_2 <92%	SaO_2 <92%
Peak flow 33–50% of predicted	Peak flow <33% of predicted
Too breathless to talk/feed	Hypotension
Respiratory rate >30 breaths per minute (>5 years old)	Exhaustion confusion or coma
Respiratory rate >50 breaths per minute (2–5 years old)	
Heart rate >120 beats per minute (>5 years old)	Silent chest poor respiratory effort or cyanosis
Heart rate >130 beats per minute (2–5 years old)	

Initial treatment

Salbutamol is the first line treatment for asthma. In those with mild/moderate attacks with oxygen saturations over 92% on air, 10 puffs of a salbutamol inhaler via a spacer can be used, thus limiting side effects. In those with acute severe or life-threatening asthma, nebulised salbutamol should be used (5 mg >5 years old, 2.5 mg <5 years old). In cases where nebulised salbutamol is given, it should be used with ipratropium bromide (250 µg >2 years old, 125 µg <2 years old). In severe cases, nebulisers can be given continuously. Magnesium sulphate 150 mg can be added to nebulised salbutamol or ipratropium and may provide added benefit in severe asthma.

Oral prednisolone should also be given in a dose of 1 mg/kg or if oral medication cannot be tolerated intravenous hydrocortisone 4 mg/kg can be used.

Further management

In cases where children are not responding to initial treatment, further management includes a salbutamol bolus intravenously. This is 15 µg/kg up to a maximum dose of 250 µg (5 µg/kg under 2 years of age). Magnesium sulphate can also be administered in a dose of 40 mg/kg up to a maximum dose of 2 g. Aminophylline intravenously is another alternative. Following these a salbutamol (1–5 µg/kg/min) or aminophylline (1 mg/kg/h) infusion can also be considered.

Ventilatory support is indicated in those with poor respiratory effort, decreased consciousness, inadequate oxygen saturations or worsening arterial blood gases. These patients need their breathing assisted with bag-valve-mask ventilation while preparations are made to intubate them.

Assuming the patient's clinical condition allows it, each intervention should be followed by a period of time to assess the patient's response to it.

Investigations

Other than a full set of observations (which are mandatory), additional tests that should be considered are:
- Peak flow measurements to help assess the severity of the asthma attack and monitor the response to treatment
- Arterial blood gas (ABG) in cases where there is a poor response to initial treatment to assess ventilation. Serial ABGs may be useful
- Chest X-ray will be useful in cases with a poor response where pneumonia or a pneumothorax needs to be excluded – though for pneumothorax ultrasound will provide quicker information

Scenario

A phone call has alerted you that a 6-year-old boy is arriving with severe shortness of breath. There is an experienced staff nurse to help you in the resuscitation area. Prepare your team and manage the child.

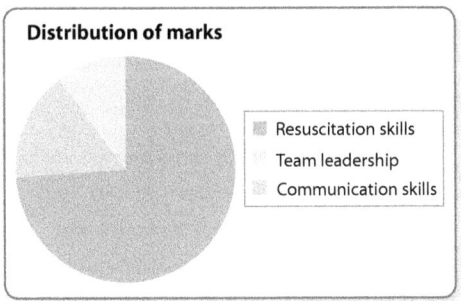

Initial patient observations

(As the patient is assessed during the scenario these observations will be provided by the nurse)

Airway	Patent
Breathing	Respiratory rate 50 breaths per minute, wheeze bilaterally, using accessory muscles, not speaking
	Oxygen saturations 84% on air. 92% on high flow oxygen

Circulation	Heart rate 140 beats per minute, 60/42 mmHg, capillary refill time 3 seconds
Disability	Glasgow coma score 14 (eyes 4, verbal 4, motor 6). Sweaty and tired
	Blood sugar 7.2 mmol/L
Exposure	Temperature 37°C

Arterial blood gas:

pH	7.15
pCO_2	7.0 kPa
PO_2	10 kPa
HCO_3	18 mmol/L
Base excess	−6 mEq/L
Lactate	4 mmol/L

Guidance on scenario

The child will arrive in respiratory distress and without an adult. If additional help is called a second competent nurse arrives but the paediatrician is unavailable. The paediatric intensivist is with another sick patient and will be coming soon.

The child will not be able to speak and has features of life-threatening asthma. The child does not respond to initial treatment with nebulisers. The candidate will be required to gain intravenous access and initiate appropriate intravenous treatment with steroids, magnesium and salbutamol or aminophylline. Towards the end of the scenario the child will be tiring, if a blood gas was sent earlier the results will now be available (as above). When the critical care doctor arrives they will want to try further bronchodilators. The candidate must explain why the patient needs intubation/ventilation and negotiate an appropriate plan.

Mark sheet	Achieved	Not achieved
Introduces self to staff nurse		
Confirms skills and experience of nurse		
Performs correct calculations		
Calls for additional help		
Performs appropriate ABCDE assessment with appropriate basic interventions		
Initiates appropriate bronchodilator therapy		
Recognises patient's poor response to treatment		
Contact/bleeps paediatric intensivist for urgent review		
Continues nebuliser therapy		
Gains intravenous access		
Takes blood and sends appropriate samples with venous or arterial blood gas		
Escalates medical therapy with appropriate medication in safe doses		
Interprets blood gas correctly		
Correctly states to intensivist that child needs intubation and ventilation as has responded poorly and is tiring		
Makes appropriate plan		
Requests a chest X-ray		

Cont'd...

Cont'd...

Mark sheet	Achieved	Not achieved
Delegates tasks to other staff appropriately		
Comments on need to contact/involve parents		
Global mark from examiner		
Global mark from parent		

Alternative scenarios

Agitated patient: the 12-year-old patient is scared, drowsy and uncooperative with their initial assessment or initial management. They are hypoxic and hypercapnic. They will require sedation followed by intubation and ventilation prior to additional medical therapy

Pneumothorax: a 13-year-old with asthma arrives with sign of severe asthma with minimal air entry bilaterally. They deteriorate after initial treatment and have no breath sounds on the left side of their chest with only minimal air entry contralaterally. They require immediate management of a pneumothorax as well as escalation of the medical therapy for the underlying asthma

Suggested reading

British Guideline on the Management of Asthma. British Thoracic Society and Scottish Intercollegiate Guidelines Network, 2016.

8.4 Paediatric advanced life support

On recognising an unresponsive child in a hospital setting, the first person present must call for help. The airway should then be opened using appropriate manoeuvres:
- Head tilt/chin lift (in those without a neck injury)
- Jaw thrust

Following these manoeuvres, if adequate respiration does not begin, five rescue breaths should be given. These breaths are adequate if the chest is seen to rise with each of them. If at this point normal breathing does not begin and there are no signs of life, a central pulse should be palpated (femoral, carotid or brachial). If a pulse is absent for 10 seconds or the child is bradycardic (heart rate <60 beats per minute) with no signs of life or reaction to ventilation, chest compressions should begin. Chest compressions should not be delayed if there is uncertainty about the presence of an adequate pulse or signs of life. Chest compressions should be over the lower half of the sternum and compress the chest by one third of its depth.

In infants chest compressions can be performed in two ways:
1. The hands can encircle the chest so the thumbs are placed on the lower half of the sternum. Compressions are then delivered by squeezing and flexion of the thumbs. This technique requires two rescuers as too much time is required for repositioning with only a single rescuer
2. The alternative which may be better suited to the ED setting is for chest compressions to be delivered by two fingers placed on the lower half of the sternum

In children the heel of either one or both hands can be used, depending on the force required to compress the chest adequately.

Current guidelines recommend compressions and ventilations are delivered in a 15:2 ratio. The desirable rate for compressions is 100–120 per minute.

Once good quality compressions and ventilations are underway the next priority is to ensure that both a definitive airway and intravenous (or intraosseous) access are secured. Once intubated, compressions can continue uninterrupted and ventilations can be given at a rate of 10–12 each minute.

On-going high quality basic life support as described above is essential and must continue in two minute cycles. However additional management depends on what rhythm is identified and whether it is non-shockable [asystole or pulseless electrical activity (PEA)] or shockable [pulseless ventricular tachycardia (VT) or ventricular fibrillation (VF)].

In all cases where ongoing resuscitation is required it is vital to establish a definitive airway, this should be done early but in the case of a shockable rhythm should not delay defibrillation. Current guidance is to spend no more than one minute attempting intravenous access before opting for intraosseous access. The team leader must ensure ventilations and chest compressions are well coordinated and performed to a high standard with minimal delays. Once a definitive airway is placed the ventilations and compressions can continue independently of each other.

Non-shockable rhythms

In these cases adrenaline should be given as soon as possible (intravenous or intraosseous in a dose of 0.1 mL/kg of 1:10,000 (10 µg/kg) adrenaline).

After each two-minute cycle of cardiopulmonary resuscitation a rhythm check should be performed and if the rhythm is consistent with a cardiac output a pulse check should also be performed. If the rhythm is asystole or there is no pulse a further two-minute cycle should begin. Adrenaline should be administered in the same dose every two cycles (or 4 minutes). During the two-minute cycles reversible causes for the cardiac arrest should be considered and treated as appropriate.

Shockable rhythms

If pulseless VT or VF are identified, a shock of 4 J/kg should be given using a defibrillator and followed (without delay) by continuation of chest compressions. After each two-minute cycle of cardiopulmonary resuscitation, a rhythm check should be performed, if the rhythm remains shockable, a further shock should be given in the same dose, again followed by chest compressions.

If cardiopulmonary resuscitation has continued until a third shock is delivered, it should be followed by both adrenaline (0.1 mL/kg of 1:10,000) and amiodarone (5 mg/kg) via the intravenous or intraosseous route. These drugs can both be given again after a fifth shock, and from this point on adrenaline should be given after every second cycle.

During the two-minute cycles reversible causes for the cardiac arrest should be considered and treated as appropriate.

Reversible causes of cardiac arrest

Detailed knowledge of the management for reversible causes of cardiac arrest is required. During ongoing cycles of resuscitation each reversible cause should be considered and excluded if irrelevant, or the correct treatment should be initiated.

Hypoxia	Toxins
Hypovolaemia	Tamponade (cardiac)
Hypo-/hyperkalaemia	Tension pneumothorax
Hypothermia	Thromboembolic

Scenario

You are expecting a 5-year-old boy to arrive via ambulance in two minutes. He has been pulled out of a swimming pool and is unresponsive. He was last seen five minutes earlier. Prepare your team for the child's arrival. You have two experienced staff nurses and a junior ED trainee to help you initially.

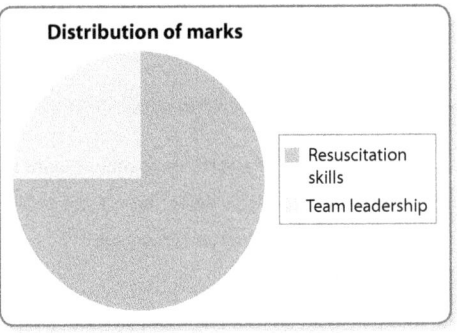

Distribution of marks
- Resuscitation skills
- Team leadership

Initial patient observations

(As the patient is assessed during the scenario these observations will be provided by the nurse)
Airway   Oropharyngeal airway, vomit on face and in airway

Breathing	Apnoeic
	Trachea central, percussion note resonant and equal bilaterally
	Bag-valve-mask ventilation good air entry bilaterally
Circulation	Absent central pulse
Disability	Glasgow coma score 3, pupils 3 mm equal
	Blood sugar 5.0 mmol/L
Exposure	Temperature 34°C

Guidance on scenario

On arrival the rhythm is pulseless electrical activity (PEA). The airway has been soiled with vomit and a definitive airway is required early. If help is called a paediatrician and a critical care doctor will arrive after the child has arrived. Intravenous access is unsuccessful and the candidate is expected to request intraosseus access. After several cycles of resuscitation, assuming the correct technique and doses of adrenaline have been used the patient will regain a pulse. If they have not been intubated they will have respiratory distress and be hypoxic until their airway is protected. A blood gas will not be available as it cannot be done with an intraosseous (IO) sample. They will also get progressively cooler and if they have not been warmed the candidate will be prompted to do so when they refer the patient to critical care.

The patient will also arrive with both their parents who are extremely distressed as the gate to their swimming pool had been left open. They repeatedly ask if their child is going to be OK.

Mark sheet	Achieved	Not achieved
Introduces self to team		
Confirms skills and experience of team and allocates roles		
Calls for paediatric cardiac arrest team		
Performs correct calculations		
Confirms cardiac arrest and performs rhythm check with defibrillator		
Commences cardiopulmonary resuscitation with correct ratio of compressions to ventilations, ensures good quality CPR		
Requests intraosseous access		
When anaesthetist arrives (if help called for) asks for child to be intubated as soon as possible		
After intubation allows asynchronous compressions and ventilations		
Asks for a naso-/oro-gastric tube to be inserted to decompress the stomach		
Correctly follows non-shockable algorithm		
Considers reversible causes		
Asks for blood gas if not done so earlier		
Recognises presence of a pulse and stops cardiopulmonary resuscitation		
Reassesses ABCDE appropriately		
Asks for patient to be warmed		

Cont'd...

Cont'd...

Mark sheet	Achieved	Not achieved
Hands patient over to intensivist when they arrive		
Makes appropriate plan for ongoing care		
Interacts with parents appropriately, delegates staff member		
Global mark from examiner		
Global mark from team		

Alternative scenario

Overdose: a 3-year-old girl has collapsed and been brought to the ED. She was staying at her grandparents house while her parents went away for the day. Her grandmother arrives with her. When assessed the rhythm is pulseless VT. After a single shock her rhythm has changed to a broad-complex tachycardia and she is acidotic. When her airway is assessed she vomits some of her grandfather's antidepressant tablets.

8.5 Management of a child choking on a foreign body

There is a clear algorithm for how to manage a situation where a child is choking on a foreign body. Some interventions depend on the size/age of the child, as described below.

If a foreign body is clearly visible in the mouth it should be removed. Caution should be used not to push any object further into the upper airway.

Three possible scenarios may arise. The child may have an:

- Effective cough: this is the case if they are able to speak or take a breath between coughs. In these cases, the child should be encouraged to continue coughing as this is the most effective way to relieve any obstruction. In many cases the obstruction will be cleared. If, however, the child deteriorates the following interventions should be performed
- Ineffective cough and normal conscious level: in this scenario the management involves five back blows followed by five chest or abdominal thrusts in an attempt to dislodge a foreign body. Five firm blows or thumps should given using the heel of the hand across the patient's back. In an infant the back blows can be delivered while they are lying prone across the caregiver's forearm or thigh. A larger child can be leaned across a lap or simply leaned forwards while standing

If the back blows have had no effect infants should receive five chest thrusts and older children five abdominal thrusts. Chest thrusts can be given with the infant supported by a forearm or thigh. They are delivered in the same way as chest compressions but at a rate of one per second. Abdominal thrusts for older children are performed with the child standing or kneeling. The caregiver moves behind the child and may need to kneel down themselves. They then place a fist below the xiphisternum and place their other hand on top of the fist. Both hands are then sharply pulled back and upwards into the abdomen. This is repeated five times. A similar procedure can also be performed with a child lying down on his/her back. These interventions should be repeated with regular assessments until the obstruction is relieved or the patient deteriorates and becomes unconscious

- Ineffective cough and decreased conscious level: in this scenario, the caregiver should call for help and again check the airway and, if possible, remove any foreign body. They should then administer five rescue breaths and begin cardiopulmonary resuscitation using 15 compressions to two ventilations

Scenario

A junior doctor who is new to your department has asked you how to deal with a child who chokes on a foreign body. Teach them how to manage such a scenario using the manikin provided.

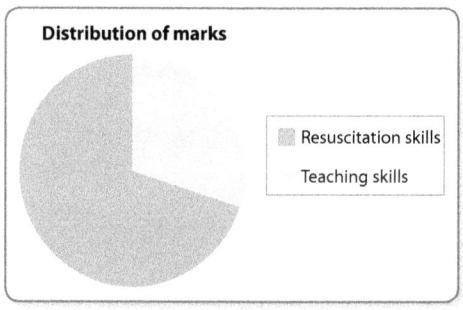

Distribution of marks
- Resuscitation skills
- Teaching skills

Guidance on scenario

This station requires knowledge of a simple algorithm that candidates should be familiar with. It requires knowledge of the recommended treatment and good teaching skills. As such it is a test of whether a candidate can adhere to basic principles and good teaching technique.

Mark sheet	Achieved	Not achieved
Introduces self to junior doctor		
Enquires about level of previous experience and knowledge		
Asks about anything specific they want to learn		
Sets and agrees on appropriate learning objectives		
Correctly explains management algorithm		
Demonstrates opening the airway and looking for a foreign body		
Demonstrates back blows		
Demonstrates abdominal thrusts		
Demonstrates chest thrusts		
Allows junior doctor to practice techniques		
Comments on and corrects junior doctor's technique where appropriate		
Checks if junior doctor has any questions or concerns		
Answers questions appropriately		
Agrees a plan for on-going learning		
Is non-judgemental and facilitates learning		
Global mark from examiner		
Global mark from junior doctor		

Alternative scenario

Inhaled toy: a 4-year-old girl was playing with a soft rubber toy. She took it from an older sibling and pretended to swallow it. She was seen to choke and collapse. On her way to hospital she has very noisy breathing and a weak cough. On arrival after initial manoeuvres to clear her airway she becomes hypoxic and has a pulseless electrical activity (PEA) cardiac arrest. The object cannot be cleared and she requires a needle cricothyroidotomy and ongoing advanced life support.

8.6 Paediatric seizures

Candidates must be familiar with an appropriate algorithm for the management of paediatric seizures in the acute setting such as that described in the Advanced Paediatric Life Support (APLS) guidelines. Specifically, this guideline is for children having tonic-clonic seizures in status epilepticus (i.e. seizure activity for 30 minutes without any episodes of recovery during that time). This forms the basis for the stepwise management of seizures in the ED and is outlined below (If seizure activity does not respond to treatment the clinician should proceed to the next management step):

1. **Benzodiazepines:** Once there has been seizure activity for 5 minutes these should be administered. If a patient arrives by ambulance it is possible that paramedics (or parents) may have already done this. The options are:
   - Intravenous lorazepam (0.1 mg/kg)
   - Buccal midazolam (0.5 mg/kg)
   - Rectal diazepam (0.5 mg/kg)
2. **Benzodiazepines:** If the child is still fitting 10 minutes after the initial dose was given it is advised that a further dose should be given. It is recommended that this is intravenous lorazepam. If no intravenous access has been gained it is recommended that the lorazepam is given by the intraosseous route. In total only two doses of benzodiazepine should be given
3. **Phenytoin/phenobarbitone:** If the child is still fitting 10 minutes after the second dose of benzodiazepine senior assistance must be called for. An infusion of phenytoin should be given in a dose of 20 mg/kg over 20 minutes. If the child is already taking phenytoin this should be 20 mg/kg of phenobarbitone over 20 minutes. Alternative drugs that may be used with specialist input are levetiracetam or sodium valproate

    Rectal paraldehyde can also be given while the phenytoin/phenobarbitone is being prepared. The dose is 0.4 mL/kg of paraldehyde mixed with an equal amount of olive oil (but this should not delay the phenytoin infusion)
4. **Thiopentone:** If 20 minutes have passed since the beginning of step 3 and the seizure is ongoing a rapid sequence induction with thiopentone will be required. A short acting muscle relaxant should be used. An alternative to RSI with thiopentone is to first try midazolam intravenously in a dose of 0.1 mg/kg, however, a decision to further delay RSI must be guided by the clinical state of the patient

Though terminating the seizure is a fundamental part of this scenario candidates must remember to consider and manage potential causes for the seizure. Common possibilities are hypoglycaemia, meningitis or poisoning. It would be easy for a candidate who knows the above algorithm to fail this scenario for forgetting to check a child's blood sugar or for not acting upon a fever and a purpuric rash. These considerations should be dealt with as part of a standard ABCDE evaluation of the patient. In addition if there is clinical evidence of raised intracranial pressure the child should be positioned with a 20° head up tilt, pCO_2 should be maintained in the normal range and hypertonic saline or mannitol may also be administered.

Scenario

You are notified that the paramedics are arriving soon with a 2-year-old child who has been fitting. They have just administered a dose of rectal diazepam but it has had no effect. You have a staff nurse and a junior doctor to help you.

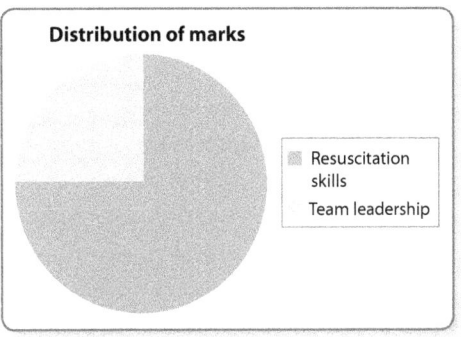

Distribution of marks
- Resuscitation skills
- Team leadership

Initial patient observations

On arrival in the department the chid has stopped fitting.
(As the patient is assessed during the scenario these observations will be provided by the nurse)

Airway	Self-maintained
Breathing	Respiratory rate 8 breaths per minute, oxygen saturations 90%
Circulation	Heart rate 150 beats per minute, capillary refill time 4 seconds
Disability	Unresponsive to pain, pupils equal and reactive, Blood sugar 2.2 mmol/L
Exposure	Temperature 39.6°C, mottled, no rash or injuries

Guidance on scenario

During the initial assessment the child will requiring bag valve mask ventilation. If the candidate requests or wants to perform an RSI they will be told the equipment and additional help are on the way. The child begins to twitch and then have a further tonic-clonic seizure. The child's mother becomes very upset and needs a member of staff to calm her. The child must be treated in a stepwise fashion to stop the ongoing fitting. Intraosseous access will be required. They must also be treated for sepsis and hypoglycaemia. If called early additional help will not arrive until later in the scenario. If the above management is delivered the patient will stop fitting. When the critical care doctor arrives the candidate is expected to handover and ask to proceed to RSI as the child is still requiring bag mask ventilation and only responsive to pain.

Also in this scenario the mother will be crying and asking questions, particularly when vascular access is gained.

Mark sheet	Achieved	Not achieved
Introduces self to staff nurse		
Confirms skills and experience of nurse and junior doctor		
Performs correct WETFLAG calculations		
Introduces self to parent and takes relevant history		

Cont'd...

Cont'd...

Mark sheet	Achieved	Not achieved
Administers high flow oxygen		
Performs appropriate initial assessment		
Asks additional doctor to perform bag valve mask ventilation		
Calls for additional help (paediatrician/intensivist)		
Gains intraosseous access when intravenous access unsuccessful		
Aspirates and flushes intraosseous needle to confirm position		
Administers intraosseous lorazepam in correct dose		
Administers phenytoin infusion in correct dose		
After seizure stops reassesses child appropriately		
Administers crystalloid fluid bolus		
Administers appropriate antibiotic in correct dose		
Corrects blood sugar		
Hands patient over to paediatrician/critical care		
Plans for RSI		
Explains events and treatment to mother		
Delegates a staff member to support mother		
Global mark from examiner		
Global mark from parent		

Alternative scenario

Head injury: a 6-year-old boy is being brought to the department having been found in the garden patio area fitting in the evening. He has no past medical history. On arrival he is still fitting. He is found to have a large haematoma in the right parieto-occipital area and a dilated unreactive pupil. He must have his airway protected with full neuroprotective measures initiated prior to transfer to the CT scanner.

8.7 Paediatric septic shock

The airway should be managed appropriately with high flow oxygen applied in all cases before proceeding with the standard ABCDE assessment.

The immediate management for shock is to gain intravenous or intraosseous access. Ideally take samples for baseline investigations including blood sugar, blood gas, full blood count, urea and electrolytes, liver function tests, C-reactive protein, clotting studies, group and save (or crossmatch if needed) and blood cultures.

Once access is gained normal saline boluses should be given in a volume of 20 mL/kg followed by reassessment for signs of improvement in the patient's haemodynamic state. If two such boluses have been given and signs of shock are ongoing a critical care assessment for intubation and ventilation must occur. In cases of cardiogenic shock or where raised intracranial pressure is suspected it is advisable to use fluid more cautiously in 10 mL/kg boluses.

An antibiotic such as cefotaxime 50–80 mg/kg should be administered by the intravenous or intraosseous route. Local guidelines may vary and candidates should be familiar with what they would use and be able to justify their choice. Under the age of 3 months add an antibiotic such as amoxicillin to cover for Listeria. Other suspected conditions will require alternative appropriate antibiotics (toxic shock syndrome, neutropenia, hospital acquired infection).

Hypoglycaemia and sepsis often go hand in hand, and hypoglycaemia (blood sugar below 3 mmol/L) must be excluded. If the patient is hypoglycaemic this should be corrected by 2 mL/kg boluses of 10% dextrose.

In suspected septic shock it is advisable to call for additional help and paediatric specialist support early. Further management may require central access, inotropes and mechanical ventilation. These procedures are always safest if planned in advance by staff who have had time to prepare, rather than in a rush once it is clear the patient is not responding adequately to treatment.

Scenario

You have been informed that a 3-year-old child who is very drowsy is arriving by ambulance. Prepare to manage the child in your resuscitation area. There are two experienced staff nurses and a junior doctor available to help you.

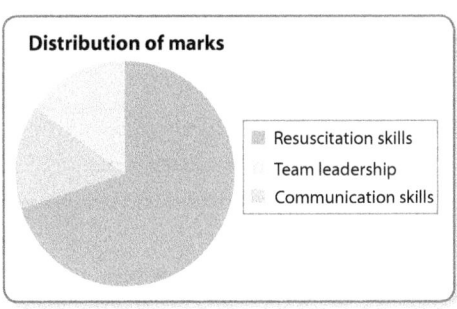

Initial patient observations

(As the patient is assessed during the scenario these observations will be provided by the nurse)

Airway	Maintained
Breathing	Respiratory rate 60 breaths per minute. Clear lung fields bilaterally Oxygen saturations 90% on air

Circulation	Heart rate 180 beats per minute. Capillary refill time 5 seconds
	Blood pressure 54/32 mmHg
Disability	Responsive to pain (crying), decreased tone.
	Blood sugar 2 mmol/L
Exposure	Temperature 39°C. Purpuric rash on legs

Guidance on scenario

A basic (but thorough) ABCDE assessment without any omissions is vital to pass this station. If the candidate does not ask about blood sugar or temperature, these vital facts will not be provided to them. Likewise if the child is not exposed the rash will not be seen. During the initial assessment prior to the first bolus of fluid the patient will no longer have a pulse. The pulse will return after two cycles of advanced life support and a dose of adrenaline. The child's physiology will further improve after two boluses of crystalloid. Additional treatment for sepsis and hypoglycaemia is also required prior to the arrival of a critical care team.

Mark sheet	Achieved	Not achieved
Introduces self to nurses		
Confirms skills and experience of nurses		
Performs correct calculations		
Takes relevant history of events from paramedics		
Checks patient's airway		
Performs appropriate initial assessment with basic interventions		
Recognises nature of illness and calls for paediatric help early		
Coordinates good quality CPR in correct ratio		
Gains intravenous or intraosseous access and sends appropriate blood samples		
Administers adrenaline in correct dose		
Reassesses after return of pulse		
Gives bolus of normal saline		
Checks blood sugar and corrects it appropriately		
Gives correct dose of appropriate antibiotics		
Reassesses appropriately and gives further normal saline bolus		
Requests critical care support		
Delegates tasks to other staff appropriately		
Hands over to critical care doctor and makes appropriate plan		
When father arrives is sensitive to him		
Explains events and treatment to father		
Delegates a staff member to support father		
Global mark from examiner		
Global mark from mother		

Alternative scenario

Toxic shock syndrome: a 14-year-old girl arrives in the department. She is febrile, drowsy, hypotensive and has an unusual rash. The scenario will suggest toxic shock. The collateral history from her mother is that is healthy and growing normally and recently started having periods. She must be treated along normal sepsis guidelines, will require critical care support and must have a tampon removed.

8.8 Paediatric supraventricular tachycardia

Supraventricular tachycardia (SVT) arises relatively commonly in early childhood and can present with haemodynamic instability and signs of shock. Particularly in young children who cannot describe any symptoms it may be tolerated for a long time. Once myocardial oxygenation and function is compromised there may be a seemingly quick deterioration. SVT is a regular narrow complex tachycardia. It can be differentiated from sinus tachycardia by several characteristics:

- Unlike sinus tachycardia SVT commonly results in a heart rate over 220
- During SVT there is no beat-to-beat variation in the heart rate
- The presence in the history of other features likely to cause shock is more likely to result in sinus tachycardia than SVT. Immediate management involves moving the child to the resuscitation area, calling for additional help, applying high flow oxygen, monitoring and beginning an ABCDE assessment

Initial treatment for SVT should be vagal stimulation to attempt cardioversion. This can be done by:

- Unilateral carotid sinus massage
- A Valsalva manoeuvre such as blowing into a syringe to move the plunger
- Stimulating the diving reflex by immersing an infant's face in ice cold water for 5–10 seconds

If these procedures are ineffective or the child is displaying signs of shock the next treatment option is intravenous adenosine through a large peripheral cannula followed by a flush of normal saline. The dose of adenosine is initially 100 µg/kg. If unsuccessful, further incremental boluses can be given at 2-minute intervals of 200 µg/kg, 300 µg/kg (maximum dose if under 1 month old) and then 400–500 µg/kg up to a maximum dose of 12 mg.

In a shocked child if intravenous access is likely to cause delay or proves difficult, direct current (DC) cardioversion is the treatment of choice. Children responsive to pain should be sedated or anaesthetised. Initially a synchronised shock of 1 J/kg should be delivered. If unsuccessful this should be repeated at 2 J/kg. If unsuccessful this should be repeated after intravenous amiodarone in a dose of 5 mg/kg.

In a stable child where adenosine has been unsuccessful the case should be discussed with an appropriate specialist before further treatment.

Scenario

You are informed that an ambulance is arriving with an unwell 1-year-old and his mother. The crew has said the child appears drowsy, pale and clammy. You have an experienced staff nurse, a nursing student and a junior ED trainee available to help you. Prepare to manage the child on arrival.

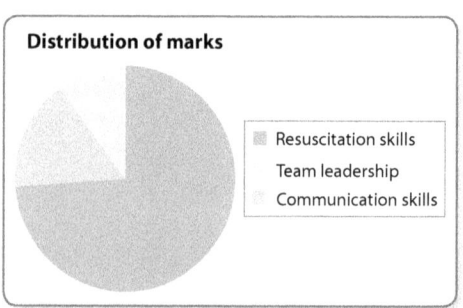

Distribution of marks
- Resuscitation skills
- Team leadership
- Communication skills

Initial patient observations

(As the patient is assessed during the scenario these observations will be provided by the nurse)

Airway	Maintained
Breathing	Respiratory rate 50 breaths per minute.
	Clear lung fields bilaterally
	Oxygen saturations 96% on air. 100% on high flow oxygen
Circulation	Heart rate 250 beats per minute (**Figure 8.8.1**).
	Blood pressure 65/30 mmHg
	Capillary refill time 2 seconds
Disability	Glasgow coma score 15. Alert
	Blood sugar 4.8 mmol/L
Exposure	Temperature 37°C. Mottled skin

Figure 8.8.1 Initial rhythm strip.

Guidance on scenario

The patient is suffering from SVT (a rhythm strip will be provided to the candidate). Initially the child is haemodynamically stable but the rhythm does not respond to vagal manoeuvres or adenosine. The child will deteriorate and the candidate must recognise this and proceed to synchronised DC cardioversion. The patient will cardiovert to sinus rhythm after a second synchronised shock. Further assistance will not be available until the end of the scenario. A specialist will arrive towards the end of the scenario and take a handover for the child. If back in sinus rhythm at this point they will ask if the child can be observed in the ED and then be discharged home.

The child's mother will be present throughout the scenario. She will initially be distressed but if managed appropriately will settle and be anxious but cooperative and asking occasional questions.

Mark sheet	Achieved	Not achieved
Introduces self to team		
Calls for additional help in resuscitation room		
Confirms skills and experience of team and allocates roles		
Performs correct calculations		
Takes handover from crew		
Reassures mother but is not distracted by her distress		
Performs appropriate initial assessment with basic interventions		

Cont'd...

Cont'd...

Mark sheet	Achieved	Not achieved
Asks for defibrillator and rhythm strip		
States likely diagnosis is SVT		
Attempts vagal stimulation/diving reflex		
Gains intravenous access (takes samples for appropriate blood tests including a blood gas and a blood sugar)		
Attempts cardioversion with adenosine in correct doses		
Notes deterioration in child, reassesses and prepares for DC cardioversion		
Uses appropriate safe sedation		
Administers synchronised shocks safely and at correct energy		
Reassesses patient appropriately, recognises cardioversion to sinus rhythm		
Hands patient over to paediatrician when they arrive		
Does not agree to facilitate discharge from ED		
Communicates sensitively with mother		
Explains events and treatment to mother		
Delegates a staff member to support mother		
Global mark from examiner		
Global mark from team		

Alternative scenario

Cardiac arrest: the above child has been in SVT for a prolonged period of time. They decompensate rapidly into a pulseless broad complex tachycardia. The parents are present and must have the situation explained while the team achieve IO access, perform CPR and deliver defibrillation.

8.9 Paediatric trauma

Trauma cases should be managed with a standard ABCDE approach with appropriate interventions at each step. This stepwise approach minimises the possibility of a candidate missing a vital step or intervention. Depending on the size and skillset of the trauma team provided it is, however, completely acceptable to ask colleagues to perform different tasks simultaneously. Details on how to perform relevant procedures have been discussed in chapter 6 and many of the principles related to trauma management are also discussed in chapter 9.

In terms of fluid resuscitation in paediatric trauma, current guidelines advise warm crystalloid fluid or blood should be given in boluses of 10 mL/kg. This is to prevent sudden increases in blood pressure which may displace clots and lead to additional blood loss. Depending on the nature of the injuries it may be appropriate to use blood products from the beginning of resuscitation efforts. Once 20 mL/kg of crystalloid has been administered, blood should be used for further resuscitation efforts. Tranexamic acid should be administered in a dose of 15 mg/kg.

Appropriate analgesia must also be given. The correct dose of morphine is 80 μg/kg below 1 year old and then 100 μg/kg. This dose should be titrated to the child's pain and used with caution in patients with a decreased level of consciousness. Fentanyl, ketamine, paracetamol and nitrous gas may all be useful in the correct clinical setting. Femoral nerve block should also be considered when appropriate.

In cases where significant injuries are suspected an appropriate trauma team should be called early. They can assist with early interventions and help plan for any further investigations and treatment the patient may need.

Scenario

An ambulance is shortly arriving with a 7-year-old girl who has been hit by a car. She has multiple injuries. Prepare your team to manage the patient. There is one ED staff nurse available to assist you.

Distribution of marks
- Resuscitation skills
- Team leadership

Initial patient observations

(As the patient is assessed during the scenario these observations will be provided by a team member)

Airway	Oropharyngeal airway
Breathing	Respiratory rate 40 breaths per minute.
	Oxygen saturations 76% on air. 88% on high flow oxygen
	Decreased air entry on right side. Hyper-resonant to percussion
	Trachea deviated to left
Circulation	Heart rate 140 beats per minute. Blood pressure 65/60 mmHg.

	Capillary refill time 4 seconds
	Abdomen soft, non-tender. No guarding
	Pelvis stable. Deformed and swollen right thigh
Disability	Glasgow coma score 7 (eyes 2, verbal 2, motor 4)
	Right frontal haematoma, right pupil 5 mm, left pupil 3 mm both reactive
	Blood sugar 6.4 mmol/L
Exposure	Temperature 35°C.

Guidance on scenario

The staff members available in this scenario are competent at many tasks but need to be directed as to what needs doing. The patient has a decreased level of consciousness with a head injury and a tension pneumothorax. Achieving a definitive airway and decompressing the right side of the chest are both priorities. If a right thoracostomy is performed without intubation and positive pressure ventilation commenced within a few seconds the patient will arrest. The patient's observations will improve further once they receive 10 mL/kg of blood and have their femur placed in a traction splint.

If performed FAST will not demonstrate any free fluid. If these tasks are all completed the patient's observations will stabilise. The candidate will then be expected to initiate neuroprotective measures and agree a plan with the neurosurgical specialist.

Mark sheet	Achieved	Not achieved
Introduces self to team		
Calls for additional help in resuscitation room/trauma call		
Confirms skills of team members and allocates roles		
Performs correct calculations		
Takes appropriate handover from paramedics		
Facilitates appropriate primary survey with basic interventions		
Ensures intravenous/intraosseous access and appropriate blood sampling		
Requests early RSI and definitive airway		
Coordinates right chest thoracostomy with RSI – must use chest drain if thoracostomy significantly earlier than RSI		
Reassesses and allows completion of primary survey		
Administers bolus of crystalloid or blood in appropriate volume		
Requests traction splint for suspected femoral fracture		
Administers mannitol or hypertonic saline in appropriate dose		
Commences neuroprotective measures		
Asks for FAST scan		
Reassesses patient appropriately		
Plans for appropriate imaging of patient		
Contacts neurosurgical specialist and makes plan		
Delegates tasks to other staff appropriately		
Agrees further plan for patient with specialists		
Global mark from examiner		
Global mark from team		

Alternative scenario

Motorcross accident: a 12-year-old boy on a motorbike has collided with a tree. He was 'messing around' after a racing event so had taken his helmet off. He has facial injuries which will require a surgical airway. He has bruising across his abdomen and a deformed right femur. He will require treatment for haemorrhagic shock and a femoral splint before transfer to CT.

8.10 Neonatal duct dependent circulation

Following birth the ductus arteriosus normally closes. In cases where it does not close there is significant circulatory compromise. However in cases where there is congenital disease the result can be a duct dependent circulation. Affected neonates present with signs of compromise when the ductus arteriosus begins to close. These congenital anomalies can be divided into two groups which will present differently:

1. Duct dependent systemic blood flow (or left sided obstructive lesions including aortic stenosis, coarctation of the aorta, transposition of the great arteries). These children present with breathlessness, inability to feed, a grey discolouration and cardiogenic shock. As a result of poor organ perfusion they have a severe metabolic acidosis
2. Duct dependent pulmonary blood flow (or lesions obstructing pulmonary flow including pulmonary stenosis/atresia and tetralogy of Fallot). These cases present with cyanosis that does not correct with additional oxygen, though they display relatively little respiratory distress until they decompensate

These patients are often in shock and profoundly unwell. The initial management will need to address all causes of shock/cyanosis including investigations and treatment for sepsis. Certain features, however, will suggest a cardiac cause for their presentation:

- Tachycardia disproportionate to respiratory effort
- Cyanosis that does not correct with supplementary oxygen
- Raised jugular venous pressure
- Gallop rhythm
- Enlarged liver
- Cardiomegaly on chest X-ray
- Absent femoral pulses

Prostaglandin (not to be confused with prostacyclin) is given by infusion and will prevent the ductus arteriosus from closing. It can, however, cause hypotension and apnoea so suitable specialists should be involved in the care from as early as possible. It is not unusual for these patients to need intubation and mechanical ventilation. Prostaglandin will prevent duct closure and stabilise the patient until diagnostic investigations and definitive management can be arranged.

Scenario

An ambulance is shortly arriving with a 4-day-old girl who is pale and 'appears unwell'. You are in the resuscitation room with one experienced staff nurse. Prepare for and manage the patient.

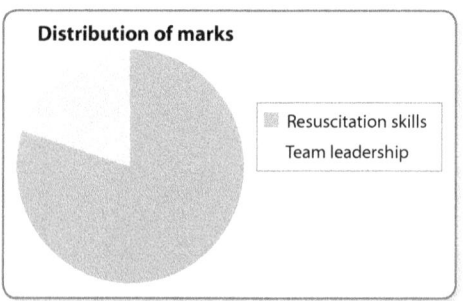

Distribution of marks: Resuscitation skills, Team leadership

Initial patient observations

(As the patient is assessed during the scenario these observations will be provided by the nurse)

Airway	Clear
Breathing	Respiratory rate 60 breaths per minute. Good air entry bilaterally
Circulation	Heart rate 180 beats per minute Capillary refill time 4 seconds Absent femoral pulses
Disability	Floppy, responsive to pain Blood sugar 4.2 mmol/L
Exposure	Temperature 36.4°C Pale with grey lips, no rash

Guidance on scenario

The candidate may recognise that the child is an age when a congenital abnormality may present. There will be no improvement with oxygen, fluid and antibiotics. At this point, the candidate is expected to recognise the diagnosis and initiate the correct treatment. Without this the patient will fail to improve. Specialist input is required early to guide the correct dose and critical care should also be called as there is a risk of the patient deteriorating further.

Mark sheet	Achieved	Not achieved
Introduces self to nurse		
Confirms skills and experience of nurse		
Calls for paediatric specialist help		
Performs correct calculations		
Takes initial history from paramedics		
Checks airway and applies oxygen		
Assesses breathing (auscultates, checks respiratory rate, checks oxygen saturation)		
Assesses circulation (heart rate, capillary refill time)		
Checks bilateral brachial and femoral pulses		
Gains intravenous/intraosseous access and sends appropriate samples		
Gives appropriate crystalloid bolus		
Gives appropriate antibiotics		
Assesses disability and exposes patient		
Reassesses patient – recognises no response to oxygen or fluid		
Considers potential diagnoses- calls for help from paediatric cardiology and critical care		
Asks for chest X-ray		
Asks for prostaglandin infusion		
Aware of side effects of prostaglandin infusion		
Hands patient over to paediatrician when they arrive		
Makes appropriate plan for ongoing care		
Global mark from examiner		
Global mark from nurse		

Alternative scenario

There are few alternatives to this scenario. Whatever subtle variations there may be, the expectation will be to treat initially for shock or hypoxia and once the patient is seen not to respond the diagnosis can be made with appropriate treatment initiated.

8.11 Newborn baby resuscitation

It is vital that an emergency physician is aware of the guidelines for resuscitating a newborn baby. Though it is not a regular event for a child to be born in the ED it is not unheard of, but few staff will be familiar with the necessary steps to take.

The first step, if there are any concerns is always to call for help. Following this the immediate priority is to dry the baby and keep it warm by wrapping it in a towel and providing a hat and a radiant heater. When a baby is allowed to become cold it is at greater risk of hypoglycaemia, acidosis and not surviving. If the baby is in need of resuscitation the cord can be clamped and cut early. Otherwise this can be delayed until after complete delivery has been achieved.

Three areas of the child's status must be assessed to decide on the requirement for resuscitation:

1. **Breathing**: It is normal for a newborn to take 60–90 seconds to establish a normal breathing pattern. If they remain apnoeic or gasping with ineffective breathing initial resuscitative measures are required
2. **Heart rate**: This should be over 100 beats per minute. It is best assessed by auscultation over the cardiac apex or using an appropriate oxygen saturation monitor (with the trace correlated to clinical findings)
3. **Tone**: Inadequate tone/floppiness suggests the child may have become hypoxic or be unconscious

Colour is not part of the formal assessment however can be representative of the degree of perfusion and oxygenation

When there are no concerns in these areas a baby can be considered to be healthy. If there are any concerns (e.g. abnormal respiration, a slow heart rate, reduced tone or a bluish discolouration) the baby should be stimulated gently. If they do not respond their airway should be opened and cleared. If there is still no adequate response the baby should receive five inflation breaths to stimulate lung expansion and breathing. If the child is initially apnoeic or has an absent pulse or bradycardia, and is blue, pale or floppy their airway should be opened and five inflation breaths delivered.

The airway should be managed with the head in a neutral position. This may require a towel under the shoulders and neck and may require a jaw thrust. Suction should also be used to clear any secretions.

The initial five breaths delivered to a baby are called inflation breaths. Their purpose is to assist with alveolar expansion and the replacement of lung fluid with air. These are sustained breaths lasting 2–3 seconds each. They should ideally be delivered using a pressure limiting device and soft mask that covers the nose and mouth. As the first of the five breaths displaces lung fluid the chest may not expand. If the heart rate rises and is maintained over 100 beats per minute these breaths have been successful. Ventilatory support can continue at 30–40 breaths per minute until regular breathing has been established. Initial resuscitation should normally be performed with air due to toxic effects of excess oxygen.

Chest compressions should be started if the heart rate remains slow (<60 beats/minute) after 30 seconds of ventilation. These are best delivered by encircling the baby in both hands so the thumbs lie on the baby's sternum and the fingers on the baby's back.

Compressions should then be delivered to one-third of the depth of the chest in a ratio of three compressions to one ventilation. The heart rate should then be reassessed every 30 seconds. Once it is above 60 beats per minute and rising, compressions can be stopped with the ventilations continuing until effective breathing begins or the child is placed on a ventilator.

If there has been no improvement and prior to administering drugs airway, breathing and chest compressions should all be reassessed and optimised. Drugs are to be used if there is still an inadequate heart rate after lung inflation and chest compressions; they should be administered by an umbilical venous line (or an intraosseous line if needed). The umbilical vein is the single large dilated vein next to two constricted arteries.

- Adrenaline can be given as per the normal paediatric resuscitation guidelines in a dose of 0.1 mL/kg of 1:10,000 adrenaline (approximately every 4 minutes)
- Sodium bicarbonate should be given in cases with no cardiac output or a sustained profound bradycardia in a dose of (1–2 mmol/kg) 2–4 mL/kg of 4.2% solution
- If hypoglycaemia is suspected 2.5 mL/kg of 10% dextrose should be given followed by an infusion of 10% dextrose
- Naloxone (200 µg intramuscularly) is not to be used for acute resuscitation. It can however be considered if there are concerns regarding respiratory depression in cases where the mother received opiates prior to delivery

Scenario

You are informed an ambulance is arriving in a few minutes with a woman who is about to give birth. One of your colleagues is going to assess the mother when they arrive and you will lead a team to assess the baby. You have an experienced nurse and junior doctor to help you.

Initial patient observations

(As the patient is assessed during the scenario these observations will be provided by the nurse)

Airway	Clear
Breathing	Respiratory rate 0
	No respiratory effort
Circulation	Auscultated heart rate 40 beats per minute
Disability	Unresponsive/floppy
	Blood sugar 3.0 mmol/L
Exposure	Temperature 36°C

Guidance on scenario

The candidate is expected to call for help early and a paediatric registrar and critical care doctor will arrive.

The neonatal life support algorithm must be commenced and run appropriately with the candidate demonstrating the required knowledge. The child will have meconium in their mouth. They will require brief suctioning, on-going ventilation, umbilical vein cannulation, chest compressions, a dose of adrenaline and dextrose. With each of these steps of treatment they will show gradual signs of responding but still require on-going management.

Mark sheet	Achieved	Not achieved
Introduces self to team		
Confirms skills and experience of team and delegates tasks		
Calls for paediatric arrest team		
Prepares appropriate equipment		
Performs correct calculations		
Dries baby and makes efforts to keep it warm		
Cuts cord (already clamped by paramedics)		
Performs appropriate initial assessment		
Delivers five initial inflation breaths		
Reassesses baby		
Continues ventilatory support		
Confirms chest rising		
Commences chest compressions with acceptable technique		
Knows correct ratio of compressions to ventilations		
Coordinates vascular access, states technique when prompted		
Checks blood sugar		
Administers adrenaline		
Makes appropriate plan for ongoing care		
Delegates tasks to other staff appropriately		
Global mark from examiner		
Global mark from team		

Alternative scenario

As with the previous section there are very limited variations to how this scenario could be presented. The scenario and management are for a very specific patient group and there are very limited variations in how the case can be managed. Candidates should ensure they are familiar with the algorithm and all associated procedures.

8.12 Paediatric stridor

Knowledge of the causes, assessment criteria, and emergency management will be expected when faced with a scenario of paediatric airway obstruction (**Table 8.12.1**).

A 'pre-alert' message may be provided. As described in the introduction to this chapter you should make any necessary calculations and then brief and organise your team. If it is clear that further help will be needed, make the decision to call for help early. Communicate with the team, patient and parent often to ensure clarity and confidence as to what is happening.

A working diagnosis and management plan should be clarified as early as possible based on the presentation, clinical findings and any history that may be provided. Sharing this knowledge will mean the whole team have a shared understanding of what the problem is, and what tasks are required of them. The necessary interventions can then be made, followed by reassessment and further escalation as required.

Table 8.12.1 Differentiating features of common causes of stridor

Differentiating feature	Croup (common)	Epiglottitis (rare)	Foreign body obstruction (rare)
Onset	Acute	Acute	Sudden
Typical age	6 months to 5 years	2–7 years	Any age, typically younger
History	Runny nose, barking cough	Fever, sore throat, dysphagia	Parent or care giver may have seen or heard the incident
Stridor	Harsh	Soft, may be absent	May be absent
General condition	May be alert or show signs of respiratory distress	'Toxic' – pale, poorly perfused, drooling and febrile	Unwell, distressed, coughing

Approach to epiglottitis

The priority is to arrange for the airway to be secured quickly and safely. Contact an anaesthetist and alert theatres early to arrange a gas induction. In the meantime avoid distressing the child because agitation and crying may precipitate airway obstruction. Likewise do not place tongue depressors or instruments in the mouth. Be prepared for progression of the condition and sudden deterioration. Have the difficult airway trolley at hand: A needle cricothyroidotomy may be required if the child cannot be ventilated.

Steps/interventions to perform as appropriate

- Supplemental oxygen may be necessary regardless of the cause. This may be provided by a non-rebreathe mask or to drive a nebuliser. Depending on the child's age and level of distress it may be appropriate to simply hold the mask in front of them and waft the oxygen or nebuliser as applying it to their face may distress them further
- Assessing the severity of the underlying illness depends on work of breathing and how 'toxic' the child appears (how deranged their physiology is). Is there any stridor at rest or only when distressed? Is the child alert, interacting and engaging in play, or exhausted and quiet?

- Drugs
  - Nebulised adrenaline – use 1:1,000 concentration (i.e. 1 mg/mL) in a dose of 0.4 mL/kg, maximum 5 mL at a time. This starts to work within minutes and lasts for approximately 2 hours. The need for repeated doses may indicate higher severity of illness
  - Nebulised budesonide – 2–4 mg nebulised budesonide starts to act within 30 minutes.
  - Oral steroids – dexamethasone 0.15–0.6 mg/kg (maximum 8 mg) or prednisolone 1 mg/kg if dexamethasone is not available. If the child vomits and does not tolerate any steroids, nebulised steroids should be adequate
  - Antibiotics are not indicated for suspected croup. Though necessary, they are not an immediate priority in epiglottitis
- Airway intervention – Candidates need to ensure a secure airway. The probability of requiring an emergency airway intervention is higher in suspected epiglottitis
- Chest X-ray and lateral neck soft tissue X-ray – consider imaging if there is a wider differential diagnosis, such as foreign body obstruction, pneumonia or a retropharyngeal abscess, and the patient is well enough to tolerate the procedure

Scenario

You are informed that an ambulance is bringing in 14-month-old who has a cough. Her parents called the ambulance because they were worried about her noisy breathing.

Assess the child and perform interventions as necessary. You have a trained nurse with you.

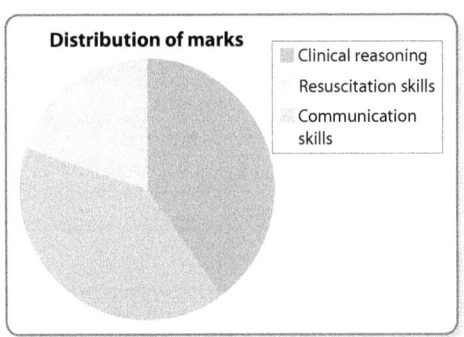

Initial patient observations

(As the patient is assessed during the scenario these observations will be provided by the nurse.)

Airway	Stridor
Breathing	Respiratory rate 60 breaths per minute. Bilaterally decreased air entry
	Tracheal tug and intercostal recession. Oxygen saturations 88% on air
Circulation	Heart rate 150 beats per minute
	Capillary refill time 4 seconds
Disability	Alert but looking tired
Exposure	Temperature 37.4°C

Guidance on scenario

There are no features suggestive of epiglottitis and the cough will be described as 'harsh' or 'barking'. The diagnosis will not be certain. The patient will vomit if given oral steroids. They will tolerate nebulised adrenaline which has no significant effect. They will begin to tire and their work of breathing will increase while their oxygen saturations begin to slowly drop. The child will require intubation. Though a plan should be made for unsuccessful intubation the procedure will be successful. Additional medical help will be available if called early. As well as providing the appropriate care, the candidate will have to address the mother's concerns.

Mark sheet	Achieved	Not achieved
Introduces self to nurse		
Confirms skills and experience of nurse		
Performs correct calculations		
Performs appropriate initial assessment with basic interventions		
Administers steroid in appropriate dose		
Administers nebulised adrenaline in appropriate dose		
Administers nebulised steroid when child vomits		
Recognises lack of response – calls for additional help if not already done		
Completes initial assessment and reassessment		
Coordinates safe RSI and intubation		
Administers appropriate antibiotics		
Obtains appropriate imaging (Chest X-ray and possible neck X-ray)		
Makes further plan for management		
Explains events and treatment to mother		
Global mark from examiner		
Global mark from parent		

Instructions for parent

Maya has been unwell for last 2 days. It started with a fever and cough. She did not have her dinner and was crying in the evening. You gave her paracetamol. She managed to go to sleep after that. She started coughing 2 hours after going to bed and seemed very distressed.

Maya was born at 30 weeks' gestation. She is relatively fit and well. Her immunisations are up to date. She goes to a day care centre three times a week.

You are worried for your daughter and want to know what will happen next. You are reassured if the doctor or a member of staff explain what they are thinking and doing. If you are not spoken to you remain very upset throughout the scenario and keep interrupting the team.

Alternative scenario

Epiglottitis: the child arrives and is febrile, sitting up and drooling. They are hypotensive but conscious. There is no theatre available for the child as an emergency laparotomy just began. A judgement call must be made as to when to intervene. The candidate is expected to facilitate cautious early assessment and coordinate immediate assessment by the paediatric, anaesthetic and ENT teams. The patient will deteriorate requiring immediate airway management in the ED.

Chapter 9

Trauma presentations

9.1 Introduction
9.2 Burns
9.3 Cardiac tamponade and ED thoracotomy
9.4 Haemothorax and pneumothorax
9.5 Head injury
9.6 Trauma in pregnancy
9.7 Haemorrhagic shock
9.8 Threatened airway
9.9 Traumatic cardiac arrest

9.1 Introduction

A trauma-related resuscitation scenario is very likely to appear in the exam. The ABCDE style approach as taught on traditional trauma courses, along with organising and leading a trauma team, should be well practised in advance. As well as reading this introduction candidates are encouraged to read and reflect on the discussion of non-technical skills in the introduction to this book.

The team leader's role is very important when managing trauma teams. The team leader should prepare the team for the arrival and management of the patient, take confident decisions, direct interventions and liaise with specialties to arrange definitive management. They are also responsible for ensuring the trauma team do not get distracted by their individual roles but work together to expedite definitive life-saving treatment.

Though it is true that in real life an ABCDE approach oversimplifies how interventions are performed in real-life trauma situations, the emphasis for the candidate is to demonstrate a logical and methodical approach. Candidates, and senior clinicians in general, must be aware of the cognitive load they place on themselves and be their own judge of how many actions should happen at once. The two priorities are to assess the patient providing life-saving interventions as quickly as possible but secondly to ensure this is done as accurately as possible at the first attempt. A balance between thoughtful clinical assessment and speed is required. If a large competent trauma team is available, we recommend distributing roles so tasks like airway assessment, application of monitoring, primary survey and IV access happen simultaneously. However, it is still helpful to talk through the findings in an ABCDE style to ensure nothing is missed, and then return to this after each intervention and if the patient deteriorates. In cases where the team available is smaller it will be more appropriate to use a more stepwise approach. Marks will always be available for the overall impression the candidate makes and how well they structure and use the skills of their trauma team.

Preparing for the patient's arrival

Standard pre-hospital information will normally be provided. For the purpose of the OSCE scenarios in this chapter information is provided in an age, time of injury, mechanism, injuries, signs and treatments received (ATMIST) format. Criteria to activate a trauma team in most EDs are relatively standardised. They are commonly based on the mechanism, injuries present or the patient's physiology (**Box 9.1.1**). If a decision is made that the trauma team is required they can be alerted prior to the patient's arrival, be briefed on the situation and be prepared for the patient. Often in the exam additional staff may not be on hand immediately thus forcing the candidate to manage the situation with less experienced staff.

Consider the following: Do you need to contact the trauma surgeon, the anaesthetist, and interventional radiologist? Have you got enough space in your resuscitation room? Do you need to prepare for any interventions which can be anticipated (e.g. intravenous fluids, blood, massive transfusion, chest drain, thoracotomy, etc.)? What are the skills each member of the trauma team possesses (ask them what they are able to do)? Have you assigned roles to team members (**Figure 9.1.1**)? Does everyone know who the team leader is?

Introduction 9.1

Box 9.1.1 Typical trauma team activation criteria

- **Mechanism**
  - Road traffic accident, ejection of the patient from the vehicle
  - Bicyclist, motorcyclist or pedestrian hit by vehicle > 30 miles per hour
  - Fall > 5 m
  - Age > 70 years old with chest injury
  - Another death in the same incident
- **Injuries**
  - Obstructed airway
  - Injury to two or more body regions
  - Fracture of two or more long bones
  - Suspected spinal cord injury
  - Amputation of limb proximal to the wrist or ankle joint
  - Penetrating injury to head, neck, torso or proximal limb
  - Burns > 15% body surface area in adults or >10% in children or airway burns
- **Physiological signs**
  - Systolic blood pressure < 90 mmHg or heart rate > 130 beats per minute
  - Respiratory rate < 10 or > 30 breaths per minute
  - Decreased GCS or seizure acivity

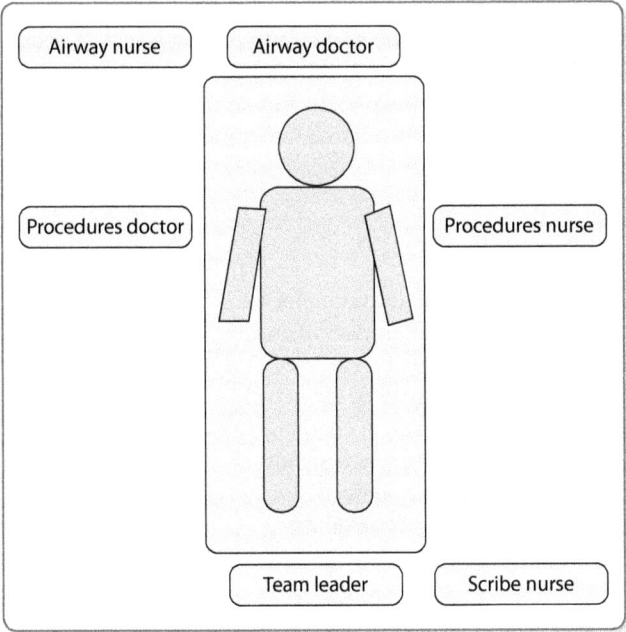

Figure 9.1.1 Trauma team positions.

On the patient's arrival

While traditional trauma courses provide the standard of care for managing a trauma patient, they offer a vertical approach where things happen one after the other. This is valuable to focus on an ABCDE style of assessment and necessary interventions. However, in the ED, where additional assistance is available, a horizontal approach is required, where assessment, intervention and decisions are taken simultaneously. Whenever possible it is advisable to:
- Know the team members by name and let others know your name and role
- Keep a hands-off approach when directing the team. If the team leader is involved directly in patient management there is nobody overseeing the whole situation
- If appropriate listen to the handover for 30 seconds prior to touching the patient. This gives everyone a chance to listen to the history
- Ensure smooth running of the resuscitation, and take decisions once adequate information is available
- Form a plan and communicate it with the team members
- Display assertive, polite and clear communication, a willingness to listen, an ability to keep an open mind and the confidence to involve the required specialties at the right time
- If the situation is not moving in the right direction, be prepared to reboot the team. Ask everyone to stop and offer each member of staff clear instructions on the task you would like them to perform

Figure 9.1.1 depicts a commonly used arrangement when managing trauma teams. Having agreed their tasks beforehand, an airway doctor (intensive care unit or ED) normally performs an assessment of the airway, while the 'procedures' doctor (ED or surgical) performs an assessment of BCDE, and later a secondary survey. Both relay the information to the trauma team leader.

Prior to commencing the station, review the scenario and be clear on whether the main area being tested is your resuscitation skills or team leadership skills. If the emphasis is on your resuscitation skills, you are expected to assess the patient and perform interventions. However, if the emphasis is on team leadership, adopt a hands-off approach where you focus on directing the trauma team effectively.

Alternative scenarios

At the end of each of the following extended resuscitation stations, we have included one or more alternative scenarios. These contain a brief summary of an alternative presentation and may contain guidance on what interventions will be required. This is to encourage candidates to consider the variety of scenarios they may be faced with and prepare for them.

Candidates should expand on this further and think of challenging scenarios that could appear in the exam. Having done so it is important to rehearse how each of those scenarios should be dealt with. The more alternatives that are practiced, the less chance there is of being confronted with a case the candidate feels unprepared for.

Suggested reading

Au EH, Holdgate A. Characteristics and outcomes of patients discharged home from the Emergency Department following trauma team activation. Injury 2010; 41:465–469.

9.2 Burns

The initial management priorities are the same as for any other trauma patient. Specific issues to consider are airway burns, inhalational injury, hypovolaemia and identifying any other life-threatening injuries. It may be necessary to measure or estimate the body surface area (BSA) involved as an initial guide to resuscitation. If relevant, remember to consider systemic effects of electrical and chemical burns.

Airway

Airway burns should be suspected with burns in enclosed spaces where inhalation of steam and hot gases can take place. Burns to mouth, nose and pharynx, singed nasal hair, sputum containing soot, productive cough, change of voice, hoarse brassy cough, croup-like breathing and stridor are signs of airway burns.

Urgent airway control with intubation is required if airway burns are present or strongly suspected as the clinical condition is likely to deteriorate.

Breathing

Burn injury can compromise respiration. Inhalation of products of combustion, especially carbon monoxide and cyanide can cause poisoning resulting in reduced level of consciousness. Oxygen helps to eliminate carbon monoxide, rapidly reducing its half-life. All major burns patients should receive 100% oxygen through a humidified non-rebreathing mask on presentation, particularly if the patient is clinically unwell or if carbon monoxide poisoning is suspected or confirmed.

Full thickness circumferential burns of the chest can also cause mechanical breathing restriction due to the inelasticity of burnt tissue and oedema produced by the burn and fluid resuscitation. This can require a chest escharotomy (division of the burnt eschar into the subcutaneous fat but not into fascia or muscle). Longitudinal incisions are made down each mid-axillary line to the subcostal region and joined up by a chevron incision running parallel to the subcostal margin creating a mobile breastplate that moves with ventilation (**Figure 9.2.1**). Limb escharotomies may also be required for circumferential burns impairing circulation.

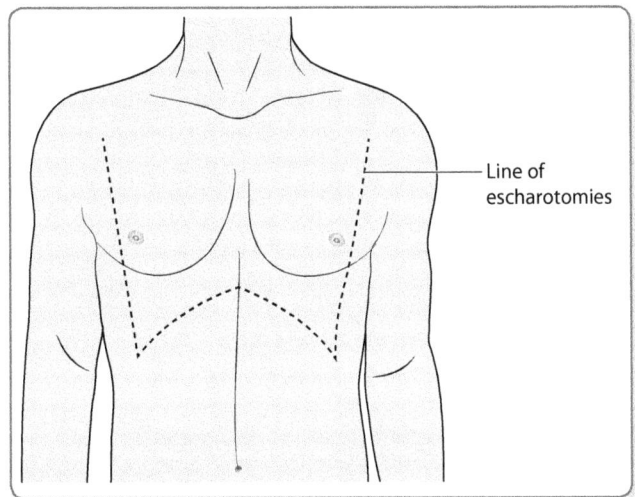

Figure 9.2.1 Chest escharotomy.

Escharotomies are best done with electrocautery in theatre, as they tend to bleed. They are an urgent procedure, and delay to theatre may mandate they are performed in the ED. They should be discussed with the local burns unit and performed under instruction if required.

Circulation

Burns cause release of inflammatory mediators, causing vasodilatation and loss of fluid from the intravascular compartments. In adults >15% and in children >10% BSA burns, can cause severe hypovolaemia without any bleeding.

Start fluid resuscitation as per the Parkland formula, which is 4 mL of crystalloid per kilogram body weight per percent of body surface area involved. Give half the calculated volume in the first 8 hours (from the time of the injury) and the subsequent half over the next 16 hours. Add maintenance requirements to this in children.

Estimating the burn area

Two commonly used methods to quantify the burn surface area are Lund and Browder charts (**Figure 9.2.2**) and the rule of nines (**Figure 9.2.3**). When estimating the burn area, ignore simple erythema, and if possible distinguish between superficial and deep burns.

An alternative simple technique for smaller burns is to measure them using the palmar surface of the patient's hand (including the fingers) to estimate the area covered. The palmar surface roughly equates to 1% of an individual's own body surface area.

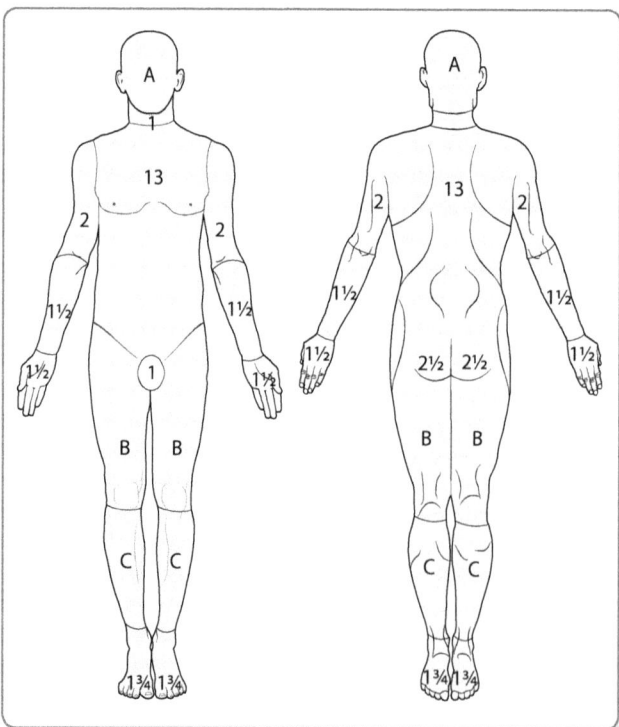

Figure 9.2.2 Lund and Browder chart.

Relative percentage of body surface area affected by burn						
Area	Age 0	1 years	5 years	10 years	15 years	Adult
A = ½ of head	9 ½	8 ½	6 ½	5 ½	4 ½	3 ½
B = ½ of thigh	2 ¾	3 ¼	4	4 ½	4 ½	4 ¾
C = ½ of lower leg	2 ½	2 ½	2 ¾	3	3 ¼	3 ½

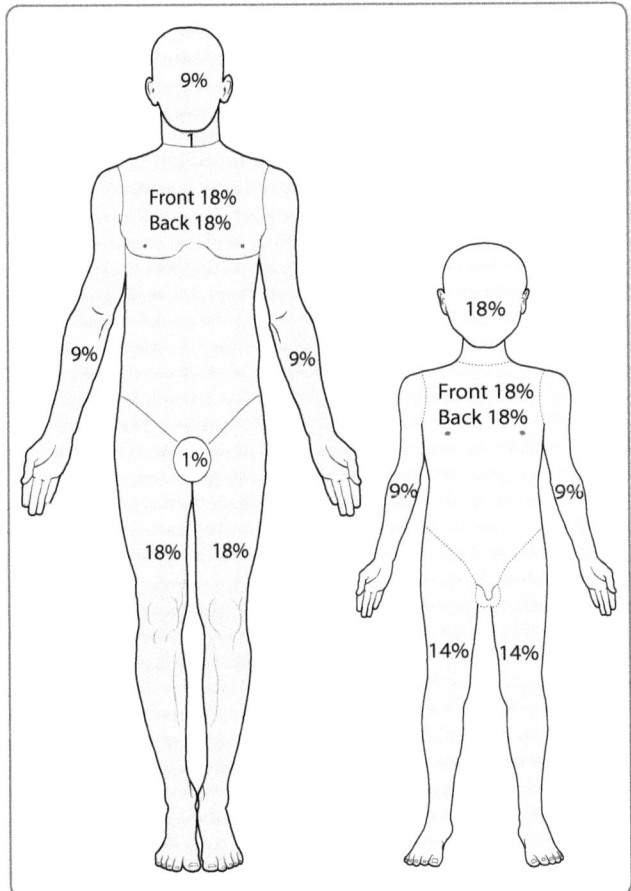

Figure 9.2.3 Rule of nines (adult and paediatric).

Identify other life-threatening injuries

Depending on the history it is advisable to have a high level of suspicion for additional internal injuries and fractures. Do not assume a patient has no other injuries as it would be easy to overlook these and attribute abnormal physiology to a burn injury.

Electrical and chemical burns

These burns may cause cell damage and breakdown. Particularly in the case of electrical burns the pathology may not just be at the site of the burn. Ask yourself: Does the patient have an arrhythmia? What is the potassium and creatine kinase? Extensive muscle injury leading to compartment syndrome and long bone fractures can be a feature of electrical burns. Some chemicals can produce systemic toxicity, e.g. hydrofluoric acid causing severe hypocalcaemia.

Dressing major burns

Once the surface area and depth of a burn have been estimated, the burn wound should be washed, and loose skin removed. Blisters should be deroofed, except for palmar blisters (painful), unless these are large enough to restrict movement. The burn should then be dressed. For an acute burn which will be referred to a burn centre, cling film is an ideal dressing as it protects the wound, reduces heat and evaporative losses, and does not alter the wound appearance. This will permit accurate evaluation by the burn team later. Flamazine should not be used on a burn that is to be referred immediately, since it makes assessment of depth more difficult.

Scenario

You are the senior ED doctor in a District General Hospital. The nearest burns centre is a 60-minute drive away. The ED nurse has taken a pre-alert call and provides you with the **ATMIST**:

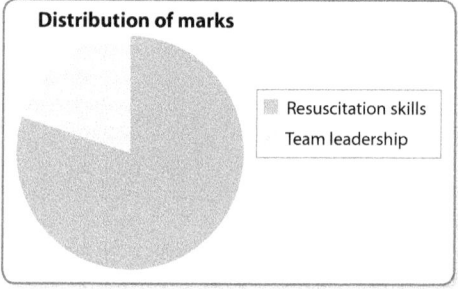

Distribution of marks
- Resuscitation skills
- Team leadership

A – 48-year-old male
T – 90 minutes earlier
M – Truck driver, involved in a high speed MVA, single vehicle against a large tree.
Fire developed in the cabin where he was trapped by confinement. The rescue services put out the fire, but he remained trapped for 60 minutes.
I – Burns to face, anterior neck, chest and upper back
S – Pulse 140, blood pressure 100/60 mmHg, GCS 13 E3, V4, M6
T – Intravenous cannulation, normal saline 500 mL, 5 mg morphine

Estimated time of arrival in the ED is 2 minutes. You have one nurse to help you.

Initial patient observations

(As the patient is assessed during the scenario these observations will be provided by the nurse)

Airway	Facial burns, hoarse voice, cough
Breathing	SaO_2 86% on Hudson mask, respiratory rate 28 breaths per minute, bilateral mild wheeze, bilateral equal air entry
Circulation	Heart rate 130 beats per minute, blood pressure 100/54 mmHg

Disability	Distressed, Glasgow coma score 13 (eyes 3, motor 6, verbal 4)
	Blood sugar 9.2 mmol/L
Exposure	Temperature 36°C
	No C-spine precautions.
	Full thickness burns to face, anterior neck and circumferential chest
	Body surface area involved approximately 40%

Guidance on scenario

The OSCE will test a candidate's knowledge of burns and how to manage a burns patient. The patient will be in severe pain preventing cervical spine immobilisation. It is expected that the candidate will treat pain with suitable analgesia and protect the cervical spine.

There is no response to the trauma call – the nurse tells you an emergency laparotomy has just begun upstairs. Only an experienced but junior airway doctor will be available quickly (if a candidate chooses to call no help and instead manage the airway there will be no doctor available to perform other tasks). If they choose to do this the nurse may suggest calling the trauma team or an anaesthetist. Once available the airway doctor will not take the initiative but will follow any directions they are given. They however suggest not intubating the patient and just observing the airway. If the airway is not secured the patient will develop stridor which will gradually get worse. A full primary survey with appropriate initial management is then expected.

The patient needs early intubation and becomes hypotensive requiring fluid resuscitation. After intubation the airway doctor will state that the patient is difficult to ventilate and requires escharotomy. If chest or pelvis X-rays are requested they will be provided and will look normal. Operating theatre escharotomy will require early planning – early notification may allow thoracic escharotomy in OT before deterioration, while delay will necessitate preparation for escharotomy in ED. Towards the end of the scenario an intensive care consultant arrives.

Mark sheet	Achieved	Not achieved
Introduces self to the nurse appropriately		
Asks to put out a trauma call		
Confirms team member experience and skills		
Assigns appropriate roles to team members		
Asks everyone to wear personal protective equipment		
Anticipates airway problems and asks to check airway and difficult airway trolley		
Takes appropriate handover from ambulance crew		
Ensures cervical spine is immobilised safely throughout		
Asks for monitoring to be attached		
Ensures stepwise ABCDE assessment		
Identifies facial burns and circumferential chest burns		
Administers high flow oxygen and pain relief		

Cont'd...

Mark sheet	Achieved	Not achieved
Recognises risk to airway and possibility of requiring escharotomy		
Does not agree with anaesthetist when they suggest observing the airway		
Facilitates safe rapid sequence induction and intubation		
Identifies difficult ventilation on BVM or high airway pressure with low TV on ventilator with need for escharotomy.		
Requests escharotomy in theatre or prepares for this in department		
Proceeds with primary survey appropriately		
Asks for burns to be covered as soon as possible		
Starts intravenous fluids – plans to calculate as per Parkland's formula		
Asks for another cannula to be inserted and appropriate blood samples to be taken		
Asks for blood gas to consider CO or cyanide poisoning		
Safely starts patient on ventilator and identifies difficult ventilation		
Asks anaesthetist to place arterial line for invasive monitoring		
States need to arrange for appropriate imaging (CT scan)		
States need to do a log roll – checks for burns/injuries on the back		
Estimates burn surface area – circumferential chest, neck and face = 40% BSA		
Estimates body weight and starts fluid as per Parkland's formula		
Asks for catheter to measure urine output		
Plans to call burns centre for transfer		
Hands over to intensive care doctor when they arrive		
Global score from examiner		
Global score from team		

Alternative scenarios

Difficult airway: there is a delay in patient presentation which leads to failure of intubation attempt and requirement for a surgical airway which will also be difficult due to swelling and possible lower airway burns.

Cyanide poisoning: the patient presents from a fire in a plastics and textiles warehouse with a reduced level of consciousness and a raised lactate on blood gas. The clinical findings will be consistent with those of cyanide poisoning in acute burns. They will require early airway management, cutaneous burns management and treatment for poisoning with Dicobalt edetate or Hydroxocobalamin (Cyanokit) should be initiated.

Shocked patient: the patient may be shocked from a non-burns related injury. They may have a tension pneumothorax or have bleeding from an intra-abdominal or pelvic injury. They may not respond to initial burns-focused management. A FAST scan and initiation of a blood transfusion and/or application of a pelvic binder may be required for the scenario to progress. The key message being that the burns should not distract from additional traumatic injuries.

Suggested reading

Burns and scalds. Clinical knowledge Summaries. National Institute for Care and Health Excellence, London 2017.
Baird J. Electrical Injuries. RCEM Learning. RCEM London, 2014.
Matthews J, Atwal R. Major Trauma – Burns. RCEM Learning. RCEM, London, 2017.

9.3 Cardiac tamponade and ED thoracotomy

In traumatic cardiac tamponade there is no indication to perform needle pericardiocentesis. Pericardiocentesis is likely to fail as the blood within the pericardium is clotted. The patient will need a thoracotomy, either in ED or theatre, depending on their physiological state.

Cardiac tamponade should be suspected in a patient with penetrating chest trauma with a wound in or near the central chest 'box' (i.e. between the nipples and from the level of the clavicles to the xiphisternum).

Clinical signs are difficult to identify, and the patient is treated according to their physiology. An eFAST scan is a good initial investigation, but these may be falsely reassuring as the amount of fluid may be small and it may accumulate further after the scan. If the patient is haemodynamically stable with a relevant penetrating chest injury, it is preferable to perform an exploration and thoracotomy in theatre under controlled conditions. If the patient loses cardiac output in the ED a resuscitative thoracotomy by an emergency physician is indicated. With a patient in extremis and unfit for transport to theatre the procedure may also be performed in the ED by an experienced surgeon.

Generally fluid resuscitation should be minimal in penetrating injuries, with the desired end-point being the presence of mentation and a palpable radial pulse. However with an isolated cardiac tamponade judicial blood or fluid boluses may increase preload temporizing the patient for a few minutes while suitable equipment/staff are arranged.

Emergency department thoracotomy technique

This is indicated in the presence of a penetrating chest injury when the patient has lost cardiac output within approximately the last 10 minutes. The aim is to relieve any tamponade by incising the pericardium and controlling bleeding from any cardiac wounds that are identified. Procedures to control bleeding from the lung hilum, aortic compression and internal cardiac massage are also possible but unlikely to be successful unless performed by an experienced specialist.

- If the patient with a penetrating chest injury suffers a cardiac arrest the first step is to perform bilateral thoracostomies. These will relieve a tension pneumothorax. The landmarks are the same as for chest drain insertion. Using a blade and then blunt dissection the pleural cavities are decompressed
- If tension pneumothorax was not the cause of the cardiac arrest and cardiac output is not restored, extend both thoracostomies to the sternum by cutting through the intercostal muscles between two ribs
- Cut through the sternum with heavy scissors or a Gigli saw
- Keep the chest open with a rib spreader or an assistant who holds the chest wall away from the thoracic cavity
- Expose the pericardium and lift it up with forceps. Incise the pericardium longitudinally in the midline with blunt dissection and scissors up to the root of the aorta
- Remove any blood clot and examine the heart for any wounds. The anterior surface of the heart is formed by the right ventricle and this is likely to be the chamber with a salvageable injury

- Methods to close a wound include:
  - Suturing
  - A Foley's catheter can be used to stop bleeding from a wound by placing it within a wound, then inflating the balloon with 10 mL saline. The catheter must be clamped to prevent blood flowing out of the heart
  - A stapler may also be used to close any wounds
- Definitive management will require a cardiothoracic or trauma surgeon with support from the intensive care/anaesthetic teams

Scenario

You are the senior ED doctor in a District General Hospital.

The ED nurse has taken a pre-alert call and provides you with the **ATMIST**:

A - 32 male
T - 15 minutes earlier, arriving in the ED in 2 minutes
M - Attempted suicide, the patient stabbed himself with a 6-inch kitchen knife
The patient removed the knife at the scene.
I - Isolated stab wound to the left anterior precordium
S - Pulse 120 beats per minute, blood pressure 80/50 mmHg, GCS 15 (E4, V5, M6)
T - Intravenous cannulation, 5 mg morphine

Estimated time of arrival in the ED is 2 minutes. You have two nurses and two doctors (one with airway skills) to help you.

Distribution of marks
- Resuscitation skills
- Team leadership

Initial patient observations

(As the patient is assessed during the scenario these observations will be provided by the nurse)

Airway	Patent
Breathing	Respiratory rate 38 breaths per minute
	Clear chest
	Oxygen saturation 100% on high flow oxygen
Circulation	Heart rate 150 beats per minute, blood pressure 60/30 mmHg
	Distended neck veins
Disability	Distressed, Glasgow coma score 13 (eyes 3, verbal 4, motor 6)
	Blood sugar 9.0 mmol/L
Exposure	Temperature 37°C

Guidance on scenario

Having assessed the patient, the candidate is expected to recognise cardiac tamponade and the need for urgent thoracotomy ideally in theatre. If a cardiothoracic surgeon is paged, they will not answer immediately. The candidate should explain that if the patient suffers a cardiac arrest from cardiac tamponade, he requires immediate emergency thoracotomy and then prepare for this procedure.

The patient will become progressively more hypotensive and tachycardic. If a FAST scan is requested a doctor will perform it and see fluid in the pericardium. The patient will deteriorate and suffer a cardiac arrest. After the patient arrests the candidate is expected ensure the patient has a definitive airway secured and to perform a thoracotomy. There will be a right ventricular injury that requires closure. Once this is done, if the patient has also received an adequate volume of blood they will achieve ROSC. They will need to be reassessed and preparation made for immediate transfer to the operating theatre.

Mark sheet	Achieved	Not achieved
Introduces self to the nurse appropriately		
Asks to put out a trauma call		
Confirms team member experience and skills		
Assigns appropriate roles to team members		
Asks everyone to wear personal protective equipment		
Anticipates thoracic injuries and plans appropriately		
Anticipates major haemorrhage and plans appropriately		
Takes brief handover from ambulance crew		
Asks for appropriate monitoring to be attached		
Facilitates primary survey and eFAST and basic interventions		
Recognises pericardial fluid on ultrasound, diagnosing tamponade		
Calls cardiothoracic team for assistance/urgent thoracotomy		
Recognises potential for emergency thoracotomy		
Reassesses ABCD noting falling GCS and blood pressure		
Fluid/blood boluses in appropriate volume		
Diagnoses cardiac arrest		
Performs thoracotomy with correct technique		
Closes RV incision		
Reassesses ABCDE from beginning		
Hands patient over to anaesthetist and cardiothoracic surgeon		
Prepares for transfer to theatre		
Global score from examiner		
Global score from team		

Alternative scenarios

Blunt trauma: arrest in blunt trauma is highly unlikely to be due to cardiac tamponade. Emergency thoracotomy by an emergency physician is unlikely to be successful without clinical or ultrasound evidence of cardiac tamponade. There are rare occasions where an experienced specialist may undertake this procedure in blunt trauma though current data suggests a good outcome is very rare.

Interventions of value may be a 'hilar twist' to prevent bleeding from the lung or hilar vessels, or compressing the aorta to prevent more distal haemorrhage while further definitive management is coordinated.

Tamponade with a knife in situ: the patient presents in extremis with the knife protruding from the chest wall. Whether to remove the knife prior to thoracotomy is a judgement call and there is no right answer. If the patient has a pulse pre-arrest, the knife should remain in position as removal from a vessel could precipitate exsanguination. If the knife interferes with the procedure after cardiac arrest it should be removed to prevent additional injury to the patient and proceduralist. If the patient was unstable but continued to have a cardiac output transfer to operating theatres should be considered.

Suggested reading

Lloyd G. Thoracic Trauma. RCEM Learning. RCEM, London 2017.

9.4 Haemothorax and pneumothorax

Massive haemothorax, tension or open pneumothorax and flail chest are life-threatening chest injuries that should be identified and treated as part of the primary survey. Consider the use of ultrasound to confirm the presence/absence of lung sliding. However, it is not necessary to use ultrasound if it will delay an intervention if, based on the clinical information available, the intervention is going to be inevitable.

Tension pneumothorax

Accumulation of air in the pleural cavity with positive intrathoracic pressure is a tension pneumothorax. This produces severe respiratory distress and shock due to compression of mediastinal structures, reduced venous return and a reduced cardiac output.

Clinical findings
- Agitated, dyspnoeic patient
- Reduced air entry on the affected side
- Tachycardia and hypotension
- Hyper-resonant chest wall on the same side
- Tracheal deviation is a late sign

Immediate decompression is required. A cannula can be inserted in the second intercostal space in the mid-clavicular line or in the fifth intercostal space within the safe triangle. This will relieve the tension temporarily until a chest drain is inserted. A thoracostomy can also be performed in a matter of seconds and the decision as to which is most appropriate depends on the patient's ventilatory status and how quickly available the equipment for each procedure is.

Open pneumothorax

Any external wound in the chest wall communicating with the pleural space makes respiratory effort extremely inefficient as air moves selectively through the wound rather than the trachea. Sometimes the wound can act as a one-way valve leading to accumulation of air in the pleural space and leading to a tension pneumothorax.

Clinical findings
- Chest wound may be sucking in air with each breath
- Reduced air entry on ipsilateral side
- Subcutaneous emphysema may be present
- Respiratory distress, hypoxia, tachypnoea

Initial treatment is to cover the chest wound with a one-way valve/seal of which there are several types available. If not available, apply an occlusive dressing over the wound (e.g. Jelonet or Opsite dressing). Taping only three sides of a dressing to create a one-way valve is possible but no longer recommended as this is rarely effective. A chest drain will be required. The wound will then need definitive exploration and management in theatre.

Massive haemothorax

This is blood in the pleural cavity leading to shock and hypotension. This can result from blunt or penetrating chest injuries and depending on the exact nature of the injury will present with a varying degree of haemorrhagic shock and ventilatory failure.

Clinical findings
- Hypoxic, tachypnoeic patient
- Tachycardia, hypotension
- Reduced air entry on the side of injury
- Dullness to percussion
- FAST may suggest the presence of blood
- Chest X-ray may show a 'white-out' lung on the affected side, or a large fluid collection. Changes can be more subtle in a supine trauma patient as the blood is distributed through the hemithorax.

Treatment requires gaining intravenous access and volume resuscitation. A chest drain must be placed on the affected side, ideally of a large calibre (28–32 Fr). If there is immediate return of >1500 mL of blood or >200 mL/h, this is an indication for urgent thoracotomy. Surgical chest exploration with control of bleeding is the definitive treatment.

If a haemothorax is suspected during the initial ABCDE assessment of a patient, candidates must bear in mind that haemorrhage may be severe. Therefore, when a haemothorax is suspected as part of the B (breathing) candidates are advised to acknowledge the need for a chest drain and ask for equipment to be prepared but continue on to C (circulation) and ensure adequate intravenous access and blood products prior to placing any chest drains.

Flail chest

This is when two or more ribs are broken at two or more sites, leading to a section of chest wall moving with the intrathoracic pressure rather than the rest of the chest wall. This part of the chest wall may move paradoxically, inwards with inspiration and outwards with expiration. This condition is also almost always associated with an underlying lung contusion. Paradoxical chest movement reduces efficiency of breathing and combined with a lung contusion results in hypoxia, respiratory distress and severe pain.

Clinical findings
- Paradoxical chest movements
- Subcutaneous emphysema
- Chest wall bruising
- Crepitus
- Pain in chest wall, dyspnoeic patient, shallow breathing

Treatment requires adequate pain control which may include patient-controlled analgesia or a thoracic epidural. The patient may also need ventilation and management in an appropriate high dependency area.

Scenario

You are the senior ED doctor in a District General Hospital. The ED nurse has taken a pre-alert call and provides you with the **ATMIST**:

A – 19-year-old male
T – 10 minutes earlier
M – Assaulted and stabbed with a knife in the right anterior chest
I – Isolated stab wound with bubbling wound to the right anterior chest
S – Pulse 120 beats per minute, blood pressure 90/50 mmHg, respiratory rate 30 breaths per minute, oxygen saturation 94% on high flow oxygen, GCS 15
T – Needle decompression of right hemithorax, intravenous cannulation, 5 mg morphine

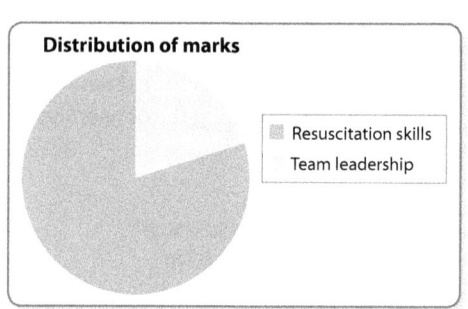

His estimated time of arrival in the ED is 2 minutes. You have two competent junior doctors and a trained nurse to help.

Initial patient observations

(As the patient is assessed during the scenario these observations will be provided by the nurse)

Airway	Patent
Breathing	Respiratory rate 45 breaths per minute, with severe respiratory distress
	Sucking right anterior 2 cm wound
	Cannula in right second intercostal space
	Absent breath sounds right chest, tracheal impalpable as neck/chest swollen with surgical emphysema
	Oxygen saturation 84% on high flow oxygen
Circulation	Heart rate 150 beats per minute, blood pressure 66/40 mmHg
Disability	Distressed, Glasgow coma score 13 (eyes 4, verbal 4, motor 5)
	Blood sugar 12.0 mmol/L
Exposure	Temperature 37°C, no other injuries

Guidance on scenario

The clinical signs will indicate a right-sided tension pneumohaemothorax which must be treated urgently. The prehospital needle-decompression is blocked or has dislodged. The candidate may repeat the needle-decompression which will release air and blood. If an eFAST scan may be performed by the candidate, it will show a large haemothorax, loss of lung sliding and no pericardial effusion. They may start blood product resuscitation while preparing further interventions. If a thoracostomy is performed there will be air and significant blood loss from the site. When placing a chest drain the candidate will be asked by the junior doctor to talk them through the procedure. The candidate will be expected to administer appropriate quantities of blood and blood products while also activating the major haemorrhage pathway. Once decompression and transfusion are both achieved the haemodynamic state of the patient will slowly improve. If the quantity of blood from the drain is not recognised as needing cardiothoracic intervention the patient will gradually deteriorate and become increasingly haemodynamically unstable until staff comment on the amount of blood that has been drained. The cardiothoracic surgeon will arrive quickly if called and initially suggest a thoracotomy in the ED, but the candidate is expected to state this should be done in theatre.

Mark sheet	Achieved	Not achieved
Introduces self to the nurse appropriately		
Asks to put out a trauma call		
Confirms team member experience and skills and assigns roles		
Asks everyone to wear personal protective equipment		
Anticipates/activates major haemorrhage pathway		
Performs/facilitates appropriate ABCDE assessment		
Ensures full exposure and identification of wounds is a priority		
Does not delay chest decompression for eFAST scan		
Decompresses tension pneumothorax		
Covers stab wound in appropriate manner		
Ensures adequate intravenous		
Sends appropriate blood samples and a cross-match request		
Commences resuscitation with appropriate blood products		
Facilitates right-sided chest drain insertion away from injury		
Directs procedure correctly		
Completes primary survey, excludes other sites of haemorrhage		
Recognises quantity of blood in drain (Immediate 1600 mL)		
Asks for cardiothoracic surgeon to be contacted immediately		
Continues resuscitation with massive transfusion		
Hands patient over to cardiothoracic surgeon appropriately		
Does not agree to thoracotomy in ED but in theatres		
Global score from examiner		
Global score from team		

Alternative scenarios

Cardiac arrest: the patient presents with chest trauma and suffers a cardiac arrest with clinical findings suggesting either a tension pneumothorax (or bilateral tension pneumothoraces) or haemorrhage – the patient may arrest prior to treatment being initiated in the ED. This should prompt immediate treatment of the likely reversible causes with bilateral thoracostomies (injured side first) and, if no response, progression to thoracotomy with rapid initiation of massive transfusion of blood products. Chest compressions have no value in this situation until these reversible causes are addressed (see Section 9.9).

Second knife wound in the neck: the patient presents with signs consistent with an uncomplicated haemothorax without circulatory compromise. There is a neck wound concealed by a cervical spine collar that may not be noticed unless the collar is removed (otherwise the patient will develop stridor). There will be an arterial wound, expanding haematoma and airway compromise requiring intubation.

Suggested reading
Lloyd G. Thoracic Trauma. RCEM Learning. RCEM, London 2017.

9.5 Head injury

Severe head injuries are defined as those where the patient has a Glasgow coma score (GCS) ≤8. However, clinically patients with a GCS between 9–13 with agitation, alcohol or drugs on board are often a bigger challenge. This is because the decision-making process is less clear cut and it can prove difficult to gain support from additional specialists to secure a patient's airway. In addition any severe injury to the head should also prompt a high suspicion for cervical spine injury.

If a decision is made to intubate a patient, prior to this being done you should attempt to check their GCS and perform a brief neurological examination to document any deficit. This provides useful information for when the patient is reassessed at later intervals and cannot be done once a neuromuscular blocking agent has been given.

A vital role for the emergency physician in managing head injured patients is to prevent secondary brain injury from hypoxia, hypotension and rising intracranial pressure (ICP). Such patients will need airway control, with interventions to control ICP and their mean arterial pressure (MAP).

Neuroprotective measures in the head injured patient are based on the principle that good management of the 'ABC' clinical parameters will minimise any subsequent 'D' pathology. The ultimate priority is to maintain adequate oxygenation and perfusion of the brain.

- Intubate early for airway control
- Avoid hyper-/hypotension on rapid sequence induction
- Maintain adequate oxygenation to avoid hypoxia
- Optimise ventilation to maintain an end tidal CO_2 of 4–4.5 kPa or 30–35 mmHg to maintain cerebral perfusion
- Do not hyperventilate the patient
- Maintain sedation with short-acting agents
- Maintain cerebral perfusion pressure (CPP)
  - Remember CPP = MAP-ICP
  - Maintain the MAP at >90 mmHg. Haemorrhage control and correcting hypovolaemia may be needed
- Control ICP by:
  - Reverse Trendelenburg position: 30° head-up tilt
  - Avoid neck ties on endotracheal tubes and once intubated apply cervical collars loosely or consider only using blocks to protect the c-spine
  - Early CT to detect haematoma and expedite early neurosurgical intervention
- In the case of clinical deterioration or unilateral pupillary dilatation, reduce ICP with:
  - Intravenous mannitol (0.5 to 1 g/kg of 20% solution)
  - Hypertonic saline (this is available in varying concentrations and must be dosed accordingly) – it may be preferable to mannitol in patients with haemorrhage as unlike mannitol it will contribute to intravascular volume resuscitation
  - Hyperventilation – reduces pCO_2 and causes intracerebral vasoconstriction – it may be used as a very short-term measure to reduce ICP but is likely to increase ischaemia

Scenario

You are the senior ED doctor in a Major Trauma Centre. The ED nurse has taken a pre-alert call and provides you with the **ATMIST**:

A – 33-year-old male
T – 30 minutes earlier
M – Construction worker, hit by the falling debris whilst working. He was not wearing a hard hat. He was initially unrousable when assessed by co-workers
I – Bleeding from the left ear, boggy swelling in left parietal region. Bruised right upper quadrant of abdomen
S – Pulse 120 beats per minute, blood pressure 130/70 mmHg, Glasgow coma score 11 (eyes 3, verbal 3, motor 5)
T – Intravenous cannulation, normal saline 500 mL, 5 mg morphine

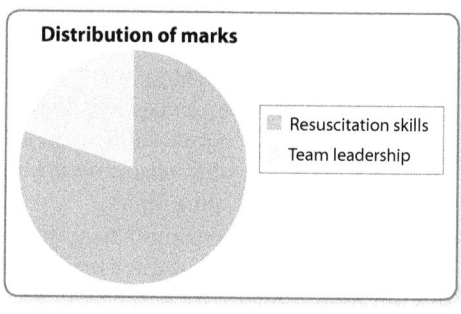

Estimated time of arrival in the ED is 2 minutes. You have one nurse and a junior doctor to help you.

Initial patient observations

The patient arrives with observations as described by the ambulance crew. As the patient is assessed during the scenario the patient gradually deteriorates with observations suggestive expanding intracranial haematoma. After intubation these observations are as follows:

Airway	Patent, no blood in airway
Breathing	SaO_2 100% on oxygen, respiratory rate 8 breaths per minute, clear chest with equal air entry
Circulation	Heart rate 130 beats per minute, blood pressure 70/50 mmHg
Disability	Glasgow coma score 5 (eyes 1, verbal 1, motor 3) Right pupil 2 mm and reactive, left pupil 5 mm unreactive Blood sugar 7.3 mmol/L
Exposure	Temperature 37°C Bruised right upper quadrant with guarding, no penetrating injury

Guidance on scenario

The patient arrives without cervical spine immobilisation or high flow oxygen applied. A rapid sequence induction (RSI) and intubation is required. If they do not do so the breathing becomes slower and noisier as the GCS gradually falls. The candidate is expected to notice a blown pupil on the injured side and initiate urgent neurosurgical intervention and temporising measures for raised ICP. The airway doctor states he is going to use 150 mg of propofol for the induction. The candidate is expected to challenge this appropriately and explain the need to ensure neuroprotective measures and avoiding hypotension.

If performed a FAST scan will indicate free fluid in the abdomen. If a transfusion with appropriate blood products is not commenced the patient's haemodynamic parameters will continue to deteriorate. The patient must be referred to the neurosurgical and general surgical teams who will attend immediately. When the neurosurgical registrar attends if the blood pressure is not adequate he will be irate and state the MAP must be higher. If the blood pressure has improved the surgical registrar will instead suggest permissive hypotension until a CT is performed. After discussion it will should be agreed to transfer the patient to CT prior to theatre with both surgical teams involved.

Mark sheet	Achieved	Not achieved
Introduces self to the nurse appropriately		
Asks to put out a trauma call		
Confirms team member experience and skills and assigns roles		
Asks everyone to wear personal protective equipment		
Anticipates difficult airway (C-spine precautions)		
Ensures cervical spine is immobilized safely throughout		
Asks for appropriate monitoring and oxygen		
Facilitates appropriate primary survey		
States need for rapid sequence induction		
Activates major haemorrhage pathway		
Coordinates preoxygenation and preparation for RSI		
Ensures safe and appropriate drugs/doses are used throughout		
Confirms safe intubation		
Arranges ongoing safe ventilation of patient		
States neuroprotective measures (normocarbia, head up tilt, maintaining systolic, avoiding neck tie – states at least 3)		
Ensures transfusion of appropriate blood/products		
Administers hypertonic saline in appropriate dose		
Contacts neurosurgeons and general surgeons		
Appropriate discussion when general surgeon suggests permissive hypotension		
Negotiates appropriate plan with surgical teams		
Arranges immediate CT		
Global score from examiner		
Global score from team		

Alternative scenarios

Agitated head-injured patient: the patient has a GCS >8 and is confused and non-compliant with treatment and spinal precautions. The candidate is expected to recognise the patient requires sedation for assessment and has a high risk of deterioration. If RSI is attempted the patient will not tolerate intravenous cannulation or pre-oxygenation. The candidate is expected to gain control of the patient with appropriate titrated sedation and coordinate a complex situation prior to initiating RSI.

Shocked patient: the patient has an associated chest injury from the falling excavator arm with haemothorax and hypotension. The candidate should simultaneously initiate chest drain and massive transfusion. The candidate should discuss the blood pressure target for resuscitation. A target MAP of 90 mmHg is still suggested for neuroprotection (as well as other normal neuroprotective measures); however, this may be unachievable and greatly exacerbate bleeding. Urgent surgical control of haemorrhage is required.

Facial trauma: the patient was hit in the face by the falling excavator arm and has Le Forte III fractures with severe airway haemorrhage. The candidate should recognise this as a very difficult airway, with risk of large volume haemorrhage and aspiration. Intubation preparation should include extra suction and planning for early use of an LMA in the event of failure to intubate (to minimise aspiration from Bag-valve-mask ventilation) with adequate preparation for a surgical airway. Facial packing with nasal epistats, bite blocks and a cervical spine collar may be required.

Suggested reading

Head Injury. Clinical knowledge Summaries. National Institute for Care and Health Excellence. London, 2016.
Blackham J, Kendall J, Roland. Cervical Spine Injury. RCEM learning. RCEM, London, 2017.

9.6 Trauma in pregnancy

The approach to a pregnant patient with major or minor trauma will for the most part follow standard trauma resuscitation guidelines. However, there are some important additional points that will be required or anticipated:
- Knowledge of physiological changes during pregnancy
- Awareness that there may be a difficult airway, delayed gastric emptying and an increased risk of gastro-oesophageal reflux with the potential for aspiration
- A raised diaphragm, requiring a higher position for chest drains
- Difficult abdominal assessment due to enlarged uterus
- Requirement to involve obstetricians early
- Potential for blood loss within the uterus – beware if tender and larger than expected for dates
- After 20 weeks, the uterus can compress the vena cava and cause hypotension – use left lateral tilt or manually displace the uterus to the left (while maintaining cervical spine immobilisation where appropriate)
- Perimortem caesarean section in cardiac arrest
- In abdominal trauma there is a risk of fetomaternal haemorrhage (FMH). In a woman with a rhesus negative blood group, there is a possibility the fetal blood is rhesus positive, and therefore FMH can cause autoimmunisation of the mother. To prevent this, anti-D must be administered. Current guidelines recommend:
  - <20 weeks' gestation – 250 IU as an intramuscular injection in the deltoid muscle
  - >20 weeks' gestation – 500 IU and the Kleihauer test (to identify a FMH of >4 mL in case more anti-D is needed)
  - Third trimester of pregnancy – 1500 IU and Kleihauer test (to check any FMH of >4 mL in case more anti-D is needed)
  - Fetal monitoring may be considered (though initial priority is maternal care)

Management

Trauma in pregnancy is managed like any other trauma and we should always remember the best outcome for the fetus is dependent upon optimal management of the mother.

Deterioration with cardiac arrest should initially be managed as any other traumatic cardiac arrest (see section 9.9). Additional pregnancy specific interventions are manual uterine displacement and left lateral tilt (15–30 degrees) to increase venous return and preparation for a perimortem caesarean section if there is no cardiac output within 3 minutes. This is a resuscitative procedure primarily aimed at improving maternal survival. Best outcome for fetus is achieved if delivery is achieved within 4–6 minutes of cardiac arrest.

Resuscitative hysterotomy is performed via midline incision from the xiphisternum to symphysis pubis. After skin and muscle dissection, the peritoneum and uterus should also be incised vertically, with the uterine incision extended with scissors to the fundus. The fetus and placenta should be delivered, and uterine massage and compression applied.

Scenario

You are the senior ED doctor in a district general hospital. The ED nurse has taken a pre-alert call and provides you with the **ATMIST**:

A – 32-year-old female
T – 60 minutes earlier
M – Road traffic accident. Head-on collision at 40 mph, wearing a seat belt
I – Bruising to the chest and abdomen from the seat belt
S – Pulse 120 beats per minute, blood pressure is 100/70 mmHg, respiratory rate 28 breaths per minute, and GCS 15
T – She is on a spinal board with a cervical spine collar. No venous access. Entonox for pain relief

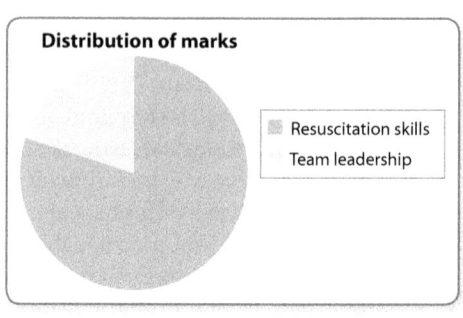

Estimated time of arrival in the ED is 2 minutes. You have one nurse and a junior doctor to help you.

Initial patient observations

(As the patient is assessed during the scenario these observations will be provided by the nurse)

Airway   Patent
Breathing   Respiratory rate 32 breaths per minute, decreased air entry left lungfield, pain on palpation of left clavicle and sternum
              Oxygen saturation 92% on high flow oxygen
              Resonant left hemithorax to percussion
Circulation   Heart rate 130 beats per minute, blood pressure 80/40 mmHg, EFAST positive for free fluid (and absent left lung sliding)
Disability   Glasgow coma score 15
              Blood sugar 9.6 mmol/L
Exposure   Temperature 37°C
              Chest and abdominal bruising from seatbelt, abdominal tenderness with guarding, 32-week's gestation palpable uterus

Guidance on scenario

The candidate is expected to demonstrate knowledge of the issues specific to trauma in pregnancy. The patient will have an exquisitely tender sternum and severe abdominal pain. The FAST scan will be positive. The candidate is expected to decompress the left hemithorax, resuscitate the patient with uterine displacement, blood products, activate an MTP and arrange urgent transfer to theatre for laparotomy. The obstetrician will not be able to arrive until the end of the scenario. An appropriate discussion should be had about appropriate radiological imaging. Given the severity of injuries a trauma CT is likely to be the most appropriate choice, though another alternative would be plain radiographs of the cervical spine, chest and pelvis followed by ultrasound of the abdomen or laparotomy (depending on the patient's haemodynamic state).

Mark sheet	Achieved	Not achieved
Introduces self to the nurse appropriately		
Asks to put out a trauma call		
Calls obstetrician to ED immediately		
Confirms team member experience and skills and assigns roles		
Asks everyone to wear personal protective equipment		
Anticipates need for and ensures left lateral tilt/uterine displacement		
Anticipates need for O negative blood and activation of major haemorrhage protocol		
Ensures cervical spine is immobilised safely throughout		
Asks for appropriate monitoring to be attached		
Manages patient's pain adequately		
Coordinates appropriate ABCDE assessment		
Performs eFAST and identifies chest and abdominal pathology		
Recognises need for and oversees chest decompression managment		
Obtains adequate intravenous access and sends appropriate blood samples		
Transfuses blood/blood products in appropriate volume, uses major transfusion pathway		
States need for Kleihauer test and anti-D		
Makes reasonable plan for imaging prior to theatre (Chest X-ray must be done post chest drain)		
Hands patient over to surgeon and obstetrician appropriately when they arrive		
Global score from examiner		
Global score from team		

Alternative scenarios

Cardiac arrest despite resuscitation: candidates should manage this as a traumatic cardiac arrest (chapter 9.9). In addition there should be manual uterine displacement and/or left lateral tilt applied, whilst preparing for a further manoeuvres. If return of spontaneous circulation is not achieved following bilateral thoracostomy and maximum major transfusion resuscitation for 3 minutes, candidates should proceed to a resuscitative hysterotomy and describe the technique. Delivery within 5 minutes of cardiac arrest will result in good outcomes for mother and baby.

Placental abruption: the patient presents with severe lower abdominal pain, an increase in fundal height with a tense uterus and vaginal bleeding. The FAST is negative with no other injuries on primary survey. Candidates should recognise placental abruption, resuscitate with blood products as required and arrange urgent obstetric assessment for probable caesarean section.

Suggested reading

Harris M. Abdominal trauma. RCEM Learning. RCEM, London 2013.

9.7 Haemorrhagic shock

Hypovolaemia must always be considered and excluded as the cause of shock in a trauma patient. A systematic approach is required to find the source of any bleeding. 'On the floor, or five more', is a useful mnemonic in this situation.
- On the floor:
  - External haemorrhage
- Five more:
  - Chest
  - Abdomen
  - Pelvis
  - Long bones
  - Retroperitoneum (bleeding at this site is difficult to detect clinically and requires a high degree of suspicion not to go unrecognised)
- Bleeding causes acidosis, hypothermia, and coagulopathy. This lethal triad will form an irreversible cycle of decline without effective resuscitation. Crystalloid resuscitation alone dilutes existing clotting factors, worsening perfusion, causing further acidosis and coagulopathy
- The basis of damage control resuscitation is to minimise the impact of the 'lethal triad'. The process begins in the ED and continues into the operating theatres and critical care. It comprises of three principles:
  1. Permissive hypotension
  2. Early haemostatic resuscitation
  3. Damage control surgery

Resuscitate with blood products to a MAP of 65 mmHg according to massive transfusion policy. (The target blood pressure depends on many factors such as the nature of the injury, the presence of a concurrent head injury, the patient's physiological state, physiological reserve and likely normal blood pressure). This involves rapid warm transfusion of red cells, platelets and FFP to counter the lethal triad. Attempt to control bleeding as soon as possible and in most circumstances the patient is likely to need to be transferred to the operating theatre. Though CT scanning prior to theatre provides additional information it is not appropriate to scan patients who are haemodynamically unstable. This decision is a judgment based on the clinical state of the patient, the suspected injuries and the practicalities of obtaining a CT in the department in question. In cases of significant haemorrhage after trauma, tranexamic acid is also recommended. The normal adult dose is 1 g intravenously as an initial bolus followed by a further 1 g as an infusion.

Targets in major transfusion are:
- Maintain temperature over 35°C
- Maintain pH >7.2, with base excess <6, lactate <4 mmol/L
- Ionised calcium >1.1 mmol/L
- Platelets >50×10^9/L (or 100×10^9/L in head injury)
- Fibrinogen >1 g/L

FAST is a useful investigation, as it is quick to perform, reproducible and can be performed frequently. It should only be performed when it will influence the next step in clinical decision making. It can detect fluid in peritoneal, pericardial and pleural cavities, but not the retroperitoneum.

Patients can bleed considerably from small wounds like scalp lacerations. Control external haemorrhage with direct pressure and a bandage. Tourniquets used judiciously also help to prevent blood loss, always record the time of application.

An extended FAST scan or chest X-ray performed as part of primary survey should demonstrate a haemothorax. However, a small amount of bleeding can be missed. If there is blood loss of over 1500 mL or 200 mL/h for 3 hours a patient should be referred trauma or cardiothoracic surgeons for consideration of a thoracotomy.

A suspected pelvis fracture will need a pelvic binder at the level of the greater trochanters which may reduce/stabilise it. Leave it in place until a pelvic fracture has been excluded. The treatment of choice is angiographic embolisation of the offending vessel, and if this is not possible open pelvic packing will be required. This needs to be followed by definitive stabilisation of the fracture.

Splint long bone fractures and maintain bone alignment. Use traction in femoral fractures to reduce the potential space and control bleeding. Definitive surgery will be performed later.

Scenario

You are the senior ED doctor in a district general hospital. The ED nurse has taken a pre-alert call and provides you with the **ATMIST**:

A – 18-year-old male
T – 20 minutes earlier
M – Road traffic accident. Motorcyclist head on collision with car at 60 km/h wearing helmet and protective clothing
I – Right leg externally rotated
S – Pulse 140 beats per minute, blood pressure is 80/40 mmHg, respiratory rate 32 breaths per minute, and GCS 15
T – He is on a spinal board with a cervical spine collar and pelvic binder, no IV access

His estimated time of arrival in the ED is 2 minutes. You have a full trauma team to assist you.

Initial patient observations

(As the patient is assessed during the scenario these observations will be provided by the nurse)

Airway	Patent
Breathing	Respiratory rate 34 breaths per minute
	Bilateral equal air entry, oxygen saturation 86% on air, 100% on high flow oxygen
Circulation	Heart rate 140 beats per minute, blood pressure 80/40 mmHg
Disability	Glasgow coma score 15 (eyes 4, motor 6, verbal 5)
	In pain, blood sugar 10.6 mmol/L
Exposure	Temperature 33.3°C
	Abrasions to right side of abdomen, externally rotated right leg
	Pelvic binder at level of anterior superior iliac spines

Guidance on scenario

A trauma team will be present. They will be competent but will look to the team leader for direction as to what tasks they should perform. The patient will obviously be shocked. The clinical findings that will be identified are a tender abdomen with guarding, pelvic disruption and an externally rotated right leg. The cervical spine must be protected, IV access must be achieved and a major transfusion commenced. The patient should receive ongoing volume resuscitation and should have the pelvic binder repositioned. A FAST scan will be positive in all areas of the abdomen and suggestive of a large volume of intra-abdominal blood. If performed a chest X-ray will be normal and a pelvic X-ray will demonstrate a disrupted pelvis. If the patient is managed correctly their systolic blood pressure will be around 80 mmHg with a MAP of 65 and will very slowly continue to fall. The candidate is expected to continue to resuscitate the patient, refuse requests for CT imaging and arrange for the patient to be transferred to theatre with ongoing major transfusion and the orthopaedic and general/trauma surgeons. If explored there will not be suitable facilities for interventional radiology to be involved.

Mark sheet	Achieved	Not achieved
Introduces self to the team appropriately		
Confirms team member experience and skills and assigns roles		
Asks everyone to wear personal protective equipment		
Asks for O negative or positive blood, activates major haemorrhage protocol and primes rapid transfuser/blood warmer		
Prepares ultrasound machine for FAST scan		
Takes appropriate handover from ambulance crew		
Ensures cervical spine is immobilised safely throughout		
Asks for appropriate monitoring to be attached		
Facilitates ABCDE assessment with appropriate basic interventions		
Identifies primary problem is haemorrhage		
Ensures 2 or more large bore IV vascular access, with blood samples sent including cross match		
Initiates volume resuscitation with appropriate blood products in appropriate quantities		
Administers tranexamic acid in correct dose		
Manages patient's pain adequately		
Uses Bair hugger and blood warmer		
Arranges chest and pelvic X-ray (Open book Pelvic fracture)		
Repositions pelvic binder over greater trochanters and tightens		
Recognises patient's failure to respond to resuscitation and too unstable for CT imaging		
Contacts appropriate surgeons for immediate review of patient		
Hands patient over to surgeons with plans for immediate theatre		
Global score from examiner		
Global score from team		

Alternative scenario

Complicated team dynamics: the scenario will be as above with clinical findings of a unilateral haemothorax, a FAST scan with positive abdominal findings and a rotated very poor quality pelvic X-ray. The patient will be shocked and be very slowly responding to interventions. The consultant trauma surgeon will be present and want the patient to go for a CT as he feels it is a risk to commence a laparotomy if the primary bleeding is elsewhere. The consultant anaesthetist will think the patient should stay in resus and continue being resuscitated and the other ED staff will feel the patient should go straight to the operating theatre. The candidate will be forced to discuss the options with the senior consultants present and quickly agree a plan.

Suggested reading

The CRASH-2 Collaborators. Effects of tranexamic acid on death, vascular occlusive events, and blood transfusion in trauma patients with significant haemorrhage (CRASH-2): a randomised, placebo-controlled trial. Lancet 2010; 376:23–32.

Harris M. Abdominal Trauma, 2013.

Dutton RP. Haemostatic resuscitation. Department of Anaesthesia and Critical Care, University of Chicago. Br J Anaesth 2012; 109:i39–i46.

9.8 Threatened airway

Direct injury to the face, maxillofacial structures, neck and larynx can disrupt the normal anatomy and cause a primary airway problem that will need to be addressed immediately. Severe head injury causing loss of airway reflexes, or a chest injury necessitating ventilatory support, will also require the airway to be secured. Suspected cervical spine injury can complicate the matter further due to the need to protect the cervical spine. It is advisable to seek expert help early and keep the difficult airway trolley at hand.

Facial trauma has the potential to cause massive airway haemorrhage which can cause life-threatening shock, aspiration with ventilation impairment and make laryngoscopy extremely difficult. Such a patient should be intubated with extra suction available and with the team briefed for failure and prepared for an immediate surgical airway. Head down tilt at the time of laryngoscopy may allow flow of blood out of the mouth and allow a better view. If intubation fails in these circumstances LMA rescue ventilation is preferred to BVM ventilation as it can prevent further aspiration whilst preparing for a second attempt or surgical airway.

In a scenario with a primary airway problem, anticipate the airway problem early. A plan in the form of airway manoeuvres, suction, achieving a definitive airway and a plan for a failed attempt to secure the airway should be the focus of interventions. If all other measures fail be prepared to secure a surgical airway in the form of a surgical cricothyroidotomy.

A simple way to perform a surgical airway is with a scalpel, finger, bougie technique. Standing to the side of the patient, the thyroid cartilage is gripped with the non-dominant hand with the index finger palpating the cricothyroid membrane. The membrane is incised in the transverse plane with a scalpel in the dominant hand, and the finger from the gripping hand is placed through the membrane. The bougie follows alongside the finger and is used to railroad a standard size 6 ETT.

It is important to remember that induction drugs have the potential to cause life-threatening hypotension in shocked patients. Drug doses should be reduced and major transfusion resuscitation should be initiated prior to intubation when required.

If there is ongoing facial bleeding the face should be packed with nasal epistats, bite blocks and a hard cervical spine collar. Together these tamponade further bleeding until definitive management.

Scenario

You are the senior ED doctor on a night shift in a district general hospital. The ED nurse has taken a pre-alert call and provides you with the **ATMIST**:
A – 30-year-old female
T – 15 minutes earlier
M – Cycling, she lost balance and went off the side of the road into a wall

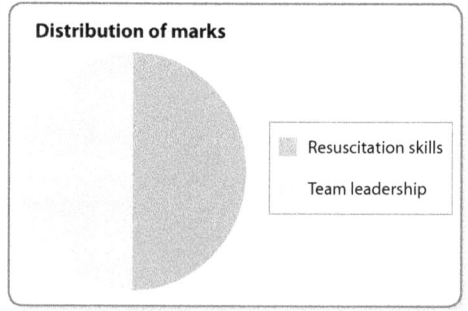

Distribution of marks

- Resuscitation skills
- Team leadership

I - Facial injuries and neck pain
S - Pulse 110 beats per minute, blood pressure is 110/70 mmHg, respiratory rate 24 breaths per minute, GCS 15
S - The cervical spine has been immobilised, one IV cannula has been placed and morphine given

Her estimated time of arrival in the ED is 2 minutes. You have a senior anaesthetic trainee and two trained ED nurses to help. The remaining trauma team is busy with an unstable patient that has also just arrived.

Initial patient observations

(As the patient is assessed during the scenario these observations will be provided by the nurse)

The patient is wheeled on a trolley with four paramedics. She is strapped to a spinal board on which she has been rolled onto her side to allow for blood trickling out of her mouth. She could not tolerate being flat as there was too much blood.

Airway	Facial injuries, avulsed teeth, blood in mouth, noisy breathing, choking
Breathing	Respiratory rate 28 breath per minute
	Bilateral equal air entry, oxygen saturation 84% on air, 90% on high flow oxygen
Circulation	Heart rate 110 beats per minute, blood pressure 90/64 mmHg
Disability	Distressed, Glasgow coma score 12 (eyes 3, motor 5, verbal 4)
	Blood sugar 9.2 mmol/L
Exposure	Temperature 36°C
	Grazes to limbs, no other injuries found

Guidance on scenario

From prior to the patient's arrival the candidate is expected to prepare for a significant airway problem. When the scenario begins it will not be possible to continue the primary survey until the airway has been dealt with. If the candidate attempts to do so the patient will deteriorate from an airway and ventilation point of view and the team will state, they are concerned about the airway. The patient will not be able to lie supine as they are panicking and there is on-going bleeding into their mouth. If left in this position they desaturate quickly. Ideally the patient will receive the RSI while on their side and be laid flat at the last moment possible.

The anaesthetic trainee is experienced enough to manage an airway and perform intubation and is prepared to intubate the patient but after two attempts, is unsuccessful. An LMA if attempted partially ventilates the patient but the oxygen saturations slowly drop. If asked to perform a cricothyroidotomy the anaesthetist says they will need the candidate to talk them through the procedure. It is acceptable for the candidate to perform the procedure or provide guidance for the anaesthetic trainee. If the remaining primary survey is undertaken there will be no concerning clinical findings. The patient's haemodynamic state will normalise with 4 units of blood. If the face is not packed the team will prompt the candidate by commenting on ongoing blood loss. Towards the end of the scenario the senior anaesthetist will arrive (as will the ENT or maxillofacial surgeon if previously called).

Mark sheet	Achieved	Not achieved
Introduces self to the team appropriately		
Asks to put out a trauma call		
Confirms team member experience and skills and allocate roles		
Asks everyone to wear personal protective equipment		
Anticipates difficult airway, discusses a plan		
Asks for difficult airway equipment		
Takes appropriate handover from ambulance crew		
Takes measures to protect cervical spine as much as possible		
Asks for appropriate monitoring to be attached		
Recognises need for airway protection		
States need for RSI		
Makes plan to attempt orotracheal intubation		
Makes plan for failed intubation including surgical airway		
Asks for appropriate drugs		
Commences blood transfusion		
Pre-oxygenates patient adequately		
Recognises desaturation and doesn't allow further attempt at laryngoscopy		
States need for surgical airway		
Correctly performs/describes surgical cricothyroidotomy		
Ensure adequate oxygenation/ventilation		
Secures airway		
Takes steps to manage facial bleeding with packing		
States need for completion of primary survey		
States need for CT (brain/face/cervical spine as a minimum)		
Hands over to senior anaesthetist or surgeon when they arrive		
Global score from examiner		
Global score from team		

Alternative scenarios

Severely agitated patient: candidates should recognise that head injury, hypoxia, extreme discomfort and pain may prevent the patient from lying for assessment or co-operating with treatment. The candidate is expected to gain control of the patient with sensible titrated sedation. The team will need to be briefed with a plan to then secure an anticipated difficult airway.

No recognisable facial anatomy: candidates are expected to prepare for an immediate surgical airway. Paradoxically, easy intubation may still be possible through a mobile deformed face and it is acceptable to attempt. Further examination will identify several other injuries which will need standard interventions.

Shock with facial injury: the patient with severe facial injuries will have haemodynamic shock and respiratory failure. Candidates should recognise that severe haemorrhage can occur into the lungs from facial injury. After intubation, resuscitation with a massive transfusion protocol is required, with referral for urgent embolisation of bleeding facial arteries. Whilst awaiting theatre it is appropriate to tamponade bleeding with facial packing in the form of nasal epistats, bite blocks and a semi-rigid cervical collar.

Suggested reading

Bhanderi N. Floating in the Face of Danger: MaxFax injuries in the ED, RCEM Learning. RCEM, London. 2016.
DAS guidelines for the management of unanticipated difficult airways. Difficult Airway Society. London, 2015.

9.9 Traumatic cardiac arrest

There is a clear algorithm for the management of traumatic cardiac arrest. The cause of traumatic arrest is usually hypovolaemia or obstructive shock with a beating healthy heart.

For this reason, chest compressions in traumatic arrest are likely to be ineffective and at worst can cause or worsen thoracic injuries whilst distracting attention from treating obstructive or haemorrhagic shock. In patients with obvious and significant trauma it is normal practice, therefore, to omit chest compressions at least until reversible causes have been corrected. It is often necessary to explain this rational to members of the team who may not understand the rational for not performing chest compressions in a cardiac arrest.

The focus instead should be on the rapid correction of reversible causes. In trauma the primary causes to identify and correct are; hypovolaemia, hypoxia, tension pneumothorax and tamponade. The traditional 4 H's and 4 T's of non-traumatic arrest may apply if there was a medical (non-traumatic event) that precipitated the trauma.

The treatment protocol for treating these reversible causes in traumatic cardiac arrest is often referred to as a '**HOT** drill', which stands for:
- Hypovolaemia:
  - Stop external haemorrhage, and ensure correct pelvic binder application
  - Transfuse rapidly with warmed blood products using a major transfusion protocol
- Oxygenate:
  - ETT (or LMA) with 100% oxygen with no PEEP
- Tension and tamponade:
  - Immediate bilateral thoracostomies to treat potential tension pneumothorax
  - Clamshell thoracotomy in penetrating chest trauma

Traumatic arrest management should be initiated quickly and aggressively because without a return of circulation in 20 minutes there is virtually no survival in traumatic arrest.

The technique for thoracotomy is described in **section 9.3**.

Rapid open thoracic decompression of suspected tension pneumothorax is preferred to a needle (which has a high failure rate) or a formal chest drain (which is a slower process). The technique is very similar to that for inserting a chest drain (**section 6.6**). Perform a finger sweep to ensure access to the pleural cavity. This is also an opportunity to confirm if the lung is inflated/collapsed and ascertain whether or not the heart is beating. As the patient is positively pressure ventilated the open thoracostomy will not compromise respiration. A chest drain need only be inserted to drain blood or in very large patients to maintain patency of the thoracostomy.

In penetrating trauma to the chest, if there is no return of circulation with transfusion, oxygenation and bilateral thoracic decompression use the thoracostomies to complete a clamshell thoracotomy to treat potential pericardial tamponade.

Tamponade is rare in blunt trauma, so thoracotomy should generally be avoided unless tamponade is noted on ultrasound assessment.

Scenario

You are the senior ED doctor in a teaching hospital. The ED nurse has taken a pre-alert call from an air ambulance helicopter bringing in a major trauma. She provides you with the **ATMIST**:

A – 40-year-old male
T – 30 minutes earlier
M – Pedestrian hit by cyclist while crossing the road
I – Left chest wall and abdominal contusions
S – Pulse 140 beats per minute, blood pressure 60/30 mmHg, oxygen saturations 90% on high flow oxygen, respiratory rate 30 breaths per minute. GCS 8 (E2, V2, M4) prior to intubation
T – He is intubated on a spinal board with a cervical spine collar and pelvic binder correctly placed, 2 large bore cannula, 2 units of blood and 1 g Tranexamic acid given, intubated with Rocuronium 100 mg and 40 mg Ketamine

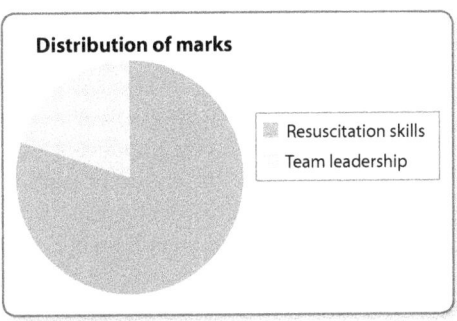

Distribution of marks
- Resuscitation skills
- Team leadership

His estimated time of arrival in the ED is 5 minutes. You have a full trauma team including an anaesthetist, a surgical registrar, a junior ED doctor and two experienced emergency nurses.

Initial patient observations

(As the patient is assessed during the scenario these observations will be provided)

Airway	Intubated, size 8.0 endotracheal tube secured at 22 cm at the teeth
Breathing	Respiratory rate 38 breaths per minute
	Reduced air entry left side, oxygen saturation 83% on high flow oxygen
Circulation	Heart rate 155 beats per minute, blood pressure not recordable
	Weak palpable carotid pulse
Disability	Glasgow coma score 3 (E1, V1, M1)
	Blood sugar 8.0 mmol/L
Exposure	Temperature 36°C
	Pelvic binder correctly positioned above the greater trochanters

The patient arrives haemodynamically unstable. He will suffer a PEA arrest during the primary survey.

Guidance on scenario

The patient has a left tension pneumothorax and abdominal injuries. During the primary survey the nurse will notice the patient has lost their pulse and will start chest compressions.

Further intravenous access will be required prior to large volume resuscitation using a major transfusion protocol. If attempted needle decompression of the chest will have no effect. The junior ED doctor has never done a thoracostomy but the surgical registrar is prepared to decompress the chest. After a decision to decompress the chest, but without specific guidance the surgeon say he needs to prepare a sterile field and will place bilateral chest drains starting on the unaffected side.

A left thoracostomy is required though bilateral thoracostomies performed simultaneously will also be effective.

The patient will regain a pulse when these are completed. He will still be haemodynamically unstable with a systolic around 70 mmHg. A FAST scan will be positive for blood in the abdomen. The patient must then be transferred straight to theatre for laparotomy. Ongoing 'major transfusion' resuscitation will be required while the transfer to theatre is arranged.

Mark sheet	Achieved	Not achieved
Introduces self to the nurse appropriately		
Asks to put out a trauma call		
Confirms team member experience and skills and allocates roles		
Asks everyone to wear personal protective equipment		
Activates MTP and primes rapid transfuser/blood warmer		
Informs team of importance of rapid transfusion and allocates one experienced nurse solely to the running the transfusion		
Informs senior surgeon of high likelihood of urgent laparotomy		
Prepares ultrasound machine for FAST scan		
Takes appropriate handover from ambulance crew		
Ensures cervical spine is protected throughout		
Ensures appropriate blood samples are sent including crossmatch request		
Administers high flow oxygen and initiates MTP transfusion		
Performs primary survey, noting chest and abdominal injuries, FAST positive		
Identifies traumatic cardiac arrest with loss of palpable pulse and reduction in $ETCO_2$ within 1 minute of starting primary survey		
Stops team performing immediate CPR and explains reasoning		
Informs team of priorities of rapid transfusion, oxygenation and bilateral chest decompression		
Notices the surgical registrar preparing chest drains and redirects to bilateral open thoracostomies		
Monitors pulses and $ETCO_2$ during resuscitation, recognising ROSC after 2 further unit blood and chest decompression		
Completes primary survey continuing rapid MTP transfusion		
Facilitates X-ray in ED: (normal pelvis, left pneumothorax on chest X-ray)		
Facilitates urgent transfer to theatre for Laparotomy		
Global score from examiner		
Global score from team		

Alternative scenario

Cardiac arrest after penetrating chest injury: candidates should complete the HOT drill including a clamshell thoracotomy treating possible right ventricular injury with cardiac tamponade.

Suggested reading

Edward M, Ashton L. Traumatic Cardiac Arrest: RCEM Learning. RCEM, London, 2015.
Lockey DJ, Lyon RM, Davies GE. Development of a simple algorithm to guide the effective management of traumatic cardiac arrest. Resuscitation 2013; 84:738–742.

EU GSPR Authorised Reprsentative
Logos Europe, 9 rue Nicolas Poussin
1700, La Rochelle, France
Phone: +33 (0) 6 67 93 73 78
E-mail: contact@logoseurope.eu

www.ingramcontent.com/pod-product-compliance
Ingram Content Group UK Ltd.
Pitfield, Milton Keynes, MK11 3LW, UK
UKHW050454150426
5217IPUK00025B/1685